T0251509

Leveraging
Consumer Psychology
for Effective
Health Communications

Leveraging Consumer Psychology for Effective Health Communications

The Obesity Challenge

Edited by
Rajeev Batra
Punam Anand Keller
Victor J. Strecher

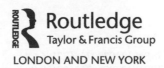

Routledge
Taylor & Francis Group

LONDON AND NEW YORK

First published 2011 by M.E. Sharpe

Published 2015 by Routledge
2 Park Square, Milton Park, Abingdon, Oxon OX14 4RN
711 Third Avenue, New York, NY 10017, USA

Routledge is an imprint of the Taylor & Francis Group, an informa business

Copyright © 2011 Taylor & Francis. All rights reserved.

No part of this book may be reprinted or reproduced or utilised in any form or by
any electronic, mechanical, or other means, now known or hereafter invented,
including photocopying and recording, or in any information storage or retrieval
system, without permission in writing from the publishers.

Notices
No responsibility is assumed by the publisher for any injury and/or damage to
persons or property as a matter of products liability, negligence or otherwise,
or from any use of operation of any methods, products, instructions or ideas
contained in the material herein.

Practitioners and researchers must always rely on their own experience and
knowledge in evaluating and using any information, methods, compounds, or
experiments described herein. In using such information or methods they should
be mindful of their own safety and the safety of others, including parties for
whom they have a professional responsibility.

Product or corporate names may be trademarks or registered trademarks, and
are used only for identification and explanation without intent to infringe.

Library of Congress Cataloging-in-Publication Data

Leveraging consumer psychology for effective health communications : the obesity
challenge / edited by Rajeev Batra, Punam Anand Keller, and Victor J. Strecher.
    p. cm.
Includes bibliographical references and index.
ISBN 978-0-7656-2717-9 (hardcover: alk. paper)
1. Obesity—Prevention. 2. Communication in medicine. 3. Health education. 4. Clinical
health psychology. I. Batra, Rajeev. II. Keller, Punam Anand. III. Strecher, Victor J., 1955–
[DNLM: 1. Obesity—prevention & control. 2. Obesity—psychology. 3. Consumer
Advocacy—psychology. 4. Consumer Health Information. 5. Health Promotion.
6. Social Marketing. WD 210 L659 2011]

RA645.O23L48 2011
362.196'398—dc22   2010022572

ISBN 13: 9780765627186 (pbk)
ISBN 13: 9780765627179 (hbk)

CONTENTS

Part III. Communication Strategy and Tactics

Part IV. Combating Obesity in Children and Young Adults

Part V. Environmental and Policy Perspectives

FOREWORD

BRIAN WANSINK

This is the newest edition in a long and impactful series of books on consumer psychology. Each book in this unique series was crafted around a single issue with pressing, real-world implications. Past editions have brought insights and solutions to topics such as measurement accuracy and psychographic segmentation. This edition tackles the pressing issue of obesity. As you will see, it does so in a creative, solution-oriented manner that is a fresh contrast to the bookshelves of obesity books that simply point out the problem without offering creative or practical solutions.

Most people know that an apple is better for them than a Snickers bar. Yet knowing does not always translate to choosing and eating. A person's choice of the Snickers bar is often viewed as a failure of either judgment or willpower.

In contrast to this view, the first two sections of this important book shine new light on why a person does not choose the apple. They show how lay theories, calorie estimation biases, and social norms can repeatedly and systematically nudge us in unhealthy directions. These chapters provide the foundation for a range of innovative solutions that follow.

In developing communication strategies and tactics for adults and children, there are two interesting ideas explored in the next two sections of the book. One is whether it is more motivating to use positive versus negative appeals (which may parallel prospect theory's view of gains and losses). A second notion is the potential power of tying messages to the consumer's identity through the use of identity signaling and through making a consumer think twice about the consistency between what they say, who they are, and what they do. Segmentation is key, and it is clearly illustrated in showing how breastfeeding appeals can be matched to personality. This offers a useful metaphor for how profile matching can be done in other contexts.

In the obesity debate, most scholars, most health practitioners, and policy-makers emphasize that the solution is either government intervention or personal responsibility. The last section of this book offers a third alternative: social marketing. It presents social marketing as a promising alternative to shrinking liberties through legislation and taxation. It shows the limitations of fixating on tobacco as a model for obesity, and it points toward the promise and the insights of win-win thinking that involves companies and consumers, policy-makers, and parents.

In the end, this book can change what you may think about the causes of obesity and what you might see as potential solutions. In a political atmosphere dominated by arguments and debates, this book offers what is needed most: fresh ideas backed by new data.

INTRODUCTION

RAJEEV BATRA, PUNAM A. KELLER, AND VICTOR J. STRECHER

This book brings together the contributions of leading research scholars in communications, consumer behavior, marketing, psychology, and public health, who met in Ann Arbor in May 2009 to share and debate ideas on how their research might be used to improve the effectiveness of obesity-fighting messages and interventions.

The book begins with two stage-setting review chapters, one each from the consumer psychology and public health research arenas. Punam A. Keller and Donald R. Lehmann report their findings from a meta-analysis of 84 relevant consumer psychology papers (involving 584 different experimental observations), investigating how 22 message, individual, and context factors interact in shaping health attitudes and behavioral intentions. They find that factors that improve health attitudes may not increase behavioral intentions and vice versa. For instance, stories about individuals seem to be very effective in shaping attitudes, while the perceived severity of communicated consequences seems important in shaping intentions. In reconciling their results, the authors suggest more research attention on "self-communication," such as the role of emotions and fantasy in determining various eating behaviors, topics covered in some of our other chapters (e.g., the ones by Mukhopadhyay, and Becheur and Valette-Florence). Keller and Lehmann also highlight the importance of context and individual differences in determining health behaviors. The second review chapter, by the American Heart Association (AHA) Council on Epidemiology and Prevention, addresses this issue by laying out the enormous range of societal and individual factors that influence the prevalence of obesity. This review allows us to map out the multiple points and levels at which interventions can be aimed, especially the urgent need for "population-based" efforts to combat the obesity epidemic. We are grateful to the AHA for allowing us to reprint this chapter; it originally appeared in their *Circulation* journal in 2008.

In the second section of the book, five chapters examine different "individual-level" or "micro" consumer factors that play a role in consumer belief-formation about how much, what, and when to eat: phenomena such as estimating how many calories a food has, or what determines our perceptions of how much self-control or self-confidence we have about food intake. Anirban Mukhopadhyay reports on research that he and others have conducted that examines the nature and malleability of consumers' "lay theories" about how much self-control they have over what they eat, how they will feel when they eat, how foods will taste if it is labeled healthy or unhealthy, and so on. He recommends that food-related messages remind consumers that their control over how they eat is quite limited—but can be increased. Alexander Chernev and Pierre Chandon next report on their many clever studies showing that consumers do not accurately estimate the calorie content of the foods they eat: they often think a food is healthy just because one ingredient of it is flagged on a nutrition label as being so (a "halo" bias), and they often underestimate the total calorie content of a pair of foods when one is factually healthy (such as a salad) but the paired item (a hamburger) is not, simply because the pair contains one lower-calorie component (an "averaging" bias). Chernev and Chandon's findings may be used for regulatory guidelines or warnings for advertisers of unhealthy foods. This chapter is followed by Kelly Geyskens describing the counterintuitive result that consumers may actually be better off if they expose themselves to strongly tempting food cues, rather than keeping away from such cues, simply because repeated exposure to unhealthy foods may make them more successful in activating the needed self-control and resistance. Informing consumers that practicing their resistance to unhealthy foods can be beneficial is a unique approach to reducing obesity. Next, Ian Skurnik, Carolyn Yoon, and Norbert Schwarz expand on the role of familiarity by investigating the effect of speed of decision-making as it relates to food choices. The inputs for speedy food choices include the degree of risk consumers face of gaining weight and their perceived ability to successfully carry out weight reduction behaviors. These findings question our basic assumptions about how much thought and planning goes into food choices. Finally, Brent McFerran, Darren W. Dahl, Gavan J. Fitzsimons and Andrea C. Morales show in a very clever manner how even the body type of the restaurant server at our table or nearby diners whose food choices we observe can affect what and how much we eat. Together, the chapters in this section offer significant insight into why consumers behave in a counterproductive manner despite being aware of healthier eating options.

From these chapters on individual perceptions and misperceptions, the book moves on to examine different communication tactics that can be used to change health attitudes and behaviors. In contrast to the prevalence of loss-frames in health communications, Daniel J. O'Keefe and Jakob D. Jensen's meta-analysis indicates that gain-framed appeals have a persuasive advantage in promoting physical activity—but not when the message concerns healthy eating. They recommend taglines such as "exercise if you want to be the right weight" instead of "if you do not exercise, you will not lose weight." Jeff Stone next leverages his expertise on hypocrisy to suggest that making consumers aware that they themselves do not practice behaviors that they preach to others—their hypocrisy—can induce cognitive dissonance and raise their motivation to act in obesity-reducing ways. The key is to encourage consumers to publicly advocate obesity-reducing actions. This is followed by a chapter by Imène Becheur and Pierre Valette-Florence in which they study whether negative emotions such as fear, guilt, and shame, which have been successful in reducing alcohol abuse, may be used to combat obesity. They conclude the answer is yes, especially for obesity communications targeting females. Taking a novel perspective on social reference group inferential processes, Lindsay P. Rand and Jonah Berger show that consumers will actually be more likely to stop following obesity-promoting behaviors—such as junk food consumption—if those behaviors are linked to dissociative reference groups. They show that particular foods are chosen, or not, not only because of their functional qualities, but also because of the social identity they communicate. Finally, using a set of results in the prescription drug compliance domain, Gary L. Kreps and his colleagues remind us of the importance of listening to consumers for barriers that need to be addressed in tailored obesity messages. The chapters in this section provide important directions for obesity health message content.

While all the chapters up to this point look at phenomena that can be applied to multiple demographic groups, the next three chapters focus on two population groups of special interest and importance, children and young adults. John J. Sailors points out that, since breastfed babies tend to be less susceptible to obesity as children and adolescents, messages aimed at mothers to encourage breastfeeding can be very important and need to take into account the women's individual characteristics—such as their level of self-monitoring—so that the message content is most relevant and persuasive. Nancy Wong and Myoung Kim then take us back to the broader set of contextual and environmental variables (some of which the AHA lists in Chapter 2) to test which environmental and community factors, parental styles, and child characteristics seem to be related to children's eating and exercise patterns and body mass index. Their structural equations model of national panel data finds that family and media factors are especially important. Concluding this section, Seung-A Annie Jin describes how avatar-based health games ("exergames") can be used to prime various aspects of teenagers' physical self in order to shape their exercise and healthy eating intentions. This chapter set describes the challenges and related solutions to addressing obesity from birth to adolescence.

The final set of five chapters looks at the crucial role of broader societal and environmental factors that interact with the individual and group-level ones that form the primary focus of most of the earlier chapters. Michael L. Rothschild, one of the best-known experts on the rationale and use of "social marketing" techniques, shows why and how social marketing principles can be used to increase the effectiveness of public health obesity interventions. The intersection of public service messages with other elements of the marketing mix, such as distribution, is highlighted in his case example on efforts to reduce drunk driving in Wisconsin. This is followed by two chapters on nutrition labeling on food packages. Brian Wansink lays out the objectives and processes used to develop and promote the new food guide pyramid, "MyPyramid," developed by the U.S. Department of Agriculture, an initiative in which he himself played a major role. Critiquing the design of such communication devices, Jason Riis and Rebecca Ratner argue that such guidelines and depictions should be made even simpler, to increase consumers' motivation and ability to follow them, and should present an alternative. The last two chapters address the role of marketing, media, and government in exacerbating or controlling obesity. Peter A. Ubel discusses some of the tensions and trade-offs between libertarianism and paternalism inherent in governmental efforts to more actively fight obesity, arriving at what he considers are the legitimate arenas in which governments should indeed intervene through policy actions. Barbara Loken, K. Viswanath, and Melanie A. Wakefield draw lessons for obesity-fighting interventions by borrowing specific guidelines from the fight against tobacco use. Among them: the important role played by explicit and implicit messages in the entertainment and news media in shaping consumer perceptions and attitudes, and thus the need to study and possibly regulate their effects.

Taken together, the chapters in this volume bring to researchers and policy-makers scores of interesting and important ideas on ways to craft obesity-fighting messages and interventions more effectively. The conclusions deserve serious consideration because they derive their strength from a variety of disciplinary paradigms, and they are all based on the highest standards of current research. It is our hope that by assembling and presenting them here we have assisted in the efforts underway to combat this major public health crisis.

The conference that led to this book, on "Leveraging Consumer Psychology for Effective Health Communications: The Obesity Challenge," was organized by the Yaffe Center for Persuasive Communication at the Ross School of Business of the University of Michigan (www.yaffecenter.org). The Yaffe Center has, as one of its goals, the facilitation and dissemination of multidisciplinary research on persuasion-relevant topics, and crafting effective messages and interventions to fight obesity seemed like a very worthwhile goal. The conference was held under the aegis of the Society for Consumer Psychology. The lead sponsor for the conference was the National Center for Health Marketing and Centers for Disease Control and Prevention (CDC) in collaboration with the National Public Health Information Coalition (NPHIC). The conference was cosponsored by the Yaffe Center for Persuasive Communication, the University of Michigan Ross School of Business, the University of Michigan School of Public Health, and Johnson & Johnson. Additional sponsorship support was provided by the Association for Consumer Research. We thank these organizations for their support and of course our distinguished and accomplished authors for their chapter contributions. We are excited to bring this important volume to you and hope that it sparks new dialogue and research on this and other public health challenges.

PART I

OVERVIEWS

CHAPTER 1

DESIGN OF EFFECTIVE OBESITY COMMUNICATIONS

Insights From Consumer Research

PUNAM A. KELLER AND DONALD R. LEHMANN

MARKETING AND OBESITY

The American Obesity Association defines obesity as a complex, multifactorial chronic disease involving environmental (social and cultural), genetic, physiologic, metabolic, behavioral, and psychological components. We believe marketing needs to be added to the factors associated with obesity. Marketing activities have a direct impact on eating habits. Americans crave and consume junk food and fast food for their convenience, price, and taste. According to its website, the McDonald's restaurant chain serves 47 million global customers every single day and potato chip sales surpassed $6 billion in the United States. Americans also overindulge on high-calorie snack foods at home, in the office, and at parties, even when they are not hungry or doing something else. Brian Wansink, director of the Cornell University Food and Brand Lab, explains why this habit leads to obesity: Generally, anything that takes our focus off the food makes us more likely to overeat.

A typical American does not understand how to eat according to standard portion sizes. Between 1970 and 2000, portion sizes exploded. Consumer packaged goods companies blew up their sizes to increase market share and provide more value to consumers. For example, the convenience store 7-Eleven sells a sixty-four-ounce soda called "Big Gulp"; it has 800 calories and is ten times the size of the soda Coca-Cola first introduced. Restaurants have also increased their portion sizes to give consumers more "bang for their buck." One order of large fries from McDonald's gives a twelve-year-old boy 24 percent of his daily calories and 35 percent of his daily fat intake. Howard Gordon, a senior vice president of the Cheesecake Factory, explains there is a wow factor in the way that the restaurant's huge portions look. Gordon notes that the Cheesecake Factory does not provide calorie information and customers ask for it "very, very rarely." Wansink explains why such large portion sizes are adding to the obesity epidemic: "Size—it matters a lot. In study after study, research shows that the larger the plate, the serving bowl, the package, or the serving utensil, the more we'll eat" (Wansink 2006).

Marketing also plays a role in encouraging sedentary behavior. In this age of booming technology more children are watching television, playing video games, and using the computer than ever before. According to the Federal Communications Commission, the average American child views over 40,000 television commercials in one year. Research shows that overexposure to advertising of high-calorie foods promotes overeating and obesity. Many of these hip, eye-catching marketing messages plug fast-food restaurants, cereal, snacks, and candy specifically targeted at children during children's shows on children's stations. When children are in school, a typical American student spends, on average, 900 hours in school and nearly 1,023 hours in front of a TV each year (Connolly 2004). Children who consistently watch TV more than four hours per day are more likely to be overweight than other children.

If we acknowledge that marketers have contributed to the obesity problem, we can take some comfort in battling the problem with insights from consumer psychology and marketing. The goal of this chapter is to facilitate the application of research to design more effective obesity communications. Unsurprisingly, numerous studies have assessed the impact of different communication strategies (e.g., level of fear arousal or framing) on participants' attitudes toward and intentions with respect to various health behaviors (see Keller and Lehmann 2008 for a related meta-analysis). While these studies are individually interesting, it is difficult to obtain an overall picture from them, much less assess in a quantitative way what the impacts are. The purpose of this chapter, therefore, is to assess the current state of knowledge in the field via meta-analysis. Two more specific goals guided our research design and analysis. First, we wanted to identify the context, message, and individual factors that increased attitudes and intentions to comply with the recommended health behaviors. Second, in order to shed light on the underlying process, we wanted to identify how well various models proposed in the literature fit the data.

OVERVIEW OF THE STUDY

We designed the meta-analysis by using two approaches. The first approach was for experts in the area to delineate the major issues that had been studied as well as relevant theories worth testing. This suggested a number of variables that could impact behavior such as number of message exposures. Second, the first author, who is familiar with the fields of marketing, psychology, and health, examined published studies to identify which theoretically interesting variables were available and what other variables were available which, upon reflection, seemed worth investigating.

We examined studies that measured the effectiveness of health communications by assessing attitudes toward the recommended health behaviors and/or intentions to comply with advocated health behaviors. We also gathered data on reported or actual behavior, although two concerns precluded similar analysis on this data: (1) the sample size was small: only twenty-four studies report behavior, and (2) there was no natural boundary on behavior similar to a finite scale for attitudes and intentions (e.g., the behavior may range from 0 to 40 cigarettes per day). We separated attitudes and intentions because we did not assume that favorable attitudes would automatically result in higher intentions. Although many studies support a positive link between attitudes and intentions to comply (Barber et al. 2005; Rah et al. 2005; Van Voorbees et al. 2005), other studies indicate a weaker link (Chandon, Morowitz, and Reinartz 2005; Chatzisarantis et al. 2004) or identify the factors that determine the strength of the relationship between attitudes and intentions (Byrne and Arias 2004; Perugini 2005). For example, the relationship between attitudes and intentions may depend on whether the attitudes are implicit or explicit (Perugini 2005).

Twenty-two study characteristics were identified as potential determinants of attitudes and intentions in response to health communications. These characteristics were divided into three categories:

1. context (3),
2. message (11), and
3. individual differences (8).

Our choice of context characteristics was guided by other meta-analytical studies (Albarracin, Cohen, and Kumkale 2003; Brown and Stayman 1992; Farley and Lehmann 1986; Peterson 2001; Sultan, Farley, and Lehmann 1990), whereas our choice of message and individual differences was guided by health communication studies in marketing, health, and psychology. We provide a brief review of each study characteristic along with more detailed descriptions of studies that have direct applications for designing more effective obesity communications.

Context Characteristics

Health Goal

Health behaviors can be undertaken for one of three reasons: a behavior can prevent the onset of a health problem (e.g., exercise), detect the development of a health problem (e.g., screening for high blood pressure), or cure or treat an existing health problem (e.g., medication for a thyroid deficiency). Health recommendations either encourage undertaking some health-related behavior, such as exercise, or discourage the continuation of unhealthy behavior, such as eating junk food. Although the literature indicates that prevention behaviors are perceived as less risky than detection behaviors (Rothman and Salovey 1997), there are limited data on different types of health goals or recommendation formats on attitude and intentions.

Study Setting

The choice of setting reflects in part whether the researcher's goal is to general-ize the theory or the specific effects obtained. If the goal is to obtain support for a theoretical position, a lab setting with a homogeneous sample such as students is often deemed appropriate. On the other hand, a field study with a relevant target sample is more appropriate if the goal is to map observed data into other research settings, for instance other populations and other health behaviors (Calder, Phil-lips, and Tybout 1981; Lynch 1982). Importantly, lab studies with homogeneous student samples may produce stronger effects on attitudes than field studies with adult samples (Peterson 2001). By contrast, stronger effects on intentions may be observed in studies designed to test applications in the field (Keller, Lipkus, and Rimer 2002).

Psychology or Marketing Journals

We include this variable as a surrogate for focus on message characteristics ver-sus context and individual differences. On the one hand, we expected a greater emphasis on attitudes as a function of message variables in marketing journals than in psychology journals. Conversely, we expected a greater number of studies on intentions as a function of context and individual differences in psychology than in marketing journals. We test here whether results generated in these two research traditions produce systematically different results once other factors are controlled for.

Message Characteristics

Message characteristics are a key controllable variable for marketing and health practitioners. Although none of those studied is unique to health or obesity, as much as possible we relied on health communication studies to inform predictions of their impact on attitude and intentions.

Level of Fear

The literature variously indicates a negative relationship (Feshbach and Janis 1953; Lipkus et al. 2001), an inverted-U relationship (Janis 1967; Sternthal and Craig 1974), or a positive linear relationship between fear and preventive behavior (Boster and Mongeau 1984; Rogers 1983; Sutton 1982). As most studies reviewed do not arouse a high level of fear, the basic conclusion from this literature is that moderate fear arousal increases protection intentions, whereas low and high fear either do not change intentions (in case of low fear) or can boomerang (in case of high fear) and lower attitudes. The literature also suggests that the effect of fear on attitudes and intentions depends on prior intentions such that high fear may be more effective than low fear for those with high prior intentions to lose weight, but the reverse may be true for people with low priors (Keller and Block 1997, 1999; Lipkus et al. 2001). One method to reduce fear arousal is to reverse the order of consequences and recommended actions (Keller 1999). Thus, obesity messages that describe ways to reduce weight prior to discussing how obesity results in higher risk of blood pressure, diabetes, and heart attacks may persuade audiences in the precontemplation or low-involvement stages, whereas leading with the health consequences may be more effective to retain audiences who have already started on a weight loss program. Together these findings suggest the need to assess prior intentions or decision-making stage to determine the appropriate level of fear or seriousness of obesity consequences in the message.

Framing

Health messages can be framed positively (e.g., "if you exercise, you will enhance your self-esteem") or negatively ("if you do not exercise, you will lower your self-esteem"). The literature indicates that intentions to engage in preventive health are generally higher when the behavior is framed in terms of its related costs (loss frames) rather than related benefits (gain frames), even when the two frames describe objectively equivalent situations (Rothman and Salovey 1997). A handful of studies show that the main effect of loss- versus gain-framed messages may depend on individual differences (prior intentions or behavior: Block and Keller 1995; Meyerowitz and Chaiken 1987; Rothman and Salovey 1997; prior involvement: Maheswaran and Meyers-Levy 1990; regulatory focus: Aaker and Lee 2001; Lee and Aaker 2004; mood: Keller, Lipkus, and Rimer 2003). These studies suggest that traditional gain frames (e.g., "take this weight loss pill and look as good as this featured model") may not persuade more involved audiences, whereas negative frames (e.g., "if you do not take this weight loss pill, you lose the opportunity to look as good as the featured model") may not persuade audiences who are not considering a weight loss program.

Level of Vividness and Base/Case Effects

Most obesity messages consider vivid presentations because material in the form of pictures, concrete information, examples of specific cases or stories, and TV presentations are more persuasive than text-only, abstract arguments, population or base-rate estimates, and print presentations (Kisielius and Sternthal 1986). For example, the Ad Council's "SmallStep" obesity campaign has a picture of a woman's waist and hips and provides concrete examples of reducing size by taking short walks during lunch hour or cooking at home instead of buying take-out meals. However, the vividness effects are reversed (Block and Keller 1997; Igartua, Cheng, and Lopes 2003) or disappear (Rook 1986) when audiences are highly involved or have different regulatory goals (Lee, Keller, and Sternthal 2010). These findings suggest that vivid materials may motivate less involved audiences to consider a weight loss regime, but additional nonvivid information on response efficacy may be necessary in more advanced decision-making stages.

Physical Versus Social Consequences

Emphasizing social consequences may be more effective than emphasizing physical consequences because they arouse less fear (Smith and Stutts 1999) and because they are more imminent. For example, the Ad Council has a radio commercial called "Date" in which the female makes fun of a dangling chin on her male date. Social consequences are especially salient among females and may unfortunately lead to alternative risky behaviors; Denscombe (2001) finds that females smoke more than males because of social identity and desire to control their weight. This book contains chapters on the effects of social norms on the persuasiveness of obesity communications (McFerran et al. 2009).

Referencing

In general, people tend to think that bad things happen to other people and not to themselves. There is considerable evidence of this optimistic bias (Menon, Block, and Ramanathan 2002; Raghubir and Menon 1998). Accordingly, health communications in which the consequences of nonadherence are directed at others (e.g., friends or family members) are more effective than when the consequences are directed at the individual. Witness the ads showing a grandmother who cannot play with a grandchild due to osteoporosis. Similar ads may be effective to control adult obesity.

Message Argument Strength

Argument strength in health messages can be attained by a variety of means, including two-sided arguments and high response efficacy information (Block and Keller 1998). Although strong arguments are more effective than weaker ones, the literature consistently shows that argument strength is more appreciated by highly involved audiences or those with previously positive attitudes (Ahluwalia 2000; Rosen 2000). Argument strength effects also seem conditional on other message factors such as level of fear (Gleicher and Petty 1992) and negative frames (Dinoff and Kowalski 1999). Interestingly, in a health context, weaker messages may be more effective if they are viewed as more reassuring (Williams-Piehota et al. 2003). Weaker arguments may be created by using social rather than physical health consequences. Given that target audiences are often less involved, social consequences such as emphasizing that bad eating habits may present a poor role model for kids might increase the effectiveness of obesity communications.

Source Credibility

The general literature indicates that source effects are strongest when the audience is not highly involved and is engaged in peripheral processing. The health communication literature indicates that a female communicator may actually increase the level of involvement (Dinoff and Kowalski 1999). However, the current animosity toward traditional health sources such as physicians, insurance companies, pharmaceutical companies, and government health associations may result in lower persuasion for obesity communications that highlight these sources. This suggests the use of female communicators outside the health profession whom less involved target audiences can relate to.

Number of Message Exposures

The health communication literature has not tested repetition effects as much as other literatures. A few studies indicate that multiple exposures are more effective than a single exposure (e.g., Dijkstra et al 1999). Recognizing the importance of obesity reminders or triggers, the Ad Council has developed a campaign called "Theatre" in which a couple carries a lump of fat with them to the movies. Similarly, the Heinz museum in Pittsburgh displays eight pounds of what looks like body fat.

Tailored Versus Standard

Recent research in health has turned to evaluating the effectiveness of communication that is tailored to the audience characteristics such as stage in decision-making (Prochaska and DiClemente 1982), using a variety of methods such as customized messages (Everett and Palmgreen 1995; Lipkus et al. 2001; Palmgreen et al. 2001), telephone counseling (Dijkstra et al. 1999), computerized messages (Brug et al. 1998), or a combination of them (Curry et al. 1995). These studies either find a change in decision-making stage (e.g., from precontemplation to contemplating the advocated health behavior, Curry et al. 1995) or no effect of tailoring when compared to a standard message (Drossaert, Boer, and Seydel 1996). A recent study by Keller et al. (2009) shows that tailored newsletters to parents of obese kids were more persuasive than standard obesity communication. Parents in the precontemplation stage were more persuaded by a message addressing their barriers (e.g., "you are only a child once" or "my child needs to grow wide so that she can grow tall"). Similarly, parents in the contemplation stage were more persuaded by a message addressed to them specifically (e.g., "I cannot serve different meals to different kids because they vary in obesity").

Emotional Level of the Message

Schwarz (1990) suggests that emotions have a functional role in directing attention and behavior. As compared to positive emotional states that signal that there is no problem, negative emotional states signal a problem-solving or prevention goal. Thus emotional obesity messages, especially those signaling a negative state, are expected to be more persuasive than unemotional ones. However, it is important to investigate the role of different negative emotions on message persuasion. Certain emotions such as sadness may result in emotional eating whereas anxiety may signal a need to reduce uncertainty and prompt responsible eating (Raghunathan and Pham 1999). Accountability or level of self-control may be another key emotional dimension for risk assessment. Passyn and Sujan (2006) indicate that some combinations of emotions, such as anxiety, fear, and hope (low accountability emotions), may result in more emotional eating than other combinations, such as fear, guilt, and challenge (high accountability emotions). In addition, some emotions may be easier to control than others (guilt vs. anger), and lack of emotional control has been found to be positively linked to risky behaviors such as overeating (Keller 2009).

Individual Characteristics

Gender

Females are likely to have more positive attitudes and intentions than males because (1) females are more concerned about health or physical consequences than males (Beech and Whittaker 2001); (2) females are more likely to engage in systematic health message processing (Meyers-Levy 1988); and (3) females are more concerned about long-term effects than males (Smith and Stutts 1999). However, these results may be limited to women who are not sad or overweight. Keller (2009) finds that, compared to males, females are more likely to regulate their sadness by engaging in risky behaviors such as compulsive eating. Furthermore, the main effect of gender on persuasion may be lost or reversed in the media's obsessions with thin female models. Smeesters, Mussweiler, and Mandel (2009) find that media exposure affects the self-esteem of overweight and underweight women. In comparison to underweight women, overweight participants ate fewer cookies and had higher intentions to diet and exercise when exposed to heavy models than when exposed to thin models.

The literature suggests it may be worthwhile to design different obesity messages for male and female adolescents. Keller and Olson (2009) find that males are more anxious than depressed because they compare their self-view to what they ought to do, whereas their female counterparts are more depressed than anxious because they compare their self-view to their ideals. Consequently, health messages that focus on self-efficacy were more effective for adolescent females, whereas messages emphasizing response efficacy were more effective for adolescent males.

Age

The literature suggests that age is positively correlated with more favorable attitudes and higher intentions to comply with healthy behaviors. Some studies have questioned the value of health communications for adolescents as they transition from letting their parents make decisions for them to being more influenced by their peers (Fruin, Pratt, and Owen 1991; Pechmann and Shih 1999). Moreover, health communications designed to increase vulnerability in young adults have been found to reduce rather than increase preventive behaviors (Greening 1997; Keller and Olson 2009).

Race

The literature suggests that nonwhites may not be as influenced by health communications as whites due to access to such communications and due to the greater influence of family and peers as well as poorer access to health care. Kumanyika and Grier (2006) find that the density of obesity-promoting advertising (food, fast food, sugary beverages, sedentary entertainment, and transportation) varied by the race and ethnicity of zip code areas, with African American zip code areas having the highest densities, Latino zip code areas having slightly lower, and white zip code areas having the lowest advertising densities. African Americans are thus exposed to food promotion and distribution patterns with relatively greater potential adverse health effects than are whites. In addition, Kumanyika and Grier (2006) show that low-income and minority children watch more television than white, nonpoor children and are potentially exposed to more commercials advertising high-calorie, low-nutrient food during an average hour of TV programming. They note that neighborhoods where low-income and minority children live typically have more fast-food restaurants and fewer vendors of healthful foods than do wealthier or predominantly white neighborhoods. They also note such obstacles to physical activity as unsafe streets, dilapidated parks, and lack of facilities.

Involvement

In general, the literature indicates involvement is positively related to attitudes and intentions. Further, involvement interacts with several other factors to determine attitudes and intentions (prior attitude: Ahluwalia 2000; prior behavior: Keller 1999; message strength: Petty, Cacioppo, and Schumann 1983). For example, people who are not enthusiastic about the recommendations may have the goal of discounting the source or the relevance of the message to them or counterarguing to refute the message claims (Ahluwalia 2000).

Prior Intentions

It is not surprising that a participant's prior intentions and related levels of attitude, familiarity, and risk perceptions have a strong moderating effect on compliance with health recommendations. Besides an obvious positive main effect on attitudes and intentions, extant evidence indicates that prior intentions interact with other factors to determine compliance (perceived risk: Block and Keller 1998; response and self-efficacy appraisals: Keller 1999). For example, Keller (1999) indicates that the people with low priors are more persuaded by a low fear appeal or when recommendations are placed before health consequences in the message.

Threat and Coping Appraisal

Health-related actions prompt an assessment of threat and coping appraisal. Threat appraisal is based on two questions: "Am I vulnerable?" and "How serious could the consequences be?" Coping appraisal is based on two different questions: "Can I undertake the action (self-efficacy)?" and "If I do, will it reduce the health threat?" (response efficacy: Bandura 1982; Maddux and Rogers 1983; Rogers 1975). Individual perceptions of the answers to these two questions determine motivation for protecting oneself from a health-related threat (Rogers 1975). Some research suggests that the ability to undertake the action is more closely associated with intentions to perform a health behavior than the other three factors (Milne, Sheeran, and Orbell 2000). Recent studies have indicated the value of providing target audiences with weight reducing plans to help then implement their goals (Escalas and Luce 2003, 2004).

Goals and Audience Personality

Several recent studies suggest that the effectiveness of health communication may be a function of audience personality and goals (e.g., Cooper, Agocha, and Sheldon 2000; Fejfar and Hoyle 2000; Gerrard et al. 2000). In particular, people with high self-esteem (Gerrard et al. 2000; Schaninger 1976), risk-seeking promotion-oriented people (Higgins 1997), and sensation seekers (Hoyle, Fejfar, and Miller 2000) feel less vulnerable and show greater resistance to health threats. The literature also suggests that personality may interact with message and context factors to determine attitude and intentions. For example, regulatory fit theory suggests that people with a promotion orientation are likely to have more favorable attitudes if they are asked to engage in healthy behavior rather than if asked to discontinue unhealthy behaviors. Similarly, a gain frame and high self-efficacy will increase intentions among promotion-oriented but not prevention-oriented people (Aaker and Lee 2001; Keller 2006; Lee and Aaker 2004). Finally, prevention-oriented audiences are more persuaded by low-level construals related to "how" to engage in obesity-reducing activities rather than the "why" or consequences of such actions, whereas this message format effect is reversed if the audience is promotion-oriented (Lee, Keller, and Sternthal 2010).

THE META-ANALYSIS

Selection of Studies

We initially searched for articles using the PsycInfo and ISI (Web of Science) databases. We also conducted some searches using the Proquest.umi.com,

Factiva, and Lexis-Nexis databases. Within these databases we used keywords (and combinations of keywords with "health" being the main topic) such as Health, Messages, Communication, Campaigns, Prevention, Marketing, Marketing strategy, Experiment, Tailoring, Healthcare, and Healthcare Industry. We searched psychology, sociology, marketing, medical, and communication sources. We also checked the bibliographies of relevant papers to obtain additional papers.

We used these three basic criteria for inclusion:

1. The study was a lab or field experiment.
2. The data were provided on intention or attitude.
3. The studies contained a message intervention.

Our search resulted in a sample of 85 papers that reported a total of 584 different observations. These observations became the data used in the meta-analysis.

Variable Coding

To enhance comparability, all scale values were converted to percent terms (i.e., a 4 on a 5-point scale, the most common scale encountered, was set to equal to $(4 - 1) / (5 - 1) = .75$. In cases where a variable was both measured and manipulated, we kept both pieces of data. We also created seven continuous variables (fear, source credibility, argument strength, vulnerability, severity, response efficacy, and self-efficacy) by converting manipulated binary variables (e.g., high fear) into scale values. To do this we used both a logical extreme value (.9) and the 95th percentile value of measured values on the variable (e.g., .81). Since the results do not vary substantially depending on which we used, we report results based on the easier-to-implement extreme value procedures (i.e., .1 vs. .9).

Several variables were combined if they were reported in only one or two studies and theoretically represented the same general factor. For example, anxiety was coded as fear, relevance and vulnerability as involvement, and drama/lecture and fast/slow music were coded as level of vividness. We also assessed whether the study had used base or case information even if this variable was not the focus of the study.

Missing Data

We dealt with missing data in two ways. First, we treated it as missing in the analysis. Second, we included the mean value for cases where data was available for three variables—age, gender, and race. The results were very similar. Therefore we used the data with means replacing missing values for age, gender, and race in all our analyses (Lemieux and McAlister 2005).

Variables Included in the Analysis

Some variables had very little data and often were assessed only in a single study. We required that at least two different papers included the variable before using it in the analysis. We also required that there be at least ten observations reported before including a variable in the analysis. This eliminated several variables of theoretical analysis interest such as message elaboration. We also controlled for when the study was done and for sample size.

RESULTS

Basic statistics on the variables that passed our screen appear in Table 1.1. These lead to several observations. First, the two dependent variables, intention ($n = 359$, 53.3 percent of the total) and attitude ($n = 243$, 33.9 percent) both have sufficient observations to analyze. Second, the predictor variables clearly form a nonfactorial (i.e., unbalanced) design. The typical study involved:

1. encouraging subjects to do something (74 percent),
2   prevention of some health consequence (73.3 percent),
3. a lab study (73.1 percent),
4. physical consequences (78.3 percent),
5. a single exposure to communication (95.8 percent), and
6. student sample (73.5 percent).

One conclusion based on our findings is that future studies would be more useful if they explored conditions that differ from this implicit norm (Farley, Lehmann, and Mann 1998).

Correlational Analysis

To get an initial sense of the data, we correlated each of the analyzed variables with the two dependent variables (attitude and intention). The results are shown in Table 1.1. Most correlations are fairly modest in size, although many are significant. Significant effects are in bold. They suggest that there are systematic differences in how attitude and intention are related to each of the categories of variables studied. Given the highly unbalanced design formed by the existing literature, however, it is difficult to draw conclusions based on these results. Therefore, we concentrate our efforts on a multivariate analysis that controls for the impact of covariates.

The Meta-Analysis Model

The basic model is of the form, *Attitudes (or Intentions)* $= B_o + \Sigma B_i X_i$ where X_i are the predictor variables identified in Table 1.1. Initially we only examined

Table 1.1

Variables Examined in the Meta-Analysis

	Reported/ Manipulated		Correlations	
	N	Percent	Attitude	Intention
Context characteristics				
Encourage behavior	432	74.0	**.23**	**−.12**
Discourage behavior	100	17.1	−.03	.05
Prevention behavior	428	73.3	.09	−.02
Detection behavior	118	20.2	**.13**	.02
Remediation behavior	31	5.3	.08	.05
Context (lab)	427	73.1	−.04	**.13**
Students	435	74.6	.08	.09
Journal: Psychology	311	53.3	.00	−.09
Journal: Marketing	117	20.0	.11	−.03
Message variables				
Low fear	32	5.5	**.16**	.02
Moderate fear	15	2.6	.07	−.02
High fear	25	4.3	**.17**	.09
Gain frame	73	12.5	−.03	−.03
Loss frame	75	12.8	−.06	−.07
Vivid	94	16.1	**−.17**	−.01
Base rate	50	8.6	−.09	−.03
Case rate	75	12.0	**.39**	.11
Referencing (self)	105	18.0	−.03	**−.13**
Social consequences	67	11.5	**−.24**	**.13**
Physical consequences	457	78.3	**.21**	.01
Female communicator	34	5.8	.06	−.01
Male communicator	15	2.6	**−.22**	**−.14**
Weak argument	13	2.2	−.02	−.06
Strong argument	13	2.2	.04	−.03
Two-sided arguments	41	7.0	**.17**	**.14**
Multiple exposures	25	4.2	**.24**	**.13**
Tailored message	23	3.9	.05	.02
Emotional message	20	3.4	.11	−.03
Individual/Context variables				
Race (white → other)	95	16.3	**−.89**	−.02
Gender (male → female)	279	47.8	**.19**	**.24**
Age	102	32.9	.17	−.05
Prior intentions	60	10.3	**.24**	**.22**
Low involvement	69	11.8	−.12	−.09
High involvement	76	13.0	−.09	.02
Low severity	24	4.1	**−.17**	−.06
High severity	30	5.1	**−.29**	.02
Low response efficacy	24	4.1	.11	−.14
High response efficacy	36	6.2	.12	−.09
Low self-efficacy	17	2.9	.12	−.03
High self-efficacy	28	4.8	.12	.04
Promotion regulatory focus	22	3.8	−.08	−.03
Prevention regulatory focus	22	3.8	−.08	−.04

Note: Significant effects in bold.

main effects. As Table 1.1 shows, we had relatively few manipulated levels for many of the variables. Further, even when not manipulated, the situation has some inherent level of fear, severity, vulnerability, response efficacy, and self-efficacy. Therefore, we used judgment-based estimates (based on two judges who separately rated and then got together to produce a consensus rating) in some of the analyses.

The dependent variables were intention and attitude, measured on 0 to 1 scales. As a consequence, the coefficients represent either the impact on intention or attitude when a particular condition existed (e.g., the message encouraged healthy behaviors) for binary variables or the impact of moving from 0 to 1 on the continuous scales.

Impacts on Attitude and Intention

We first analyzed the 243 observations where attitude was the dependent variable using OLS Regression. Because the studies used in the meta-analysis often produced multiple observations and to avoid overlooking potentially important determinants, we used a significance level of .10 versus the more conventional .05. Significant effects are in bold. The results appear in the first four columns in Table 1.2.

The regression using the manipulated values (coded .1 or .9) of the variables accounts for 67 percent of the variance ($F(42, 243) = 9.52, p < .001$). These results are displayed in the first two columns. When we replaced the manipulated variables with estimates for fear, vividness, argument strength, severity, vulnerability, response efficacy, and self-efficacy, the various predictor variables account for 53 percent of the variance ($F(36, 243) = 6.45, p < .001$).

The same procedure was used for intentions. The results are displayed in the last four columns of Table 1.2. The predictor variables account for 26 percent ($F42, 359) = 2.67, p < .001$) and 31 percent ($F(36, 359) = 3.91, p < .001$) respectively of the variance in intention when manipulated and estimated values are used. The variables explain a smaller fraction of the variance than in the case of attitudes, which makes sense, partly because it is easier to change attitude than behavior. Some coefficients are similar to those for attitude (e.g., those with high priors are more positive); several, however, are quite different.

These results are somewhat troubling. Since the attitude-to-intention link is one of the best established in the literature, it is surprising that several variables have opposite effects on these two positively correlated variables. Yet here, at least for mostly student samples, the two variables respond differently, perhaps because it is easier to have an attitude than to form a concrete intention to behave in a certain way. This is not due to the different studies used in the attitude and intention analyses since when we ran the model on the eighty-four conditions (observations) where both were mentioned, significant differences still emerged.

To see if the correlation between attitude and intention depends on character-istics of the studies not accounted for by the predictor variables, we performed a "controlled" analysis on the eighty-four conditions where both intention and attitude were reported. We computed the correlation between attitudes and inten-tions across conditions within each study and used this correlation as the dependent measure. The average correlation between attitude and intention was .65, positive as expected. Across conditions, we used this correlation to identify variables that might increase or decrease the relationship between attitude and intention. These results are displayed in Table 1.3. Both frames and messages discouraging un-healthy behavior had large dampening effects on this relationship, as did base rate information, high response efficacy, male samples, and studies in psychology. The relationship between attitudes and intentions was enhanced in field studies, student or older samples, messages containing strong arguments, detection behaviors, and health consequences directed at others.

We also ran a series of separate regressions to examine the relative impact of each of the three general categories of variables on attitudes and intentions. The results indicate that message factors ($R^2 = .38$) explain more of the vari-ance in attitudes than context characteristics ($R^2 = .13$) or individual differ-ences ($R^2 = .19$). By contrast, message factors ($R^2 = .13$) explain about the same variance in intentions as individual differences ($R^2 = .11$), and both explain more than context factors ($R^2 = .07$). Put differently, while message factors are more important than individual differences, which in turn are more influential than the context factors we studied, the relative impact of message factors is greater for attitudes than intentions.

TESTS OF HEALTH-RELATED MODELS

Much of the literature in this area has applied specific models. Therefore, we used our health communication database and meta-analysis to examine five of these models along with their related extensions:

1. fear-related,
2. protection motivation theory (PMT),
3. elaboration likelihood model (ELM),
4. prospect theory, and
5. regulatory fit.

Fear-Related Effects

The drive-reduction model developed by Hovland and his colleagues (Hovland, Janis, and Kelley 1953) is based on the view that fear motivates behavioral change. However, it may be difficult to determine the optimal level of fear: results have indicated both a negative relationship between fear and behavior (Feshbach and

Table 1.2

Main Effects on Attitudes and Intentions

| | Attitude | | | | Intentions | | | |
| | Manipulated | | Estimated | | Manipulated | | Estimated | |
	t	B	t	β	t	β	t	β
Constant		7.43		4.13		1.35		.47
Context characteristics								
Encourage behavior	**.22**	**2.08**	.05	.40	-.11	-1.20	-.30	-3.16
Discourage behavior	**.41**	**4.86**	**.18**	**1.71**	.03	.29	-.08	-.78
Prevention behavior	**-.35**	**-4.81**	-.13	-1.37	.03	.30	.02	.22
Detection behavior	.08	.84	.12	1.08	.15	1.54	**.16**	**1.71**
Remediation	**-.16**	**-1.91**	-.13	-1.31	.08	1.30	.08	1.32
Context (Lab → Field)	**-.25**	**-2.74**	-.09	-.78	**.16**	**2.01**	**.18**	**2.27**
Students → Nonstudents	.02	.24	.07	.61	.13	1.39	.17	1.95
Journal: Other → Psychology	.08	-.82	.17	1.56	.05	.55	.03	.30
Journal: Other → Marketing	-.03	-.33	**.22**	**2.12**	.01	.14	.00	.01
Message variables								
Estimated fear			-.01	-.10			.02	.45
Low fear	.04	.56			-.08	-1.21		
Moderate fear	.01	.09			-.02	-.44		
High fear	.05	.75			-.01	-.16		
Gain frame	.01	.22	.05	.71	-.04	-.78	-.04	-.80
Loss frame	-.02	-.28	.02	.27	-.08	-1.39	-.09	-1.64
Vivid	-.03	-.41	**-.23**	**-3.31**	-.01	-.17	.07	1.29
Base rate started	**.11**	**2.04**	.05	.68	.05	.79	-.03	-.42
Case of a person(s)	**.39**	**5.14**	**.40**	**5.08**	**.21**	**2.86**	.10	1.57
Referencing	.10	1.25	.13	1.57	-.11	-1.54	-.03	-.36
Social consequence	.10	1.47	-.00	-.04	**.23**	**3.33**	**.25**	**3.62**
Physical consequence	**.13**	**1.84**	.04	.42	.01	.13	-.03	-.37
Estimated source			.05	.71			-.04	-.66
Female communicator	.03	.51	**-.17**	**-2.03**	-.03	-.50	.02	.39
Male communicator	**-.19**	**-3.81**	**-.30**	**-5.25**	**-.16**	**-3.03**	**-.15**	**-2.84**

Estimated argument strength			.12	1.83			.04	.68
Weak argument	.11	1.53			-.07	-1.37		
Strong argument	.17	2.41			-.04	-.82		
Two sides of an argument	.07	1.13	-.1	1.53	.02	.22	.03	.47
Number exposures	**.16**	**2.09**	-.04	-.42	**.13**	**1.85**	.07	1.24
Tailored	.07	1.21	.06	.98	-.04	-.51	-.07	-1.03
Emotional message	**.08**	**1.75**	**.18**	**3.34**	-.03	-.50	-.07	-1.07
Individual/Context variables								
Estimated race	**-.36**	**-6.38**	**-.29**	**-4.26**	-.01	-.15	.02	.34
Estimated gender	.03	.45	.10	1.25	**.20**	**3.17**	**.16**	**2.79**
Estimated age	.10	1.30	.08	.94	-.06	-.62	-.05	-.54
Prior intentions/Behavior	.30	3.56	.29	2.82	.17	2.70	.19	3.20
Estimated involvement/Vulnerability			.04	.53			.06	1.21
Low involvement	-.13	-2.45			.03	.56		
High involvement	-.09	-1.64			.11	1.79		
Estimated severity			.05	.48			.22	3.35
Severity low	-.23	-4.70			-.01	-.09		
Severity high	-.36	-6.50			.03	.47		
Estimated response efficacy			.02	.19			.19	2.98
Response efficacy low	.08	1.71			-.12	-2.17		
Response efficacy high	.14	2.91			-.09	-1.58		
Estimated self-efficacy			.05	.83			.15	2.87
Self-efficacy low	-.03	-.64			-.08	-1.55		
Self-efficacy high	-.01	-.10			-.01	-.09		
Promotion regulatory focus	**.17**	**2.86**	.07	1.02	.06	1.09	.06	1.21
Prevention regulatory focus	**.17**	**2.84**	.07	.97	.03	.50	.03	.56
R^2		.67		.53		.26		.31

Note: Significant effects in bold.

Table 1.3

Factors Explaining the Correlation Between Attitudes and Intentions

Predictor variables	B	β	t
Constant	−.96		−.211
Context characteristics			
Encourage behavior	−.80	−.80	−1.25
Discourage behavior	**−4.62**	**−4.297**	**−9.76**
Prevention behavior	.97	.88	1.71
Detection behavior	**1.31**	**1.22**	**2.33**
Context (Lab → Field)	**2.48**	**2.60**	**3.69**
Nonstudents → Students	**4.20**	**3.57**	**5.58**
Other → Psychology	**−1.81**	**−1.57**	**−5.95**
Message variables			
Estimated fear	−.05	−.03	−.43
Gain frame	**−2.02**	**−1.25**	**−11.32**
Loss frame	**−2.02**	**−1.25**	**−11.27**
Estimated vivid	−.02	.01	.08
Base rate stated	**−1.45**	**−.90**	**−5.21**
Case of a person(s)	−.17	−.17	−.93
Referencing	.26	.15	.60
Social consequence	−.08	−.04	−.25
Physical consequence	**−.73**	**−.42**	**−1.97**
Estimated source credibility	−.23	−.10	−.72
Estimated argument strength	**1.80**	**.39**	**2.96**
Number of exposures	−.23	−.27	−1.43
Two sides of an argument	−.00	−.00	−.02
Tailored	−.01	−.00	−.04
Individual differences			
Estimated race	4.78	.29	.85
Estimated age	**.02**	**.48**	**2.43**
Prior intentions/behavior	.02	.02	.22
Estimated involvement/vulnerability	.26	.07	1.09
Estimated severity	.21	.08	.59
Estimated response efficacy	**−2.60**	**−1.01**	**−5.04**
Estimated self-efficacy	.05	.02	.30

Note: Significant effects in bold; some variables are missing due to insufficient data; wherever possible, estimates replace manipulated values.

Janis 1953), an inverted-U relationship (Janis 1967; McGuire 1968) and a positive one (Boster and Mongeau 1984; Sutton 1982). We found no support for either a linear effect (attitudes: $R^2 = .00$, $F = .05$, $p = .82$, intentions: $R^2 = .00$, $F = .72$, $p = .40$) or a quadratic effect of fear (attitudes: $R^2 = .00$, $F = .39$, $p = .68$; intentions: $R^2 = .01$, $F = 1.55$, $p = .21$) in the published data examined.

The staged fear model is based on the view that high fear prompts defensive processing among those who are not predisposed to follow the recommendations (Keller 1999). We find support for this model on intentions ($R^2 = .06$, $F = 8.18$, $p < .001$) such that the impact of high fear on intentions was more positive when people were already predisposed to follow the recommendations (Table 1.4).

Protection Motivation Theory (PMT)

Rogers's (1975, 1983) PMT model indicates increases in protection intentions as a function of the probability attached to four factors: perceived severity, vulnerability, response efficacy, and self-efficacy. Several rules for combining these factors have been identified, although a simultaneous analysis of threat appraisal (vulnerability and severity) and coping appraisal (response and self-efficacy) seems most popular (Block and Keller 1998; Witte 1998; Wurtele and Maddux 1987).

Our findings indicate that the PMT model is significant for attitudes ($R^2 = .06$, $F = 4.06$, $p < .01$) and intentions ($R^2 = .04$, $F = 3.48$, $p < .01$). All four components have a positive impact on attitudes and intentions. However, the vulnerability path is insignificant for both attitudes and intentions and the severity path is insignificant for intentions (Table 1.4). Otherwise, as predicted by PMT, an increase in these factors is significantly associated with higher attitudes and intentions. Thus, in general the model is supported.

Rather than giving all four PMT factors the same status, the ordered protection motivation model (OPM) predicts staged appraisals of first threat (severity and vulnerability) and then coping appraisal (response efficacy and self-efficacy). Our findings do not support ordered PMT. Threat appraisal is not significantly related to response efficacy ($R^2 = .01$, $F = 1.36$, $p = .26$) or self-efficacy ($R^2 = .00$, $F = .16$, $p = .85$) for attitudes. For intentions, threat appraisal is significantly related to response efficacy ($R^2 = .04$, $F = 8.02$, $p < .001$) and self-efficacy ($R^2 = .03$, $F = 4.80$, $p < .01$), but not in the predicted directions; rather than increasing coping, an increase in severity is associated with lower self-efficacy, and vulnerability is associated with reduced response efficacy.

Scherer (1984, 1988) suggests that fear arousal mediates threat and coping appraisal. We did not find support for this model since threat appraisal was not significantly related to fear arousal. Thus, we find support for PMT but not for ordered PMT or PMT mediated by fear arousal.

Elaboration Likelihood Model (ELM)

The basic premise of ELM is that there are two routes to attitude change (Chaiken, Liberman, and Eagly 1989; Petty and Cacioppo 1986). When motivation or ability to process a persuasive message is relatively high, persuasion is more likely to occur as a function of careful consideration of the arguments presented (systematic or central route processing). By contrast, when motivation or ability to process the message is relatively low, persuasion is more likely to occur as a function of simple inferences from source characteristics or message execution factors such as vividness (heuristic or peripheral processing).

Table 1.4

Tests of Health Models

	Attitudes*		Intentions*	
	B**	t	β	t
Fear drive models				
Linear effect	−.02	−.23	.05	.85
Quadratic effect	.17	.85	.24	1.54
Staged fear drive model				
Fear × Prior intentions	−.26	−.71	**.39**	**2.29**
Protection motivation theory				
Severity	**.12**	**1.96**	.08	1.44
Vulnerability	.08	1.24	.06	1.16
Response efficacy	.16	2.51	.11	2.02
Self-efficacy	.15	2.35	.12	2.25
Ordered PMT				
Severity → Response efficacy	−.11	−1.63	**.19**	**3.62**
Vulnerability → Response efficacy	.02	.33	−.09	−1.69
Severity → Self-efficacy	−.03	−.46	−.09	−1.69
Vulnerability → Self-efficacy	.02	.37	**.14**	**2.60**
Elaboration likelihood model				
Involvement × Argument strength	−.42	−1.07	−.59	−1.18
Involvement × Vivid	−.16	−.82	−.22	−.86
Involvement × Case	**−.32**	**−1.69**	.02	.12
Involvement × Base	−.25	−1.74	−.36	−2.57
Involvement × Male communicator	−.37	−1.40	−.10	−.77
Involvement × Female communicator	.21	.78	−.03	−.16
Involvement × Gain frame	−.21	−1.39	−.17	−.84
Involvement × Loss frame	−.09	−.58	−.28	−1.38

To examine ELM in a health communication context, we ran five separate regressions with main and interaction effects to test how the level of involvement impacts the influence of five message factors:

1. argument strength,
2. vividness (pictures or text),
3. base or case rate information,
4. male or female communicator, and
5. framing.

That is, we tested the main effects of estimated involvement/vulnerability and argument strength and the interaction between the two on attitudes and intentions.

Absence of support for ELM for health communications was indicated by mostly insignificant interactions. The strongest interaction was between involvement and base information and it was negative. However, of the sixteen

	Attitudes*		Intentions*	
	B^{**}	t	β	t
Prospect theory				
Loss frame × Prevention	.17	.89	−.10	−.66
Gain frame × Prevention	.02	.09	−.16	−1.06
Loss frame × Detection	−.03	−.33	−.06	−.57
Gain frame × Detection	−.08	−.83	−.18	**−1.70**
Loss frame × Encourage healthy behaviors	−.03	−.22	.18	1.20
Gain frame × Encourage healthy behaviors	−.09	−.56	.18	1.21
Loss frame × Discourage unhealthy behaviors	**−.20**	**−3.13**	−.00	−.06
Gain frame × Discourage unhealthy behaviors	**−.15**	**−2.42**	−.01	−.25
Loss frame × Consequences to self vs. others	.14	1.95	.18	2.96
Gain frame × Consequences to self vs. others	.12	1.70	.19	3.16
Regulatory fit				
Promotion focus × Encourage healthy behaviors	**−.12**	**−1.96**	−.02	−0.32
Prevention focus × Encourage healthy behaviors	−.10	−1.08	−.05	−.74
Promotion focus × Discourage unhealthy behaviors	−	−	−	−
Prevention focus × Discourage unhealthy behaviors	.20	2.51	.18	1.22
Promotion focus × Gain frame	**.31**	**2.93**	.03	.41
Prevention focus × Gain frame	.29	2.24	.12	1.97
Promotion focus × Loss frame	**.30**	**2.36**	.11	1.61
Prevention focus × Loss frame	**.36**	**2.75**	.01	.12
Promotion focus × Self-efficacy	−.21	−.86	.00	.03
Prevention focus × Self-efficacy	−.24	−1.00	**.26**	**−2.17**
Promotion focus × Response efficacy	.12	.52	−.04	−.37
Prevention focus × Response efficacy	.16	.67	**.20**	**1.70**

Note: Significant effects are in bold; *all relevant main effects were included in the model to test the interaction effects; **net effect after accounting for main effects.

interactions tested for attitude and intention, fifteen were negative (and the other was +.02). This suggests that involvement tends to decrease the positive impact of these message factors or, when the impact is negative, makes it even more negative.

Prospect Theory

Prospect theory suggests that people are more willing to accept risks when they evaluate options in terms of associated costs or losses, but avoid risks when options are described as benefits or gains (Tversky and Kahneman 1981). To examine the predicted higher persuasion in the lower risk/gain and the higher risk/loss conditions, we analyzed loss and gain frames with three sets of behaviors that might vary in level of risk: prevention (less risk) versus detection (more risk), encouraging health-affirming action (less risk) versus discouraging unhealthy behavior (more risk), and consequences that affected others (less risk) rather than oneself (more risk). We used regressions that included four main effects (e.g., gain frame, loss frame, prevention, detection) and the appropriate interaction term with framing (e.g., gain/prevention, gain/detection, loss/prevention, loss/detection) when we examined prevention versus detection.

The data do not support prospect theory. There was no significant effect of prevention/detection behaviors on attitudes ($R^2 = .03$, $F = 1.01$, $p = .43$) or intentions ($R^2 = .02$, $F = .77$, $p = .63$). The overall regression for encouraging/ discouraging health behaviors is significant for attitudes ($R^2 = .14$, $F = 4.72$, $p = .001$) but not intentions ($R^2 = .03$, $F = 1.33$, $p = .23$), whereas the reverse is true for referencing (intentions: $R^2 = .08$, $F = 5.75$, $p < .001$, attitudes: $R^2 = .03$, $F = 1.50$, $p = .19$). The impact of frames was less positive when the message discourages unhealthy behaviors and more positive when the consequences of nonadherence were directed at someone other than the recipient. These findings do not provide support for prospect theory since both frames have the same directional impact.

Regulatory Fit

According to regulatory focus theory (Higgins 1997), most people have one of two foci. People with a promotion focus seek accomplishment and growth and are more risk-seeking. In contrast, individuals with a prevention focus seek security and safety and are more risk-averse (Shah, Higgins, and Friedman 1998). People experience regulatory fit when their goal pursuit process is compatible with their regulatory focus (Higgins 2000). Regulatory fit has been observed with message frames and efficacy appraisals (promotion/gains, prevention/losses: Aaker and Lee 2001; promotion/self-efficacy, prevention/ response efficacy: Keller 2006).

We analyzed regulatory fit for three variables, encouraging health-affirming actions versus discouraging unhealthy behavior, gain versus loss framing, and low versus high response and self-efficacy. Our data indicate mixed support for regulatory fit. We found support for regulatory fit between regulatory focus and whether the message goal was to encourage or discourage behaviors, although the model fit the data on attitudes ($R^2 = .11$, $F = 5.95$, $p < .001$) better than intentions ($R^2 = .03$, $F = 1.55$, $p = .14$). Attitudes were more favorable when promotion-oriented people were encouraged to undertake health-affirming actions and when prevention-oriented people were discouraged from unhealthy actions.

Regulatory focus and message frame significantly impacted attitudes ($R^2 = .08$, $F = 2.48$, $p = .01$), but not intentions ($R^2 = .03$, $F = 1.22$, $p = .29$). Regulatory fit was not supported, as an increase in either regulatory focus (prevention or promotion) was associated with less favorable attitudes, in the presence of either a gain or loss frame. The findings for the regulatory fit model examining regulatory focus and efficacy were also mixed (intentions: $R^2 = .03$, $F = 2.18$, $p = .056$; attitudes: $R^2 = .04$, $F = 1.77$, $p = .12$). Consistent with the regulatory fit model, intentions to comply were higher when prevention-oriented people were appraising response efficacy than when they were appraising self-efficacy.

DISCUSSION

Consumer research studies provide several guidelines for the content and formatting of obesity communications. The basic overriding result is that the type of message communication used has an impact on attitudes and intentions based on a meta-analysis of 85 papers which report results in 584 different experimental conditions. Some of the most influential variables for increasing intentions are case information (i.e., a story about an individual), not using a male to communicate the message, and focusing on detection behavior. Intentions also depend importantly on a number of context and individual differences including perceived severity, response efficacy, and self-efficacy. These findings suggest that effectiveness of obesity communication may be enhanced by increasing the severity of obesity-related health consequences (e.g., heart attack vs. diabetes). In addition, using emotional stories about why and how other normal people (not physicians or other medical service providers) were successful in achieving their weight reduction goals is another recommendation for effective obesity message formatting. Looked at more closely, the results have some interesting aspects that bear further discussion.

Attitudes Versus Intentions

The context, message, and individual characteristics that best explain attitudes are not the same characteristics that best explain intentions. In general, we seem to have more control over attitudes than intentions. Health message communications are key for attitude formation, but individual and context differences compete with message factors for determining intentions to comply with the message recommendations.

With one exception (the use of cases or stories), the five characteristics that best explain attitudes do not overlap with the five factors that most influence intentions. Messages advocating prevention behaviors that evoke high severity (e.g., "eat calcium since you are at high risk for osteoporosis") to nonwhite targets are negatively related to attitudes, whereas stories discouraging unhealthy behaviors (e.g., Kim was unhappy with herself and decided she was going to stop eating high-fat snacks) can enhance attitudes. If the goal is to enhance intentions to follow recommendations, however, the best place to start would be to target a female who had high prior intentions or was already following the recommended behaviors with a story on the negative or positive social consequences of (non)adherence without using a male communicator (e.g., Kim was already considering changing her snacking habits and Oprah's story about moms who have more energy to spend time with their kids and friends increased her resolve).

Context characteristics that are associated with positive attitudes toward health recommendations such as encouraging or discouraging unhealthy behaviors have the opposite relationship with intentions. For example, people seem comfortable forming positive attitudes toward healthy behaviors, but their intentions are lower when faced with these choices. Similarly, lab studies are associated with more positive attitudes, but lower intentions. Further, several message factors have a significant effect on attitudes or intentions but not both, while only three factors have similar effects (case information and multiple exposures have positive effects, male communicator has a negative effect). There are also six message factors that influence neither attitudes nor intentions (fear, message frame, referencing, source credibility, two-sided arguments, and tailoring), which suggests placing less emphasis on these factors.

Why might someone have positive attitudes toward the advocated health behavior yet not form intentions to comply with the behavior? According to the theory of reasoned action (TRA), intentions are a function of attitude toward the behavior and subjective norms or social pressures regarding the performance of the behavior (Fishbein and Ajzen 1975). However, the TRA is based on the assumption that humans act rationally and that the behavior is under complete volitional control of the individual. In practice, individual differences (e.g., ability, motivation, knowledge, emotions) and context factors (e.g., social support, convenience) undermine volitional control (Van Hooft et al. 2005). To address this issue, Ajzen (1985) introduced the theory of planned behavior (TRB), which is an extension of TRA with perceived behavioral control that is similar to self-efficacy (Bandura 1982). Thus, attitudes may be better predictors of intentions when self-efficacy is high than when it is low (Sutton 1998).

Although attitudes and intentions have been disconnected in the past literature (Chandon, Morowitz, and Reinartz 2005; Chatzisarantis et al. 2004), our findings that they have different antecedents is news. Health recommendations may result in conflict between health and nonhealth goals. For example, smoking may be viewed as a positive means to reducing weight, but negatively related to looking attractive. Similarly, eating fish may be positively related to a health goal, but negatively related to the goal met by comfort foods.

The discrepancy between attitudes and intentions also suggests the need to incorporate additional dimensions of affect to close the gap between attitudes and intentions. For example, instead of attitudes, we might need to focus on desire. Desires imply a motivational commitment to act; attitudes do not. Desires refer to future states, whereas attitudes can apply to the past, the present, or the future. Attitudes are held or can be changed (not satisfied), whereas desires are satisfied (Oettingen, Pak, and Schnetter 2001). Since a large part of the challenge to lose weight is based on fantasizing about the ideal size, it is worth examining the consumer psychology literature on fantasy. Fantasy seduces a person to mentally enjoy the desired future in the here and now because there are no reflections on present reality that would point to the fact that the positive future is not realized (Oettingen, Pak, and Schnetter 2001). Thus a necessity to act is not induced and expectations of success are not activated or used. We should warn consumers about the downsides of fantasizing if they want to lose weight. Process goals on when, where, how (e.g., "I will eat an omelet for lunch every other day") are as important, if not more important, than outcome goals.

The effectiveness of obesity communication may be enhanced by helping consumers manage emotions. Sad people often turn to food for immediate comfort. Obesity communication needs to make people aware of the importance of making healthy food accessible when anticipating a sad situation. It is also important to disconnect food from positive emotions. One of the goals of obesity communication is to lower the audience's resistance to altering the belief that happiness cannot be found without food. Instead of rewards, message reminders need to connect food with negative associations such as physical discomfort or heartburn. Obesity communication needs to include new methods for enhancing comfort as well as cues to retrieve occasions when food was resisted. Finally, ideas about nonfood rewards for overcoming eating obstacles are needed to prevent relapse (e.g., buying a novel or planning a vacation).

Our findings also suggest that intentions may reflect trade-offs across health and other behaviors, whereas attitudes may be formed in the context of a particular health behavior. In particular, the finding that self-efficacy influences intentions, but not attitudes, suggests that even if response efficacy is high, people are not willing to consider undertaking the behavior if they do not believe they can. They may, however, compensate by engaging in other behaviors related to health or even more abstract goals. For example, feeling bad due to an unhealthy lunch may be compensated for by increased volunteer work (to feel good).

Implications for Modeling Health Communications

Our results provide insights into the process underlying message effects on attitudes and intentions. We did not find support for the fear-driven model, but we did find that the impact of high fear on intentions was more positive when people were already predisposed to follow the recommendations. The literature reviews indicating a positive linear relationship between fear and attitudes (Boster and Mongeau 1984; Sutton 1982) suggest that previous samples are likely to have included students with high priors.

Our data support protection motivation theory, but not its extensions. Lack of support for the ordered PMT is consistent with other studies indicating that severity and vulnerability have opposite effects (Sheeran and Orbell 1998). An increase in severity is associated with increased response efficacy, whereas a decrease in vulnerability is marginally associated with increased response efficacy. Further, an increase in severity is marginally associated with lower self-efficacy, whereas the impact of self-efficacy on intentions is higher when people are vulnerable. The data do not support Scherer's (1984, 1988) view that fear arousal is a mediator between threat and coping appraisal. Specifically, threat appraisal was not significantly related to fear arousal.

In general, we also did not find strong support for the elaboration likelihood model as most of the health message factors seemed to undermine attitudes and intentions when people were highly involved. In this context, two findings may be viewed as supportive of ELM. First, case materials such as stories were associated with lower attitudes in general, especially for people who were highly involved. This is consistent with the view that vivid material may distract people who want to engage in central message processing. Second, for more involved audiences, base information is associated with lower attitudes and intentions. If base information is viewed as a central cue, then, in contrast to ELM, our findings indicate that higher levels of involvement are associated with higher intentions when base information is not included in the message. These findings support ELM if base information is regarded as aggregate and/or not informative among involved audiences.

We also did not find support for prospect theory; either the type of frame was associated with less favorable attitudes in relatively high risk contexts (e.g., discourage unhealthy behaviors) or loss frames were more effective than gain frames in lower risk contexts (e.g., consequences of secondhand smoke). Unless risk assessment is reversed for consequences directed at oneself as opposed to others, this finding is the opposite of that predicted by prospect theory. Regardless, both loss and gain frames produce similar directional effects.

Our data provide mixed support for regulatory fit (Higgins 1997). Consistent with regulatory fit, attitudes were more favorable when prevention-oriented people were discouraged from unhealthy behaviors, whereas encouraging behavior did not influence them. Also, intentions were higher when prevention-oriented people were given response efficacy rather than self-efficacy information. Similar to other studies, promotion-oriented people were not as sensitive as prevention-oriented people to the health behavior or efficacy variables (Lee, Keller, and Sternthal 2010). However, any increase in regulatory focus was associated with less favorable attitudes in the presence of either frame.

The Case for Tailoring Obesity Messages

Our results indicate it is best to avoid relying on mass appeals to influence intentions to comply with health recommendations. Rather, information on gender, age, race, prior intentions, and regulatory focus of the target audience is critical in designing effective health communications. The literature indicates that as compared to males, females are more likely to make trade-offs across domains than within health domains. Furthermore, females are less likely to update their weight goals and body image standards. Females also overeat in response to and in anticipation of emotions, especially sad emotions (Dube and Morgan 1996; Keller 2009). Finally, females are more likely to control themselves out of a sense of responsibility for others. These findings highlight the need to tailor obesity communications for male and female segments.

The literature suggests that race segments may be relevant for designing message content and placement to reduce obesity. Research on social norms and parenting skills are relevant to enhancing the effectiveness of obesity communications. A study by Kumanyika and Grier (2006) identifies the need to counteract the disproportionate onslaught of fast-food marketing in minority neighborhoods. Research also indicates that non-Caucasian audiences may be more persuaded by vivid than nonvivid health communications (Keller and Lehmann 2008).

The findings from our meta-analysis may also be used to facilitate the design of effective health communications. In addition to demographic variables such as gender and race, one might use sociopsychological variables such as involvement, protection motivation variables such as perceived severity or efficacy, and self-regulation orientations such as promotion or prevention focus as a basis for segmentation. For example, elderly audiences who typically strive for the minimum acceptable health goals (i.e., a prevention focus) may be more influenced by messages that discourage unhealthy behaviors than by messages that encourage healthy eating and exercise behaviors (Keller and Lehmann 2008).

The numerous significant interactions suggest the importance of matching health communication to the target audience. Public service announcements that work for one group or segment may boomerang or be ignored by other segments. There is significant interaction between fear, prior intentions, and the coping appraisal variables. In addition, our findings indicate that response and self-efficacy have different effects on attitudes and intentions. An increase in self-efficacy is positively related to higher intentions, but intentions are even higher with the addition of high fear. By contrast, although an increase in general response efficacy increases intentions, when high fear is present, high response efficacy is associated with lower intentions. One explanation for these results is that fear can be motivating when people are confident they can undertake the recommended actions (i.e., under high self-efficacy conditions). However, high levels of fear can be a deterrent when people believe the actions may be effective (high response efficacy), but do not know whether they can implement the actions. This explanation is consistent with the finding that high response efficacy has little impact on those people with high prior intentions and actually is associated with lower attitudes among the converted. Thus, those with high prior intentions may be seeking to strengthen their beliefs on self-efficacy or on how to implement their goals rather than on whether the recommended actions are effective.

Limitations

Obviously this study has limitations. It does not examine the relationship between attitudes, intentions, and behavior. Similar meta-analyses in the nonhealth literature indicate that intentions explain no more than 50 percent of behavior and that relationship is diminished as the time gap between assessment of intentions and behavior increases (Sheeran and Orbell 1998). One approach to increase the link between intentions and behavior is to encourage people to set clear standards regarding when the intended outcome will be achieved (Gollwitzer 1990). Another method is to present people with hypothetical scenarios that describe (un)successful progress toward behavioral outcomes, measuring intentions to continue performance of the

Table 1.5

Summary of Significant Context, Individual, and Message Effects on Attitudes and Intentions

Study characteristics	Significant findings
Context effects	1. Message recommendations that encourage healthy behaviors (e.g., exercise) or discourage unhealthy behaviors (e.g., quit snacking) are positively and significantly associated with attitudes, but encouraging healthy behaviors is negatively related to intention. 2. Prevention (e.g., do not eat while watching TV) and remediation recommendations (e.g., cholesterol-reducing statins) are negatively associated with attitude, whereas detection recommendations (e.g., diabetes-related blood test) are insignificant. By contrast, detection recommendations are positively related to intention. 3. Message interventions in lab studies produce more positive attitudes than those done in the field, whereas the opposite is true of intention. 4. The use of students versus nonstudents made no difference in attitudes, but nonstudents have more positive intentions. 5. There is some indication that marketing journals report more positive attitudes than journals in other fields such as psychology, health, or communications.
Individual effects	1. Whites are associated with significantly less positive attitudes, while females have more positive intentions. By contrast, age makes no significant difference. 2. Not surprisingly, prior intentions are positively related to attitudes and intentions. 3. While estimated involvement/vulnerability makes little difference, in cases where involvement was manipulated to be either low or high, low involvement was related to less favorable attitudes and high involvement to high intentions. Either low or high severity was negatively related to attitude, but not intentions. 4. Those cases where response efficacy was manipulated had more favorable attitude and lower intentions; when estimated response efficacy was analyzed, it has a positive impact on intentions. 5. Manipulations of self-efficacy had an insignificant impact, but estimated self-efficacy had, as expected, a positive impact on intentions. 6. Manipulations of regulatory focus had a positive impact on attitude, but not intention; both promotion and prevention regulatory focus manipulations are related to more favorable attitudes.
Message effects	1. Contrary to expectations, the level of fear has an insignificant impact on attitude and an insignificant negative one on intention. 2. Gain and loss frames in health messages have little impact, although loss frames may lead to somewhat lower intentions. 3. Vivid material, such as a before-after picture of a model, appears to be associated with lower attitudes, but is unrelated to intentions.

4. Messages that contain either base (percent of the population that is obese) or case (a story about a specific person battling obesity) information are associated with more positive attitudes; case information appears to increase intentions as well.
5. Self versus other referencing (effect of obesity on oneself or close others) has no significant impact, although directionally other referencing is positively related to attitudes but not to intention.
6. Social consequences are positively related to intentions but not attitude, while physical consequences may be positively related to attitude but not intention.
7. Using both female and male communicators appears to undermine attitude, while only male communicators have a negative impact on intentions.
8. Stronger arguments enhance attitudes but not intention, while the number of exposures to a message increases both.
9. While tailored messages have no significant impact, emotional messages have a negative impact, although only significantly so for attitude.

---

behavior—for example, sticking to a diet at weight loss of three pounds in the first month, two in the second, and so on (Chatzisarantis et al. 2004).

We also were unable to examine some important variables and to test some theories due to insufficient data. In particular we were limited in our examination of the role of elaboration, recall, affective reaction to the consequences, and health recommendations. Also we could not test the health belief model or the transtheoretical model because of insufficient data.

Future studies should include more nonexperimental data; our limited data suggest that lab studies and field studies produce different results. In addition to more effectively capturing the influence of individual and context factors, field studies may provide more insights on longitudinal effects and the relationship between attitudes, intentions, and behavior. There are also the standard problems of meta-analysis. These include the possibility of omitted studies (also known as the file drawer problem) and the unbalanced nature of the design. Further, the results are aggregate and largely correlational since we do not have a model of the causal relations among all the variables.

All these problems notwithstanding, there are some interesting and potentially important results. The consumer literature and models provide specific guidelines to design more effective obesity messages. There is tremendous potential to reduce obesity via effective health communications.

REFERENCES

Aaker, Jennifer L., and Angela Y. Lee. 2001. "'I' Seek Pleasures and 'We' Avoid Pains: The Role of Self-Regulatory Goals in Information Processing and Persuasion." *Journal of Consumer Research*, 28, 33–49.
Ahluwalia, Rohini. 2000. "Examination of Psychological Processes Underlying Resistance to Persuasion." *Journal of Consumer Research*, 27 (2) (September), 217–232.

Ajzen, Icek. 1985. "From Intentions to Actions: A Theory of Planned Behaviour." In *Action-Control: From Cognition to Behaviour*, ed. J. Kuhl and J. Beckman, 11–39. Heidelberg: Springer.

Albarracin, Dolores, Joel B. Cohen, and Taren G. Kumkale. 2003. "When Communications Collide With Recipients' Actions: Effects of Post-Message Behavior on Intentions to Follow the Message Recommendation." *Personality and Social Psychology Bulletin*, 29 (7), 834–845.

Bandura, Albert. 1982. "Self-Efficacy Mechanism in Human Agency." *American Psychologist*, 37, 122–147.

Barber, Patricia, Beatriz G. Lopez-Valcarcel, Jaime Pinilla, Yolanda Santana, Jose R. Calvo, and Anselmo Lopez. 2005. "Attitudes of Teenagers Towards Cigarettes and Smoking Initiation." *Substance Use & Misuse*, 40 (5), 625–643.

Beech, John R., and James Whittaker. 2001. "What Is the Female Image Projected by Smoking?" *Psychologia*, 44 (3), 230–236.

Block, Lauren G., and Punam A. Keller. 1995. "When to Accentuate the Negative: The Effects of Perceived Efficacy and Message Framing on Intentions to Perform a Health-Related Behavior." *Journal of Marketing Research*, 32 (2), 192–203.

———. 1997. "Effects of Self-Efficacy and Vividness on the Persuasiveness of Health Communications." *Journal of Consumer Psychology*, 6 (1), 31–54.

———. 1998. "Beyond Protection Motivation: An Integrative Theory of Health Appeals." *Journal of Applied Social Psychology*, 28 (17), 1584–1608.

Boster, Franklin J., and Paul Mongeau. 1984. "Fear-Arousing Persuasive Messages." In *Communication Yearbook 8*, ed. Robert N. Bostrom, 330–375. Beverly Hills, CA: Sage.

Brown, Stephen P., and Douglas M. Stayman. 1992. "Antecedents and Consequences of Attitudes Toward the Ad: A Meta-Analysis." *Journal of Consumer Research*, 19 (1), 34–51.

Brug, Johannes, Karen Glanz, Patricia Van Assema, Gerjo Kok, and Gerard J.P. van Breukelen. 1998. "The Impact of Computer-Tailored Feedback and Iterative Feedback on Fat, Fruit, and Vegetable Intake." *Health Education and Behavior*, 25 (4), 517–531.

Byrne, Christina A., and Ileana Arias. 2004. "Predicting Women's Intentions to Leave Abusive Relationships: An Application of the Theory of Planned Behavior." *Journal of Applied Social Psychology*, 34 (12), 2586–2601.

Calder, Bobby J., Lynn W. Phillips, and Alice M. Tybout. 1981. "Designing Research for Application." *Journal of Consumer Research*, 8 (September), 197–207.

Chaiken, Shelley, Akiva Liberman, and Alice H. Eagly. 1989. "Heuristic and Systematic Information Processing Within and Beyond the Persuasion Context." In *Unintended Thought*, ed. James S. Uleman and John A. Bargh, 212–252. New York: Guilford Press.

Chandon, Pierre, Vicki G. Morowitz, and William J. Reinartz. 2005. "Do Intentions Really Predict Behavior? Self-Generated Validity Effects in Survey Research." *Journal of Marketing*, 69 (2), 1–14.

Chatzisarantis, Nikos L.D., Martin S. Hagger, Brett Smith, and Cassie Phoenix. 2004. "The Influences of Continuation Intentions on Execution of Social Behaviour within the Theory of Planned Behaviour." *British Journal of Social Psychology*, 43 (4), 551–583.

Connolly, Ceci. 2004. "Higher Costs, Less Care." *Washington Post*, September 28.

Cooper, M. Lynne, V. Bede Agocha, and Melanie S. Sheldon. 2000. "A Motivational Perspective on Risky Behaviors: The Role of Personality and Affect Regulatory Processes." *Journal of Personality*, 68 (6), 1059–1088.

Curry, Susan J., Colleen McBride, Louis C. Grothaus, Doug Louie, and Edward H. Wagner. 1995. "A Randomized Trial of Self-Help Materials, Personalized Feedback, and Telephone Counseling with Nonvolunteer Smokers." *Journal of Consulting and Clinical Psychology*, 63 (6), 1005–1014.

Denscombe, Martyn. 2001. "Uncertain Identities and Health-Risking Behaviour: The Case of Young People and Smoking in Late Modernity." *British Journal of Sociology*, 52, 157–177.

Dijkstra, Arie, Hein De Vries, and Jolanda Roijackers. 1999. "Targeting Smokers with Low Readiness to Change with Tailored and Nontailored Self-Help Materials." *Preventative Medicine*, 28, 203–211.

Dinoff, Beth L., and Robin M. Kowalski. 1999. "Reducing AIDS Risk Behavior: The Combined Efficacy of Protection Motivation Theory and the Elaboration Likelihood Model." *Journal of Social and Clinical Psychology*, 18 (2), 223–239.

Drossaert, Constance H.C., Henk Boer, and Erwin R. Seydel. 1996. "Health Education to Improve Repeat Participation in the Dutch Breast Cancer Screening Programme: Evaluation of a Leaflet Tailored to Previous Participants." *Patient Education and Counseling*, 28, 121–131.

Dube, Laurette, and Michael Morgan. 1996. "Trend Effects and Gender Differences in Retrospective Judgments of Consumption Emotions." *Journal of Consumer Research*, 23 (September), 156–162.

Escalas, Jennifer, and Mary Francis Luce. 2003. "Process vs. Outcome Thought-Focus and Narrative Advertising." *Journal of Consumer Psychology*, 13 (3), 246–254.

———. 2004. "Understanding the Effects of Process-Focused versus Outcome-Focused Thought During Advertising." *Journal of Consumer Research*, 31 (2), 274–286.

Everett, Maureen W., and Philip Palmgreen. 1995. "Influences of Sensation Seeking, Message Sensation Value, and Program Context on Effectiveness of Anti-Cocaine Public Service Announcements." *Health Communication*, 7 (3), 225–248.

Farley John U., and Donald R. Lehmann. 1986. *Meta-analysis in Marketing: Generalization of Response Models*. Lexington, MA: Lexington Books.

Farley, John U., Donald R. Lehmann, and Lane H. Mann. 1998. "Designing the Next Study for Maximum Impact." *Journal of Marketing Research*, 35 (4), 496–501.

Fejfar, Michele C., and Rick H. Hoyle. 2000. "Effect of Private Self-Awareness on Negative Affect and Self-Referent Attribution: A Quantitative Review." *Personality and Social Psychology Review*, 4 (2), 132–142.

Feshbach, Seymour, and Irving L. Janis. 1953. "Effects of Fear-Arousing Communications." *Journal of Abnormal and Social Psychology*, 48 (1), 78–92.

Fishbein, Martin, and Icek Ajzen. 1975. "Bayesian Analysis of Attribution Processes." *Psychological Bulletin*, 82 (2), 261–277.

Fruin, Donna J., Chris Pratt, and Neville Owen. 1992. "Protection Motivation Theory and Adolescents' Perceptions of Exercise." *Journal of Applied Social Psychology*, 22, 55–69.

Gerrard, Meg, Frederick X. Gibbons, Monica Reis-Bergan, and Daniel W. Russell. 2000. "Self-Esteem, Self-Serving Cognitions, and Health Risk Behavior." *Journal of Personality*, 68 (6), 1177–1201.

Gleicher, Faith, and Richard E. Petty. 1992. "Expectations of Reassurance Influence the Nature of Fear-Stimulated Attitude Change." *Journal of Experimental Social Psychology*, 28, 86–100.

Gollwitzer, Peter M. 1990. "Action Phases and Mind-Sets." In *The Handbook of Motivation and Cognition: Foundations of Social Behavior*, ed. E.T. Higgins and R.M. Sorrentino, 53–92. New York: Guilford Press.

Greening, Leilani. 1997. "Adolescents' Cognitive Appraisals of Cigarette Smoking: An Application of the Protection Motivation Theory." *Journal of Applied Social Psychology*, 27, 1972–1985.

Higgins, E. Tory. 1997. "Beyond Pleasure and Pain." *American Psychologist*, 52 (December), 1280–1300.

———. 2000. "Making a Good Decision: Value from Fit." *American Psychologist*, 55 (November), 1217–1230.

Hovland, Carl Iver, Irving L. Janis, and Harold H. Kelley. 1953. *Communication and Persuasion; Psychological Studies of Opinion Change.* New Haven: Yale University Press.

Hoyle, Rick H., Michele C. Fejfar, and Joshua D. Miller. 2000. "Personality and Sexual Risk-Taking: A Quantitative Review." *Journal of Personality*, 68, 1203–1231.

Igartua, Juan J., Lifen Cheng, and Orquidea Lopes. 2003. "To Think or Not to Think: Two Pathways Towards Persuasion by Short Films on Aids Preventions." *Journal of Health Communication*, 8, 513–528.

Janis, Irving L. 1967. "Effects of Fear Arousal on Attitude Change: Recent Developments in Theory and Experimental Research." In *Advances in Experimental Social Psychology*, vol. 3, ed. Leonard Berkowitz, 166–224. New York: Academic Press.

Juster, Frank T. 1966. "Consumer Buying Intentions and Purchase Probability: An Experiment in Survey Design." *Journal of the American Statistical Association*, 61 (September), 658–696.

Keller, Punam A. 1999. "Converting the Unconverted: The Effect of Inclination and Opportunity to Discount Health-Related Fear Appeals." *Journal of Applied Psychology*, 84 (3), 403–115.

———. 2006. "Regulatory Focus and Efficacy of Health Messages." *Journal of Consumer Research*, 33 (1), 109–114.

———. 2009. "Affect and Risk: Gender Differences." Working paper, Tuck School of Business at Dartmouth University.

Keller, Punam A., and Lauren G. Block. 1997. "Vividness Effects: A Resource Matching Perspective." *Journal of Consumer Research*, 24, 295–304.

———. 1999. "The Effect of Affect-Based Dissonance versus Cognition-Based Dissonance on Motivated Reasoning and Health-Related Persuasion." *Journal of Experimental Psychology: Applied*, 5 (3), 302–313.

Keller, Punam A., and Donald R. Lehmann. 2008. "Designing Effective Health Communications: A Meta-Analysis of Experimental Results." *Journal of Public Policy and Marketing*, 27 (2), 117–130.

Keller, Punam A., Isaac M. Lipkus, and Barbara K. Rimer. 2002. "Depressive Realism and Health Risk Accuracy: The Negative Consequences of Positive Mood." *Journal of Consumer Research*, 29 (1), 57–69.

———. 2003. "Affect, Framing and Persuasion." *Journal of Marketing Research*, 40 (February), 54–64.

Keller, Punam A., and Ardis L. Olson. 2009. "Negative Emotions and Coping Health Appraisal." Working paper, Tuck School of Business at Dartmouth University.

Kisielius, Jolita, and Brian Sternthal. 1986. "Examining the Vividness Controversy: An Availability-Valence Interpretation." *Journal of Consumer Research*, 12 (4), 418–431.

Kumanyika, Shiriki Kinika, and Sonya Grier. 2006. "Targeting Interventions for Ethnic Minority and Low-Income Populations." *Future of Children*, 16 (1), 187–207.

Lee, Angela Y., and Jennifer L. Aaker. 2004. "Bringing the Frame Into Focus: The Influence of Regulatory Fit on Processing Fluency and Persuasion." *Journal of Personality and Social Psychology*, 86 (2), 205–218.

Lee, Angela Y., Punam A. Keller, and Brian Sternthal. 2010. "Value from Regulatory Construal Fit: The Persuasive Impact of Fit between Consumer Goals and Message Concreteness." *Journal of Consumer Research*, 36 (5), 735–747.

Lemieux, James, and Leigh McAlister. 2005. "Handling Missing Values in Marketing Data: A Comparison of Techniques." *MSI Reports*, 2, 41–60.

Lipkus, Isaac M., Monica Biradavolu, Kathryn Fenn, Punam A. Keller, and Barbara K. Rimer. 2001. "Informing Women about Their Breast Cancer Risks: Truth and Consequences." *Health Communication*, 13 (2), 205–226.

Lynch, John G., Jr. 1982. "On the External Validity of Experiments in Consumer Research." *Journal of Consumer Research*, 9 (3), 225–239.

Maddux, James E., and Ronald W. Rogers. 1983. "Protection Motivation and Self-Efficacy: A Revised Theory of Fear Appeals and Attitude Change." *Journal of Experimental Social Psychology*, 19, 469–479.

Maheswaran, Durairaj, and Joan Meyers-Levy. 1990. "The Influence of Message Framing and Issue Involvement." *Journal of Marketing Research*, 27 (3), 361–367.

McFerran, Brent, Darren W. Dahl, Gavan J. Fitzsimons, and Andrea C. Morales. 2009. "I'll Have What She's Having: Effects of Social Influence and Body Type on the Food Choices of Others." *Journal of Consumer Research*, 36 (6), 915–929.

McGuire, William J. 1962. "Persistence of the Resistance to Persuasion Induced by Various Types of Prior Belief Defenses." *Journal of Abnormal and Social Psychology*, 64 (4), 241–248.

———. 1968. "Personality and Susceptibility to Social Influence." In *Handbook of Personality Theory and Research*, ed. Edgar F. Borgatta and William W. Lambert, 1130–1187. Chicago: Rand McNally.

Menon, Geeta, Lauren G. Block, and Suresh Ramanthan. 2002. "We're at as Much Risk as We Are Led to Believe: Effects of Message Cues on Judgments of Health Risk." *Journal of Consumer Research*, 28 (4), 533–549.

Meyerowitz, Beth E., and Shelley Chaiken. 1987. "The Effect of Message Framing on Breast Self-Examination Attitudes, Intentions, and Behavior." *Journal of Personality and Social Psychology*, 52 (3), 500–510.

Meyers-Levy, Joan. 1988. "Gender Differences in Information Processing: A Selectivity Interpretation." In *Cognitive and Affective Responses to Advertising,* ed. Pat Cafferata and Alice M. Tybout, 219–260. Lexington, MA: Lexington Books.

Milne, Sarah, Paschal Sheeran, and Sheina Orbell. 2000. "Prediction and Intervention in Health-Related Behavior: A Meta-Analytic Review of Protection Motivation Theory." *Journal of Applied Social Psychology*, 30, 106–143.

Oettingen, Gabriele, Hyeon-ju Pak, and Karoline Schnetter. 2001. "Self-Regulation of Goal Setting: Turning Free Fantasies about the Future into Binding Goals." *Journal of Personality and Social Psychology*, 80, 736–753.

Palmgreen, Philip, Donohew Lewis, Elizabeth Pugzles Lorch, Rick H. Hoyle, and Michael T. Stephenson. 2001. "Television Campaigns and Adolescent Marijuana Use: Tests of Sensation Seeking Targeting." *American Journal of Public Health*, 91 (2), 292–296.

Passyn, Kirsten, and Mita Sujan. 2006. "Self-Accountability Emotions and Fear Appeals: Motivating Behaviors." *Journal of Consumer Research*, (March), 583–589.

Pechmann, Cornelia, and Chuan-Fong Shih. 1999. "Smoking Scenes in Movies and Antismoking Advertisements before Movies: Effects on Youth." *Journal of Marketing*, 63 (3), 1–13.

Perugini, Marco. 2005. "Predictive Models of Implicit and Explicit Attitudes." *British Journal of Social Psychology*, 44, 29–45.

Peterson, Robert A. 2001. "On the Use of College Students in Social Science Research: Insights from a Second Order Meta Analysis." *Journal of Consumer Research*, 28 (3), 450–461.

Petty, Richard. E., and John T. Cacioppo. 1986. *Communication and Persuasion: Central and Peripheral Routes to Attitude Change*. New York: Springer-Verlag.

Petty, Richard E., John T. Cacioppo, and David Schumann. 1983. "Central and Peripheral Routes to Advertising Effectiveness: The Moderating Role of Involvement." *Journal of Consumer Research*, 10, 135–146.

Prochaska, James O., and Carlo C. DiClemente. 1982. "Stages and Processes of Self-Change of Smoking: Toward an Integrative Model of Change." *Journal of Consulting and Clinical Psychology*, 51, 390–395.

Raghubir, Priya, and Geeta Menon. 1998. "AIDS and Me, Never the Twain Shall Meet: The Effects of Information Accessibility on Judgments of Risk and Advertising Effectiveness." *Journal of Consumer Research*, 25 (1), 52–63.

Raghunathan, Rajagopal, and Michel Tuan Pham. 1999. "All Negative Moods are Not Equal: Motivational Influences of Anxiety and Sadness on Decision Making." *Organizational Behavior and Human Decision Processes*, 79 (1), 56–77.

Rah, Jee Jun, Claire M. Hasler, James E. Painter, and Karen M. Chapman-Novakofski. 2005. "Applying the Theory of Planned Behavior to Women's Behavioral Attitudes on the Consumption of Soy Products." *Journal of Nutritional Education Behavior*, 36, 238–244.

Rogers, Ronald W. 1975. "A Protection Motivation Theory of Fear Appeals and Attitude Change." *Journal of Psychology*, 91, 93–114.

———.1983. "Cognitive and Physiological Processes in Fear Appeals and Attitude Change: A Revised Theory of Protection Motivation," in *Social Psychophysiology*, ed. John T. Cacioppo and Richard E. Petty, 153–176. New York: Guilford.

Rook, Karen S. 1986. "Encouraging Preventive Behavior for Distant and Proximal Health Threats: Effects of Vivid versus Abstract Information." *Journal of Gerontology*, 41 (4), 526–534.

Rosen, Craig S. 2000. "Integrating Stage and Continuum Models to Explain Processing of Exercise Messages and Exercise Initiation among Sedentary College Students." *Health Psychology*, 19 (2), 172–180.

Rothman, Alexander J., and Peter Salovey. 1997. "Shaping Perceptions to Motivate Healthy Behavior: The Role of Message Framing." *Psychological Bulletin*, 121 (1), 3–19.

Schaninger, Charles M. 1976. "Perceived Risk and Personality." *Journal of Consumer Research*, 3 (2), 95–100.

Scherer, Klaus R. 1984. "Emotion as a Multicomponent Process: A Model and Some Cross-Cultural Data." *Personality and Social Psychology Review*, 5, 37–63.

———. 1988. "On the Symbolic Functions of Vocal Affect Expression." *Journal of Language and Social Psychology*, 7 (2), 79–100.

Schwarz, Norbert. 1990. "Feelings as Information: Implications for Affective Influences on Information Processing." In *Theories of Mood and Cognition*, ed. Leonard L. Martin and Gerald L. Clore, 159–173. Mahwah, NJ: Lawrence Erlbaum.

Shah, James Y., Tory E. Higgins, and Ronald S. Friedman. 1998. "Performance Incentives and Means: How Regulatory Focus Influences Goal Attainment." *Journal of Personality and Social Psychology*, 74 (2), 285–293.

Sheeran, Paschal, and Sheina Orbell. 1998. "Do Intentions Predict Condom Use? A Meta-Analysis and Examination of Six Moderator Variables." *British Journal of Social Psychology*, 37, 231–250.

Sheeran, Paschal, and Sheina Orbell. 2000. "Using Implementation Intentions to Increase Attendance for Cervical Cancer Screening." *Health Psychology*, 19 (3), 283–289.

Smeesters, Dirk, Thomas Mussweiler, and Naomi Mandel. 2009. "The Effects of Thin and Heavy Media Images on Overweight and Underweight Consumers: Social Comparison Processes and Behavioral Implications." *Journal of Consumer Research*, 36 (6), 930–949.

Smith Karen H., and Mary Ann Stutts. 1999. "Factors That Influence Adolescents to Smoke." *Journal of Consumer Affairs*, 33 (2), 321–357.

Sternthal, Brian, and Samuel C. Craig. 1974. "Fear Appeals—Revisited and Revised." *Journal of Consumer Research*, 1 (3), 22–34.

Sultan, Fareena, John U. Farley, and Donald R. Lehmann. 1990. "A Meta-Analysis of Applications of Diffusion Models." *Journal of Marketing Research*, 27 (1), 70–77.

Sutton, Stephen R. 1982. "Fear Arousing Communications: A Critical Examination of Theory and Research." In *Social Psychology and Behavioral Medicine*, ed. J. Richard Eiser, 303–337. London: Wiley.

———. 1998. "Predicting and Explaining Intentions and Behavior: How Well are We Doing?" *Journal of Applied Social Psychology*, 28 (15), 1317–1338.

Tversky, Amos, and Daniel Kahneman. 1981. "The Framing of Decisions and the Psychology of Choice." *Science*, 211, 453–458.

Van Hooft, Edwin A.J., Marise Ph. Born, Toon W. Taris, Henk van der Flier, and Roland W.B. Blonk. 2005. "Bridging the Gap between Intentions and Behavior: Implementation Intentions, Action Control, and Procrastination." *Journal of Vocational Behavior*, 66, 238–256.

Van Voorbees, Benjamin W., Joshua Fogel, Thomas K. Houston, Lisa A. Cooper, Nae-Yuh Wang, and Daniel E. Ford. 2005. "Beliefs and Attitudes Associated with the Intention to Not Accept the Diagnosis of Depression Among Young Adults." *Annals of Family Medicine*, 3 (1) (January/February), 38–46.

Wansink, Brian. 2006. *Mindless Eating: Why We Eat More Than We Think*. New York: Bantam-Dell.

Williams-Piehota, P., Tamera R. Schneider, Judith Pizarro, Linda Mowad, and Peter Salovey. 2003. "Matching Health Messages to Information-Processing Styles: Need for Cognition and Mammography Utilization." *Health Communication*, 15 (4), 375–392.

Witte, Kim. 1998. "Fear as Motivator, Fear as Inhibitor: Using the Extended Parallel Process Model to Explain Fear Appeal Successes and Failures." In *Handbook of Communication and Emotion: Research, Theory, Applications, and Contexts*, ed. P.E. Anderen and L.K. Guerrero, 423–450. San Diego: Academic Press.

Wurtele, Sandy K., and James E. Maddux. 1987. "Relative Contributions of Protection Motivation Theory Components in Predicting Exercise Intentions and Behavior." *Health Psychology*, 6 (5), 453–466.

CHAPTER 2

POPULATION-BASED PREVENTION OF OBESITY

SHIRIKI K. KUMANYIKA, EVA OBARZANEK, NICOLAS
STETTLER, RONNY BELL, ALISON E. FIELD, STEPHEN P.
FORTMANN, BARRY A. FRANKLIN, MATTHEW W. GILLMAN,
CORA E. LEWIS, WALKER CARLOS POSTON II, JUNE STEVENS,
AND YULING HONG [AMERICAN HEART ASSOCIATION]

Obesity is a major influence on the development of cardiovascular disease (CVD) and affects physical and social functioning and quality of life.[1,2] The proportion of adults and children who are obese has reached epidemic proportions, moving steadily away from the Healthy People 2010 goals of 15% prevalence of obesity in adults and 5% prevalence in children.[3–5] These goals may be beyond our reach for several decades to come (Figures 1 and 2).

The obesity epidemic is a major concern for the health of populations in the United States and many other nations.[6–10] Based on data from the 2003–2004 US National Health and Nutrition Examination Survey (NHANES), approximately 66 million American adults (30 million men and 36 million women) are obese and an additional 74 million (42 million men and 32 million women) are overweight. Among American children 6 to 11 years of age, an estimated 4.2 million (2.3 million boys and 1.9 million girls) are overweight; among American adolescents 12 to 19 years of age, 5.7 million (3.1 million boys and 2.6 million girls) are overweight.[11] Assuming that the same trends continue, by 2015 2 in every 5 adults and 1 in every 4 children in the United States will be obese.[12] Obesity prevalence is also rising in countries throughout the world, reaching 20% to 30% in some European countries and 70% in Polynesia (International Obesity Task Force). According to the World Health Organization, the number of overweight and obese people worldwide will increase to 1.5 billion by 2015 if current trends continue.[13] Clearly, overweight and obesity place a large public health burden on society.

From *Circulation*, 118, 424–464. Copyright © 2008 American Heart Association. Used by permission. Please visit http://circ.ahajournals.org/cgi/content/full/118/4/428 for the figures, disclosure tables, and a complete list of references.

The prevalence of some obesity-related CVD risk factors (eg, elevated cholesterol and high blood pressure) decreased in the United States during the period from 1960 to 2000, despite increased obesity.[14] Nevertheless, the prevalence of these risk factors remained higher in overweight and obese than nonoverweight individuals, despite the concomitant trend of increased use of medications to treat these risk factors. Furthermore, the prevalence of diagnosed type 2 diabetes mellitus continued to increase concurrently with increases in obesity.[14] These trends underscore the importance of curbing the obesity epidemic. Control of type 2 diabetes requires a lifetime of medical care and usually drug therapy from the point of diagnosis, with the attendant financial costs and potential adverse effects on quality of life. Pharmacological control of high blood cholesterol and hypertension likewise requires lifelong medical therapy. Even with medical intervention, increased obesity may ultimately reverse gains made with respect to declines in related CVD risk factors. Thus, there is no room for complacency in dealing with this public health problem.

It is preferable to avoid, in the first place, the excess weight gain that leads to overweight and then obesity. Effective treatment of obese individuals can substantially reduce risk factors for CVD and improve disease management,[2,15] although some effects of long-standing obesity may not be reversible[16] or readily manageable. However, even those overweight people who are able to lose weight are often unable to maintain their weight at that level, and no clear guidance currently exists on definitive strategies to achieve long-term weight loss in the population at large.[15,17] The ability of weight loss to improve overall and CVD mortality has also not been clearly established, although a study to address this question is in progress.[18]

A major emphasis on obesity prevention is needed in the population at large[19,20] to prevent the development of obesity in those adults who are still in the normal weight range and in successive generations of children and adolescents during development. Treatment will continue to be of critical importance, but treatment alone cannot curb the epidemic. Besides the limited long-term success of most obesity treatments, another factor is the limited ability to deliver enough treatment to enough people. We are already unable to deliver obesity treatment services to those who need such services, while the numbers needing treatment are rising. Health insurance seldom covers the cost of counseling for obesity, particularly the extended treatment of a year or more that is suggested to facilitate long-term weight loss.[17] The need for treatment is highest, relatively speaking, among low-income and ethnic minority populations,[21] who have a high burden of obesity, CVD, and stroke outcomes but less access to healthcare services.

This review provides a rationale for population-based obesity prevention efforts and research from a United States public health perspective. It is intended for a broad audience of health professionals, policy makers, and consumer advocates who may contribute to prevention efforts. As an overview of issues related to obesity prevention, this statement is complementary to published statements, workshop proceedings, and guidelines from the American Heart Association and other organizations that describe the effects of obesity and weight loss on CVD and its risk factors and provide guidance for obesity assessment and treatment and related lifestyle interventions[2,7,17,21–37] (Appendixes). This statement addresses the need to bring together, in one place, the various arguments for what needs to be done, and how, with respect to population-based initiatives to promote healthful eating, physical activity, and energy balance. A key goal is to motivate health professionals and others to contribute directly to broadly based obesity prevention efforts—"treating the community at large."[38] The relevance to clinicians is to describe population-based efforts needed to support and complement obesity prevention and treatment activities undertaken in day-to-day practice. Obesity prevention in the population at large is also highly relevant to obesity treatment in that it fosters social and environmental conditions that support healthful eating and active living. Such conditions are essential for all weight-control efforts.

The writing group objectives were as follows: 1) to raise awareness of the importance of undertaking population-based initiatives specifically geared to the prevention of excess weight gain in adults and children; 2) to describe considerations for undertaking obesity prevention overall and in key risk subgroups; 3) to differentiate environmental and policy approaches to obesity prevention from those used in clinical prevention and obesity treatment; 4) to identify potential targets of environmental and policy change using an ecological model that includes multiple layers of influences on eating and physical activity across multiple societal sectors; and 5) to highlight the spectrum of potentially relevant interventions and the nature of evidence needed to inform population-based approaches. The evidence reviewed includes primary sources, systematic reviews and expert reports, emphasizing articles published from June 1995 through May 2007. The population burden and health effects of obesity are described as background. Conceptual frameworks that can be used to describe and analyze prevention strategies are presented.

BACKGROUND: SCOPE OF THE PROBLEM

The Burden of Overweight and Obesity in the US Population

Adults

Overweight and obesity are generally defined using body mass index (BMI), a measure of weight relative to height that is closely correlated with total body fat content. BMI is calculated as weight in kilograms divided by height in meters squared or by dividing weight in pounds by height in inches squared and multiplying by a conversion factor of 703.[15] According to the National Heart, Lung, and Blood Institute, for adults, overweight is defined as a BMI of 25 to 29.9 kg/m^2; obesity, $\geq$ 30 kg/m^2; and extreme obesity, $\geq$ 40 kg/m^2. Measures of waist circumference or waist-hip ratio are indicative of visceral adipose tissue, or intraabdominal fat, which may be more deleterious than overall overweight or obesity in some cases. Accordingly, the National Heart, Lung, and Blood Institute Clinical Guidelines recommend the use of waist circumference in addition to BMI in clinical screening of adults. High waist circumference, defined by cutoffs of >35 inches (>88 cm) for women and >40 inches (>102 cm) for men,[15] increases the level of risk associated with a given BMI level.

Data based on measured heights and weights, which are more reliable and valid than self-report, are available from NHANES.[9] In NHANES data for 2003–2004, an estimated 66.3% of US adults ≥ 20 years of age were either overweight or obese,[9] a relative increase of 18% from the previous estimate of 56% in NHANES III (1988–1994). The estimated prevalence of obesity alone was 32.3% in the 2003–2004 NHANES, a relative increase of 40.6% from the estimated 22.9% prevalence reported in NHANES III. The prevalence of extreme obesity (BMI ≥ 40) in the 2003–2004 NHANES was 4.8%. The prevalence of obesity generally increases across adult age groups. Previously observed gender differences in obesity prevalence, at the level of BMI 30 or above, have disappeared, with men "catching up" to women between 1999–2000 and 2003–2004. However, the prevalence of extreme obesity continues to be higher in women.

Long-term trends in overweight and obesity show notable increases (from 47.4% to 66.0%, or a relative increase of 39.2%) in the percentage of persons who were either overweight or obese in the last quarter of the 20th century[39] (Figure 1). Most of the increase was attributable to increases in the prevalence of BMI ≥ 30 (obesity), whereas only minor increases occurred in the prevalence of BMI of 25 to 29.9 (overweight). The prevalence of obesity increased from 15.1% to 32.1% (a relative increase of 112.6%) for those aged 20 to 74 between the 1976–1980 NHANES and the 2001–2004 NHANES.

Children and Adolescents

For children and adolescents up to age 20 years, the term "overweight" rather than "obesity" is currently used by the Centers for Disease Control and Prevention (CDC) and generally defined as a BMI at or above the 95th percentile of sex-specific BMI-for-age values from the 2000 CDC growth charts.[40] In children and adolescents, the term "at risk of overweight" is the counterpart of overweight in adults, which the CDC defined as a BMI between the 85th and 95th percentiles. If recommendations of an expert panel convened by the American Medical Association, Health Services and Resources Administration, and CDC[41] are implemented, the terminology for children will change to align with that for adults, ie, overweight and obesity. An estimated 17% of children and adolescents 2 to 19 years of age are overweight according to the 2003–2004 NHANES.[9] Among children 6 to 11 years of age, the percentage of those considered overweight increased from 4.2% to 18.8% (a 348% relative increase) between 1963–1965 and 2003–2004. Among adolescents 12 to 19 years of age, the percentage of those considered overweight increased from 4.6% to 17.4% (a 278% relative increase) between 1966–1970 (for adolescents 12 to 17 years of age) and 2003–2004[39] (Figure 2 for recent trends).

Waist circumference percentiles based on national data are available for white, African American, and Mexican American children.[42] However, whereas clinical guidelines for obesity assessment in adults include waist circumference, the above-referenced expert committee on child and adolescent overweight[41] did not find sufficient evidence or guidance to warrant a recommendation for routine clinical use of waist circumference in children at present.

Ethnic Disparities

In adults, NHANES data indicate consistent trends of higher obesity prevalence for non-Hispanic blacks and Mexican Americans compared with non-Hispanic whites but do not provide estimates for other ethnic minority populations. Drawing on other data sources—of which some rely on self-reported weight and height and, therefore, underestimate prevalence overall or in specific demographic groups[43,44]—obesity prevalence is also higher for American Indians and Alaska Natives, other Hispanic/Latino populations, Native Hawaiians, and Pacific Islanders in comparison with non-Hispanic whites, across the adult age spectrum.[15,25,45] Depending on the ethnic group, the prevalence of obesity is higher in females only or in both males and females.[9,46–52]

In the NHANES data, extreme obesity (BMI $\geq$ 40), which is associated with particularly high levels of CVD risk and total mortality,[53] affects approximately 15% of non-Hispanic black women compared with 6% and 8% of non-Hispanic white and Mexican American women and 2% to 5% or fewer in men in these ethnic groups.[9] Among immigrants in ethnic minority populations (Hispanic/Latino, Asian American, Pacific Islander, and possibly non-Hispanic blacks), obesity prevalence typically increases with a longer duration of US residence and, in some cases, approaches rates observed among US-born residents.[54–56]

Ethnic disparities in obesity prevalence apply to both BMI and waist circumference and are accompanied by disparities in obesity-related diseases.[21] However, there are ethnic differences in the interpretation of obesity indexes.[57–60] For example, the clinical consequences of obesity are higher for people of Asian descent at lower BMI and waist circumference cut points than for whites.[60,61] A report from the World Health Organization, Western Pacific Region,[62] suggested that overweight should be defined as a BMI of 23 kg/m² or greater and obesity as a BMI of 25.0 kg/m² or greater in adults of Asian descent rather than using the respective cutoffs of BMIs of 25 and 30. A subsequent World Health Organization expert panel recognized that a range of plausible BMI cutoffs for overweight and obesity existed for these populations.[60] A more recent article[63] calls for revisions of BMI criteria for South Asians, Chinese, and Aboriginals.

Ethnic disparities in overweight prevalence are also observed in male or female children and adolescents, as in adults.[9,49,52,64–66] For example, in the NHANES data for 1999–2004, Mexican American male children and adolescents had a higher prevalence of overweight than non-Hispanic white male children and adolescents.[9] The prevalence of overweight among non-Hispanic black male children and adolescents was not materially different from that among non-Hispanic white male children and adolescents. The prevalence of overweight in Mexican American and non-Hispanic black female children and adolescents was higher than non-Hispanic while female children and adolescents. Rates of increase in overweight have been steepest in non-Hispanic black children compared with Mexican American and non-Hispanic white children and generally intermediate for Mexican American children.[67] Together with the higher prevalence of overweight in non-Hispanic black girls and Mexican American boys, these faster rates of increase indicate a particular need for preventive strategies addressed to these populations.

Socioeconomic Status and Geographic Variations

Population-based surveys show a higher prevalence of obesity in populations with lower socioeconomic status (SES), especially among white females,[68-71] although this relationship is less clear in more recent prevalence trends.[12] Patterns of SES differences in children and adolescents are complex and not consistent across age, gender, and ethnicity.[72-74] For example, in recent NHANES data, an inverse association of obesity prevalence with SES was observed in white girls, whereas higher SES was associated with higher obesity levels in African American girls.[74] Overall, SES differences in obesity are becoming less prominent in both adults and children.[12,74]

Geographic variation in obesity has been reported by state, as well as degree of urbanization. For example, interview data (ie, using self-reported height and weight data) from the 2005 Behavioral Risk Factor Surveillance System (BRFSS) survey indicate that the highest prevalence of obesity was seen in Louisiana, Mississippi, and West Virginia, whereas the lowest prevalence was seen in Colorado and Hawaii.[75] This may reflect socioeconomic differences among states.[76] Higher prevalence of obesity has been reported for rural populations compared with urban and suburban populations in the National Health Interview Survey.[77-79] For example, in 32 440 adult respondents to a 1998 National Health Interview Survey module,[78] obesity was more prevalent among adult residents of rural areas than residents of urban areas (20.4% versus 17.8%; $P = 0.0002$) and this rural-urban difference was consistent across all ethnic groups. An analysis of 2000–2001 BRFSS data showed a similar pattern but with higher prevalence (23.0% and 20.5% in rural and urban areas, respectively). Rural-urban-suburban differences in obesity and health may also reflect socioeconomic differences, with rural areas being more characterized by local poverty and lack of resources,[77] at least in part.

Health Effects of Obesity

Adults

Obesity prevention in adults can potentially have a major impact in reducing morbidity and mortality that result from the chronic effects of excess body fatness.[8,80]

The worldwide increase in obesity portends an increasing epidemic of diabetes and its serious consequences, including CVD. The American Heart Association (AHA) identified obesity as a major CVD risk factor in 1998.[81] As reviewed in a separate AHA scientific statement,[2] the impact of obesity in the pathophysiology of cardiovascular and pulmonary diseases and diabetes is well documented and has been recognized for decades.[2,82]

Weight gain after young adulthood is associated with an increased risk of CVD events and risk factors later in life independent of BMI levels. For example, in a cohort study of young adults, those who gained more than 5 lb over 15 years had unfavorable changes in CVD risk factors and higher incidence of metabolic syndrome and its components (waist, lipids, blood pressure), independent of initial BMI, than those who had stable weight.[83,84] In a 20-year follow-up of middle-aged men, risks of major CVD events and type 2 diabetes mellitus were related to excess body weight at baseline (overweight and obesity) and to weight gain.[85] Also, in the Nurses Health Study, weight gain was associated with increased risk of all-cause, coronary heart disease, and CVD mortality at any level of initial BMI.[86] The association between obesity and several diseases begins when an individual is well within the "normal" weight range. For example, in a study of >7000 middle-aged men screened in British general practices and monitored for nearly 15 years, the lowest overall mortality rate was at a BMI of 22 to 27.9; however, for a combined end point of myocardial infarction, stroke, type 2 diabetes, and death, risk was lowest at a BMI of 20 to 23.9, and all major CVD risk factors increased progressively from a BMI of <20.[87]

As shown in Table [2].1, adverse health outcomes associated with obesity are not limited to CVD.[1,59,81–166] There is a large and growing body of evidence on the other myriad health effects of overweight and obesity, based on both animal and human studies, including mechanistic studies, epidemiological studies (eg, prospective cohort and case-control studies), and clinical trials. Of the adverse medical consequences of overweight in adults, diabetes is the most strongly linked with increasing BMI.[167] For example, insulin resistance, which is associated with obesity and is a risk factor for coronary heart disease, also appears to be related to liver disease and obstructive sleep apnea.[95] Obesity increases the risk for several types of cancer, including relatively common cancers, such as breast cancer in postmenopausal women[135] and prostate cancer.[96] As shown in Table [2.]1, other relevant outcomes include osteoarthritis, gastroesophageal reflux disease, erectile dysfunction, and Alzheimer disease, as well as physical disability, employee absenteeism, impaired quality of life, and increased healthcare costs. In older adults, obesity is associated with protection against hip fracture,[168] but this protective effect on bone status does not offset the extensive array of potential adverse effects on conditions that are common in the older population.

The extensive data indicating that weight loss can reverse or arrest the harmful effects of obesity[26] are further evidence of the causal link between obesity and disease. Lifestyle intervention studies have shown the effectiveness of weight loss

Table [2.]1

Adverse Outcomes for Which Obesity Increases Risk or Complications in Adulthood

Cardiovascular diseases, diabetes, and related conditions
Coronary heart disease (CHD)
Type 2 diabetes
CHD risk factors
Type 2 diabetes
Hypertension
Dyslipidemia
Inflammation
Hypercoagulability
Autonomic nervous system dysfunction
Heart failure
Stroke
Deep venous thrombosis
Pulmonary disease (including obesity hypoventilation syndrome, obstructive sleep
   apnea)
Other outcomes*
Absenteeism from work
Alzheimer disease
Asthma
Cancer (including breast [postmenopausal], endometrial, esophageal, colorectal,
   kidney, and prostate)
Disability, physical
Erectile dysfunction
Fertility and pregnancy complications
Gallstones/cholecystitis
Gastroesophageal reflux disease
Gout
Healthcare costs
Impaired quality of life
Kidney stones
Liver (spectrum of nonalcoholic fatty liver disease)
Mortality
Obesity-related glomerulopathy
Osteoarthritis
Psychological disorders (e.g., depression, aggressive behaviors)
Surgical complications

   *Listed alphabetically. See text for relevant references.

in improving cardiovascular risk factors, including blood pressure,[156,169] insulin resistance and type 2 diabetes,[100,159] lipid disorders, and the metabolic syndrome,[26,170] in some cases lowering the incidence of hypertension or diabetes in a population at high risk for such diagnoses. Data from surgically treated obese subjects with larger weight losses than those usually observed in lifestyle trials have further confirmed the marked improvements in systolic (2 years only) and diastolic blood pressure, pulse pressure, and glucose, insulin, uric acid, triglycerides, high-density lipoprotein cholesterol, and total cholesterol levels, associated with weight loss after up to 10 years of follow-up.[153]

With respect to mortality, although controversies continue, many studies show clear, statistically significant, positive associations of BMI with CVD mortality, suggesting that obesity prevention can improve longevity. Most studies show an association between BMI in the obese range (≥ 30) and mortality.[92,106,107,140] The Look AHEAD trial[18] was initiated to specifically clarify the potential benefits of intentional weight loss on mortality. However, mortality data—even if conclusive with respect to the presence or absence of an association of obesity or weight loss with longevity—do not reflect the full spectrum of obesity-related health or quality-of-life issues (Table [2.]1).

Children and Adolescents

Events that occur at the earliest stages of human development—even before birth—may have a profound influence on risk for obesity, diabetes, CVD, and other common adult conditions and are, therefore, potentially important focal points for preventive efforts.[171] Excess weight during childhood is associated with chronic disease morbidity and adverse psychosocial effects from childhood onward and, therefore, the lifetime duration of these diseases. Obesity during childhood also increases the risk of being obese as an adult, with the attendant implications for the above-described morbidity during adulthood.

Prenatal Determinants of Obesity and Related Health Risks

Both higher and lower birth weight are correlated to later obesity-related consequences.[172] Higher birth weight is associated with larger amounts of gestational weight gain and with gestational diabetes, 2 factors also implicated in childhood obesity.[173,174] Lower birth weight is consistently associated with central fat distribution, insulin resistance, the metabolic syndrome, type 2 diabetes, and ischemic CVD.[172] Moreover, the phenotype of lower birth weight followed by higher BMI in childhood or adulthood appears to confer the highest risk of these outcomes. This pattern holds, for example, for insulin resistance among 8-year-olds in India,[175] blood pressure among Filipino adolescents,[176] the metabolic syndrome among white and Mexican American adults,[177] and coronary heart disease among Welsh men and American female nurses.[178,179] Recent studies have found that excess weight gain during childhood and adolescence appears to explain these observations.[180,181] Whether accelerated weight gain in infancy confers excess risk for these adult outcomes is controversial.[182]

Other prenatal determinants of obesity-related outcomes may span the entire "fetal supply line" from maternal dietary intake to alterations in uteroplacental blood flow, placental function, and fetal metabolism, and they may or may not have any influence on birth weight. Maternal smoking during pregnancy is one potentially

Table [2.]2

Adverse Outcomes for Which Obesity Increases Risk During Childhood

Metabolic
Type 2 diabetes mellitus
Metabolic syndrome
Orthopedic
Slipped capital femoral epiphysis
Blount's disease
Cardiovascular
Dyslipidemia
Hypertension
Left ventricular hypertrophy
Atherosclerosis
Psychological
Depression
Poor quality of life
Neurological
Pseudotumor cerebri
Hepatic
Nonalcoholic fatty liver disease
Nonalcoholic steatohepatitis
Pulmonary
Obstructive sleep apnea
Asthma (exacerbation)
Renal
Proteinuria

Source: Reference 27.

modifiable factor that appears to increase the risk for obesity and elevated blood pressure levels in offspring.[183] Smoking among women is rising in developing countries; reversal of this trend has the potential to help curb the emergence of obesity as a public health threat around the world.

Consequences of Overweight During Childhood

CVD effects of obesity during childhood are reviewed in detail in other AHA statements.[23,27] In addition to CVD morbidity, obesity can also lead to a number of other adverse health outcomes in childhood, including sleep apnea, gastroesophageal reflux, fatty liver, and orthopedic problems[27] (Table [2.]2). Evidence relating to type 2 diabetes, asthma, and psychosocial problems associated with childhood overweight is highlighted below.

Given the strong relationship of obesity and diabetes in adults, the increase in childhood obesity is likely driving the concomitant increase in rates of type 2 diabetes among children. Once considered rare in children and adolescents, referrals for type 2 diabetes now rival those for type 1 diabetes in some centers.[184] In a multiethnic, population-based study of diabetes in youth, type 2 diabetes was more common than type 1 diabetes among 10- to 17-year-olds who were black, Asian, or American Indian and almost as common among Hispanics.[185] Among 12- to 19-year-olds in the 1999–2000 NHANES, 32.1% of overweight adolescents met national criteria for the metabolic syndrome.[186] In a referral group of >400 obese children and adolescents studied in detail, elevated BMI was associated with prevalence of the metabolic syndrome, which reached 50% in the most severely obese.[187] Also, in a prospective study of nearly 2400 9- and 10-year-old girls, increased waist circumference was a robust predictor of metabolic syndrome at age 18.[188]

Although the definition of metabolic syndrome itself is controversial, childhood overweight is also related to its individual components. For example, in the Bogalusa Heart Study,[189] overweight children were 12 times more likely than their leaner peers to have high levels of fasting insulin; the relative risk was greater for whites than blacks. The race difference may reflect that independent of body fatness, blacks appear to have lower insulin sensitivity than whites.[190] Higher BMI is also associated with higher blood pressure and abnormal lipid (including higher triglyceride) levels in children and adolescents.[189,191] Girls who were overweight at age 9 were 10 times more likely than normal-weight girls to have elevated systolic blood pressure, 6 times more likely to have low high-density lipoprotein levels, and 2 to 3 times more likely to have elevated diastolic blood pressure, triglycerides, and total and low-density lipoprotein cholesterol.[192]

The association of obesity with asthma is noteworthy because asthma is the most common chronic disease of childhood. In the late 20th century, the increase in asthma incidence paralleled that of obesity.[193–196] In addition to the observation that asthmatic children can become overweight because asthma limits their physical activity, prospective studies support the hypothesis that overweight children are more likely than their peers to develop asthma. Among 3792 children and adolescents 7 to 18 years of age who were assessed annually between 1993 and 1998, those who were overweight or obese were nearly twice as likely as their leaner peers to develop asthma.[197] Data are sparse on the relation of weight status in infancy and subsequent risk for asthma but would be of interest given the recent increase in overweight among the youngest children and because the peak age incidence of asthma occurs in the preschool and school years. The results of a preliminary study suggest that increased weight for length at 6 months predicts more wheezing by age 3 years.[198] The mechanisms by which excess weight can increase the risk for asthma include the presence of inflammatory cytokines produced by adipocytes and mechanical disruption of respiration.[199]

Psychosocial problems associated with overweight in children relate to self-concept, discrimination, and excessive weight concern and overeating disorders. Even in children as young as 5 years, a weight for height exceeding the 85th percentile has been associated with impaired self-concept (eg, higher-weight 5-year-old girls having a lower perception of their cognitive ability compared with girls with lower weight status).[200] Overweight children are more likely to be teased or bullied.[201,202] Overweight adolescents are more likely than their lean counterparts to be socially isolated.[203,204] Overweight children and youth are also more likely to suffer decreased self-esteem[205,206] and more likely to be extremely concerned with their weight and engage in bulimic behaviors.[207-210] It is possible that binge eating leads to, rather than results from, excess weight gain, however.[211,212] Overweight children appear to have lower physical functioning and overall psychosocial health,[213,214] and in 1 study,[215] their health-related quality of life was similar to that of children and adolescents diagnosed with cancer.

Consequences of Childhood Overweight for Later Morbidity and Mortality

Children and adolescents who are overweight tend to remain so over time, particularly for older compared with younger children and if 1 or both parents are overweight.[216-220] Overweight adolescents may be as much as 20 times more likely than their leaner peers to be obese in early adulthood.[220] In younger children, parental obesity is a more potent risk factor than the child's own weight status in predicting whether the child will become an obese adult, whereas the opposite is true for adolescents.[220] The elevated risk of adult obesity is not limited to children who are frankly overweight. Two studies have demonstrated that children with a BMI in the 50th to 74th percentiles are substantially more likely than children with a BMI below the 50th percentile to become overweight or obese adults.[221,222] Therefore, obesity prevention must not be limited to children in the highest weight status categories.

At least 4 studies[223-226] demonstrate that adolescent overweight is associated with higher overall mortality. In these studies, males who had a higher BMI had an approximately 1.5 to 2 times greater risk of overall mortality during follow-up periods of approximately 30 to 70 years. Curiously, in 2 studies that monitored both women and men, adolescent females with a higher BMI did not have a substantially elevated risk of dying.[223,224] However, the more recent study shows that adolescent obesity strongly predicts increased mortality among women at midlife.[226]

At least 1 study indicates that weight in late adolescence is strongly related to risk of developing type 2 diabetes in adulthood. After adjusting for subsequent weight gain, 18-year-old female adolescents with a BMI >30 kg/m2 were about 10 times more likely to develop diabetes than those with a BMI <22 kg/m2.[227] Both males and females with an elevated BMI in late adolescence appear more likely than their leaner peers to develop CVD. Morrison et al[228] report 25-year follow-up data that showed an association between the presence of metabolic syndrome in children, 77% of whom had BMI at or greater than the 90th percentile, and CVD during adulthood. In the Caerphilly Prospective Study, Yarnell et al[229] studied 2335 middle-aged men who provided recalled information on weight and height at age 18. Males who were obese at age 18 were >2 times more likely than their leaner peers to have a coronary event within 14 years of joining the prospective study. Among the 508 men and women in the Harvard Growth Study,[223] those who had been overweight as adolescents were more likely than their peers to have a coronary event in adulthood or to die from CVD. Greater weight in late childhood or adolescence is also associated with higher blood pressure in adulthood.[222,230,231] Excess weight in adolescence may also increase the adult risk of conditions such as polycystic ovarian syndrome[232] or its concomitant ovulatory infertility[233] and ovarian cancer.[234,235] It is unclear whether these long-term effects of obesity in childhood stem from its longer duration or from the presence of obesity at certain critical periods for risk development.

The Case for Prevention

Overall Goals and Objectives

The goals of obesity prevention, broadly defined, include avoidance of weight gain to levels defined as overweight or obese and stabilization of weight in those who may already be overweight or obese or after weight loss.[236] Obesity prevention in childhood also has the goal of preventing obesity during adolescence and adulthood. Treatment of obese children to promote weight loss and to avoid tracking of obesity into adulthood is also a goal of obesity prevention. A focus on obesity prevention in childhood may seem particularly intuitive, because, as noted in the previous section, the process of developing obesity may begin in early life,[27,171] and arresting development of obesity in childhood has the greatest long-term payoff in years of healthy life. Preventing or reducing obesity in adulthood may be cost effective, based on the potential immediate benefits of avoiding the otherwise high prevalence of obesity-related comorbidities that develop during adulthood,[80] although the best way to determine the overall cost-effectiveness of interventions in obesity is as yet unclear.[237]

Preventive strategies for adults may include the promotion of small changes in eating and physical activity[238] or small initial weight losses to counteract expected annual weight gains or both.[239] Implicit in all obesity prevention goals are the related objectives of promoting healthful eating and activity patterns, and for children, normal growth and development, avoidance of adverse psychosocial or quality-of-life effects, and improvement in obesity-related health risk factors and outcomes.[7,19]

Achieving Individual Energy Balance to Prevent Excess Weight Gain

Prevention of excess weight gain relies on the maintenance of energy balance, whereby energy intake equals energy expenditure (in growing children and adolescents, energy expenditure plus energy for healthy weight gain) over the long term. For children and youth, this means growth and development along an acceptable weight trajectory.[240] For adults, this means maintaining a relatively stable weight across life stages, including the reproductive years, in contrast to the average progressive gain of 0.5 to 1 kg per year commonly observed in US adults.[241] A positive imbalance will increase energy storage, deposited as body fat and observed as weight gain. Although the concept is beguilingly simple, the physiological systems that regulate body weight through energy intake and expenditure mechanisms are complex, interactive, homeostatic, and still poorly understood.[8,242] Furthermore, the components of energy balance are not measured easily or with sufficient precision to be practical as a guide to help individuals maintain energy balance. Theoretically, a small persistent energy imbalance of 50 kcal per day could result in a 5-lb weight gain in 1 year (18250 kcal per year divided by 3500 kcal/lb weight gain), all other things being equal. This scenario is an oversimplification, however, because the energy cost of 1 lb of weight gain depends on the fat composition of the added weight,[243] and all things do not remain equal,[244] because, for example, energy expenditure increases with higher caloric intake and weight gain. Nevertheless, the accumulation of a constant positive energy imbalance over the long term causes weight gain, and the great ease with which this accumulation occurs in people in the United States and many other countries causes the high prevalence of obesity.[8,19]

Although prevention and treatment of obesity both rely on the same principles of energy balance, the application of the principles is quite different. For treatment of obesity, a large reduction in caloric intake of about 500 to 1000 kcal per day, along with increased physical activity, can produce a loss of approximately 8% to 10% of body weight over the relatively short period of about 6 months.[15] Although the types of low-calorie diets that best promote weight loss are the subject of current investigations,[244,245] behaviors for weight loss are focused on caloric reduction: decreasing overall food intake, reducing portion sizes, substituting lower-calorie for higher-calorie foods, and increasing physical activity. Weight loss is best accomplished by participation in a behavioral program using self-monitoring, goal-setting, and problem-solving techniques.[15,246] Motivation levels may be high for appearance reasons or if adverse health consequences and quality of-life impairments associated with obesity are readily perceived. Apparently, behaviors learned for weight loss are not sustained, however, because weight regain after weight loss is common.[247] Motivations and strategies to maintain weight after weight loss may differ substantially from those used to initiate weight loss.[248,249]

The application of energy balance principles toward prevention of weight gain and obesity is more subtle, and the results are less evident and less reinforcing than those for treatment of obesity.[250] The goal is to prevent a persistent small positive energy imbalance. To prevent obesity and weight gain, permanent lifestyle changes must be achieved and maintained over the long term and perhaps even intensified, because aging and environmental influences continue to create the conditions for positive energy imbalance. On the energy intake side of the equation, a healthy, low-energy–dense diet, along the lines of Dietary Guidelines for Americans[251] and the AHA Dietary Guidelines,[30] is recommended: rich in fruits, vegetables, and whole grains and limited in high-fat and sweetened foods with high-energy density and low nutritional value. Important strategies are reading the calorie and serving-size information on nutrition labels, requesting simply prepared foods at food establishments, and preparing and consuming appropriate portion sizes (at restaurants, a strategy is to order or consume only half-portions). Because it is unknown directly whether caloric balance is being maintained, frequent weighing helps determine whether weight is stable.[252,253] Physical activity also plays a critical role in the prevention of weight gain and obesity.[254] Current physical activity guidelines to prevent weight gain are 60 minutes per day of at least moderate-intensity physical activity,[255] which is more than the amount recommended for general health and cardiovascular function.[256] Motivation is a particularly important issue to address. There are no dramatic improvements on an individual level, because the results are no change in weight or health outcomes in contrast to the weight loss and decrease in risk factors associated with weight loss.

Achieving Energy Balance in Populations

"Population-based" obesity prevention approaches are designed to produce large-scale changes in eating behaviors and levels of physical activity to stabilize the distribution of BMI levels around a mean level that minimizes the percent who become overweight and obese, without increasing prevalence at the underweight end of the continuum.[19] Population-level obesity prevention can and should be approached not as the promotion of widespread "dieting" but rather from the perspective of promoting healthful eating and physical activity patterns and a balance between the two. This approach requires modifications of factors that shape individual choices, as well as individual habits and preferences. There is ample evidence that individual eating and physical activity behaviors are responsive to the surrounding social and physical environmental contexts both for adults and children and, thus, amenable to public health prevention interventions.[7,19,257–263] Population-based approaches are also compatible with a broad range of public health goals. For example, improvement of eating and physical activity behaviors promotes healthy growth and development in childhood and adolescence, independently of weight, protects against certain types of respiratory, musculoskeletal, and liver diseases, as well as cancer, and improves cardiopulmonary fitness and overall health and wellness. Population-based prevention approaches reach populations through a variety of routes that extend beyond clinics and traditional health services and, when prevalence is high, at a lower cost per person compared with treatment approaches.[264]

Intake-related behaviors that have been linked to obesity include frequent consumption of meals at fast-food and other eating establishments,[265–267] consumption of large portions at home and at restaurants,[268,269] consumption of energy-dense foods, such as high-fat, low-fiber foods,[270–272] and intake of sweetened beverages.[273–276] These behaviors occur in an environment in which energy-dense food is abundant, relatively inexpensive, easy to obtain, and easy to eat with minimal preparation.

Low levels of physical activity are widespread in the United States[277] and have been associated with obesity and weight gain.[278-280] In some reports, television viewing and other sedentary activities have also been related to increased body weight,[281,282] although more of the evidence relates to children.[283,284] Deficient expenditure of energy could occur not only from sedentary lifestyles, but also from physiological changes that occur with aging. With increasing age, decreases in muscle mass, resting metabolic rate, and aerobic capacity occur.[285] Also, sedentary lifestyles may indirectly result in higher energy intakes because of less ability to regulate energy balance, for example,[286] and more time and opportunity to eat. Low levels of physical activity occur in the context of an automated and automobile-oriented environment that is conducive to a sedentary lifestyle.[287]

Community design and infrastructure characteristics (sometimes referred to as the "built environment," as differentiated from naturally occurring environmental factors) have become increasingly prominent in efforts to identify population-level determinants of obesity.[288] Evidence related to several of the commonly used variables in this category is highlighted below.

Urban "sprawl" is a geographic concept that has recently been studied in relation to risk of obesity. There is some disagreement about how to define sprawl,[289] but regardless of how sprawl is defined, most agree that sprawl results in large areas of low-population density that encourage and usually require residents to drive from home to work, stores, school, and recreation facilities[290] rather than to walk or use public transportation. Several studies have examined the relation between urban sprawl and risk of obesity. For example, Ewing and associates[291] constructed a County Sprawl Index that included population density measures and block size; larger scores indicated less sprawl. Health status data, including BMI, were derived from the BRFSS and were self-reported. After adjusting for gender, age, race, education, and smoking status, residents of counties characterized by greater sprawl walked less, weighed more, were more likely to be obese, and were more likely to have hypertension. Similarly, Lopez[289] constructed a 100-point metropolitan sprawl index using the US Census and calculated it for 330 US metropolitan areas that could be linked with data from the 2000 BRFSS. After controlling for age, gender, race, individual income, and education, a significant relation was found between the sprawl index and risk for overweight and obesity. Sprawl at the state level also has been found to increase risk for obesity.[292]

Land use mix and street connectivity are other geographic concepts that also have been linked to obesity. Sprawl is characterized by less diverse land use mix and less street connectivity. Giles-Corti and colleagues[293] found that both overweight and obese adults were more likely to live in neighborhoods that lacked adequate sidewalks and proximal places for physical activity and that overweight people were more than 4 times more likely to live near a highway. Participants with poor access to recreational facilities were 1.68 times more likely to be obese.

Neighborhoods can also be described in terms of "walkability." Saelens et al[294] characterized residents as living in high-walkable (single- and multiple-family residences) and low-walkable (single-family residences) neighborhoods with comparable SES using census data. They collected data on physical activity using accelerometers, weight status, and self-reported neighborhood perceptions. Residents of highly walkable neighborhoods walked significantly more (eg, a difference of 63 minutes per week of moderate to vigorous physical activity) than residents of low-walkable neighborhoods. In addition, residents of low-walkable neighborhoods tended to report higher average BMIs and higher rates of overweight than residents living in highly walkable neighborhoods.[294]

Frank and associates[295] investigated the impact of community design and physical activity on obesity in the Atlanta metropolitan area, characterizing neighborhoods as connected or disconnected (ie, high- and low-walkable, respectively) by using land-use mix data from the county tax assessor and the 2000 census within a Geographic Information System framework. Participant data within each neighborhood were drawn from a transportation and air-quality survey, which measured individual-level factors. After adjusting for the effects of age, level of education, and individual income, a significant relation was found between land-use mix and the prevalence of obesity, although this relationship was mediated by physical activity (ie, distance walked during a 2-day period). For instance, for each single quartile increase in land-use mix, there was a concomitant 12.2% reduction (odds ratio, 0.878; 95% confidence interval, 0.839 to 0.919) in the probability of obesity.

As discussed in the next section, community characteristics that influence obesity risk in low-income and minority communities may differ from those just described. For example, communities in inner city urban areas may be very "walkable" in the sense of connectivity but offer limited opportunities for physical activity because of safety issues, a lack of affordable recreational facilities and programs, and limited access to healthy foods because of the types of food stores and restaurants that are available.

CONSIDERATIONS FOR PREVENTION IN KEY RISK SUBGROUPS

Whereas clinical preventive services are often characterized in terms of the stage of disease when the intervention occurs (ie, primary, secondary, and tertiary prevention), comprehensive public health approaches can be characterized on the basis of the population segment of interest. In the World Health Organization's obesity prevention framework,[8] whole-population approaches that target the entire community without prior screening of risk (although those at high risk are included) are termed "universal prevention." As will be discussed, whole-population approaches that are "passive" (ie, have their effects through environmental and policy changes) improve opportunities for healthful eating and physical activity without requiring deliberate actions by individuals and can be particularly useful in addressing inequities. Universal prevention approaches that rely only on changing individual behaviors directly through social marketing campaigns or community education may actually worsen disparities if they are only feasible for or attractive to relatively advantaged individuals. A combination of these types of approaches is needed.

"High-risk" approaches focus specifically on groups or individuals who are identified as being at high risk. When the focus is on groups at high risk, defined by demographic, health characteristics, or life stage, the term "selective prevention" is used in the World Health Organization framework. Focusing on specific individuals at high risk, including individuals with existing weight problems, is termed "targeted prevention." As will be discussed in a subsequent section, population approaches draw on tools and strategies from health promotion and public health to reach whole communities with educational or motivational messages or to foster environmental and policy changes that render physical and social contexts more conducive to weight control, whereas high-risk approaches often resemble treatment programs because they involve screening and follow-up at the individual level and may occur in primary care or specialized treatment settings.

Obesity prevention is important throughout the life course and for both sexes, although prevention approaches and issues may differ according to gender. Body composition (higher percent body fat) and fat distribution (generally more gynoid and less abdominal fat distribution) among females may influence the health effects of a given BMI.[296,297] Men are an important population of interest because of their higher absolute risk for obesity-related diseases and lower likelihood of seeking treatment for obesity compared with women.[17] As discussed in this section, people with mental and physical disabilities are important subpopulations for focused efforts to prevent excess weight gain.

Childbearing-Age Women

Women of childbearing age in general and particularly women who are pregnant or postpartum are of particular interest for obesity prevention during adulthood. Excess pregnancy weight gain is particularly common among women who were overweight before pregnancy and having their first child.[298] Maternal prepregnancy BMI is a strong risk factor for gestational diabetes and is a reminder that the rise in rates of obesity among girls and women of childbearing age is producing a concomitant increase in rates of gestational diabetes, which in turn will likely lead to more obesity—and thus gestational diabetes—in the next generation. This vicious cycle may well fuel the obesity epidemic for decades to come, both in the developed and the developing worlds, particularly given that perpetuation of obesity in girls may ultimately affect the gestational environments of future generations. In addition, the potential for retention of excess weight gained during pregnancy greatly increases a woman's risk of later obesity-related diseases.

Gender-Related Differences in Obesity Prevention

Compared with men, women on average are more interested in food and nutrition, eat healthier diets than men, are more likely to do the household food shopping and preparation, and are more concerned about weight and familiar with diet.

Nevertheless, obesity prevention may be more difficult for women than men. Women have lower caloric requirements than men on average and must, therefore, consume less food than men if they are to remain in energy balance.[255] This may be particularly disadvantageous for women when eating out, given that restaurant and take-home portion sizes have increased and are the same whether the customer is male or female or large or small. It appears that appetite controls in humans are more effective for avoiding hunger than preventing overeating. Experimental studies have demonstrated that the more food people are given, the more they are likely to eat.[271] Unwitting consumption of a few hundred extra calories is more detrimental to energy balance for women than men. Offsetting excess caloric intake by extra expenditure through physical activity is difficult because of the time it takes. For example, moderate activity, such as 15 minutes of walking, burns only 100 calories for an average size adult, whereas it is quite easy to consume an extra 200 or 300 calories in a much shorter time. In addition, the amount of calories expended is proportional to body size and the amount of lean tissue. A potential female advantage with respect to controlling food shopping and preparation may be offset by factors related to food preparation. Both women who work outside the home and busy homemakers may rely on convenience foods, prepared foods, or eating take out or restaurant foods, all of which are associated with higher calorie content. Depression, which is more common in women than in men,[303] has been associated with overeating and weight gain, both with respect to using food for comfort and because many antidepressants cause weight gain.[304,305] Also, stress has been associated with increased food intake, which could contribute to obesity.[306] In a recent survey, more women than men reported overeating under stress.[307]

In addition to the lower metabolism and energy expenditure associated with having higher percent body fat or a smaller body size, women are also at a disadvantage with respect to energy expenditure from a social and behavioral perspective. Leisure time or recreational activity levels are lower for females than males,[39] declining markedly in adolescence and particularly among African American girls.[308] Occupational activity levels are also lower for females.[309] Moreover, opportunities for physical activity in women are constrained by greater caregiving responsibilities and safety concerns that affect times and places available for physical activity.[310,311] Socially acceptable forms of physical activity may be fewer for women than men, particularly in some ethnic groups. Social concerns may include how exercise affects one's hairstyle or image of femininity,[312] as well as the possible displeasure of spouses or other household members, because exercise may be perceived as taking a woman away from family responsibilities.[311]

The greater concern about weight and dieting among women compared with men is well recognized and is apparently reflected in the tendency of women to participate in weight-loss programs.[17] The literature on treatment of obesity is dominated by studies in women to a much greater extent than can be explained by any gender differences in the prevalence of the problem. At any given time, nearly half of women, compared with about one third of men, are trying to lose weight, and women attempt weight loss at a lesser degree of overweight than men.[313] But dieting as such does not appear to be associated with success at preventing weight gain or obesity, perhaps because those who diet have the greatest difficulty controlling their weight or because dieting periods are interspersed with periods of overeating.

Social norms and attitudes about attractiveness differ for men and women. Slenderness has a much stronger importance for women, which appears to increase with upward mobility or high social position.[314] Social disapproval of obesity and excess weight in men is less strong, and the inverse gradient of obesity with SES, observed in women in many ethnic groups, is less predictable in men and is sometimes absent or reversed (eg, obesity may increase with increasing social position). Another reason for the higher weight concern in women is retention of weight gained during pregnancy. This may be a major contributor to lifetime weight gain among women, particularly in ethnic groups such as African American women, for whom pregnancy-associated weight gain is more marked.[315,316]

The advantages and disadvantages for men in relation to obesity prevention are the opposite of those in women. Men may be less knowledgeable about or interested in healthful diets or calorie counting than women, and men's lower participation in weight-control programs may reflect and reinforce social norms that weight-control issues are not relevant to men and not important or as important for men. Health risks for which men are more susceptible (eg, risk of heart attack) or an interest in physical fitness may attract men to weight control. Physical activity expenditure among men may also be facilitated by their greater participation in sports or higher level of occupational activity.[309] Nevertheless, sedentary pastimes, such as watching television, are popular among men, as well as among women.[317]

Adults with Mental and Physical Disabilities

People with disabilities are included in the Healthy People 2010 focus on elimination of health disparities,[3] and those with either mental or physical disabilities constitute an important audience for obesity prevention. This diverse population has higher rates of overweight, obesity, and extreme obesity than those found in the general population.[318,319] A wide variety of disabilities have an impact on diet and physical activity, with the result that many different issues must be considered when designing obesity prevention strategies. Issues affecting overweight and obesity in the disabled vary greatly with the type of disability, including effects on physical condition and appetite, physical limitations that affect the ability to participate in regular physical activity, issues regarding responsibility for food decisions, and effects of prescription drugs on intake and activity. Because the issues are different for each type of disability, only a few examples are included here.

Physical limitations have obvious effects on the ability to perform physical activity,[320] which is important in the prevention of weight gain. Physical limitations can be part of a vicious cycle in which obesity contributes to the physical limitation (eg, low-back pain, osteoarthritis of the knee, foot injuries in diabetics), which in turn affects the person's ability or willingness to perform physical activity. Depression can also be a factor.

Adults with Down syndrome have a higher prevalence of overweight and obesity than adults in the general population.[321-323] Adults with Down syndrome who live at home have higher rates of overweight and obesity than those who live in group homes.[321-323] Hypotonia (weak muscle tone) may lead to reduced physical activity and may thus contribute to the high prevalence of overweight. Overweight and obesity are also common in persons with schizophrenia and schizo-affective disorder.[324] There is some evidence that the disability itself may contribute to overweight and obesity, and it is well known that several antipsychotic drugs cause substantial weight gain.[304] Limited attempts have been made at achieving weight loss among persons with mental disabilities. When cognitive impairment is present, interventions to change behavior can raise ethical issues, such as in Prader-Willi syndrome, in which the appetite is increased and the ability to understand health consequences is decreased.[325]

Children and Adolescents

General Issues

Fetal life, infancy, childhood, and adolescence are periods of tremendous physiological changes, which may explain why some periods may be critical in the establishment of not only behaviors, but also physiological processes. As stated previously, the possibility of physiological imprinting or programming early in life suggests that there may be sensitive or critical periods in childhood when an intervention will affect lifelong physiological processes that would be more difficult to change at a later age. Reduced fetal growth is thought to be associated with central fat distribution,[326] whereas weight gain in early infancy[327] and excessive weight gain in adolescence are associated with obesity in adulthood.[216]

Eating and physical activity behaviors learned during childhood may persist into adulthood,[328-332] and food and taste preferences may be established early in life.[333,334] Thus, interventions aimed at changing behavior during this period have the potential of establishing healthy behaviors that will continue over the individual's life span. Addressing gestational determinants of childhood obesity requires prevention of obesity in women of childbearing age. Apart from associations of lower birth weight with adverse cardiovascular outcomes that have garnered much recent attention, the well-established association of higher birth weight with higher BMI in childhood and adulthood should be emphasized.[172,335] Gestational diabetes, which leads to fetal hyperinsulinemia and increased fetal growth, may cause obesity and impaired glucose tolerance as the child becomes an adult.[173] Excessive weight gain by the mother during pregnancy is also associated with a higher BMI in the child at age 3.[174] Because women are increasingly beginning pregnancy at greater weights and because excessive weight gain during pregnancy has also probably increased during the past 1 to 2 decades,[336] avoiding excess pregnancy weight gain is another potential strategy to reduce the burden of obesity-related consequences in the next generation.

Obesity prevention in the pediatric ages involves specific circumstances and considerations. Interventions aimed at this population should be adapted to the neurodevelopmental characteristics of the target age and will require expertise in child development. Because developmental changes are rapid, most behavioral interventions likely need to be targeted at relatively narrow target age groups. Because children and adolescents are generally more sensitive than adults to outside influences (parents, media, and peers), prevention interventions based on changes in the child/adolescent's environment are particularly attractive for changing behavior in this age group to achieve population-based prevention of obesity.[7]

Another aspect of obesity prevention in children and adolescents is the potential setting of the interventions. Most children attend school or go to daycare centers, where they spend a large part of their waking time, have opportunities for physical activity, and eat 1 or 2 meals. Schools and daycare centers are, therefore, ideal settings for interventions for obesity prevention in children. Schools have been used extensively[337-339] for such interventions, and there are some interventions in preschool, head start, or daycare settings.[340-343] Schools are also increasingly the setting for battles over politically charged decisions, such as exclusive contracts with beverage companies, regulation of advertising on school grounds, and community pressure on time and funding for physical education.[7] Child-specific settings, such as youth and recreational centers, have also been used for community-based interventions. Well-child visits to the primary care physician offer opportunities for pediatric obesity prevention. However, despite their dedication to preventive care, pediatric care providers are insufficiently trained to feel comfortable about implementing obesity prevention in the office[344] and are not appropriately compensated to implement obesity treatment.[345]

Children and Adolescents with Mental and Physical Disabilities

As in adults, children and adolescents with mental and physical disabilities are an important subpopulation of children who require special attention in relation to obesity prevention. Participation of children with disabilities in school and other social activities is lower than in the general population of children, and children with disabilities are more likely to be institutionalized. Such children are, therefore, less likely to be exposed to population-based obesity prevention strategies based in schools or community organizations.

Children with disabilities constitute a large but very heterogeneous population group with a variety of functional disabilities and medical impairments. In 1994, it was estimated that 12% of noninstitutionalized children and adolescents in the United States 5 to 17 years of age had some type of functional limitation, a percentage that corresponds to >6 million individuals.[346] These numbers have likely increased since 1994. Children with disabilities are overrepresented among US populations at increased risk for obesity, such as minorities and the poor.[3,346] Children with developmental disorders have a prevalence of overweight as high or higher than that of other children.[347] Many of these children with disabilities use medications that increase the risk of excessive weight gain, such as antiepileptics, antipsychotics, antidepressants, and steroids. However, although children with some types of disabilities and medical impairments are at increased risk for obesity (Down syndrome, brain cancer survivors), others are at decreased risk for obesity because of undernutrition (sickle cell anemia, cystic fibrosis). Even within the same medical impairment, for example, cerebral palsy, some patients can present with undernutrition, whereas others present with overnutrition.[348,349]

The disabilities affecting children and adolescents are heterogeneous in nature and severity, making it difficult to design a strategy that fits all children with disabilities. Because of limited mobility, communication, or learning abilities, many children and adolescents with disabilities will not be able to participate optimally in obesity prevention programs designed for the general population, and adapting obesity prevention strategies to a wide range of types and severity of disability will be a significant challenge. Existing initiatives, such as the Special Olympics, however, have been successful at increasing physical activity levels in children, adolescents, and adults with a wide range of disabilities and overcoming physical and societal barriers to sports. This could provide a model for prevention of obesity in this population.[350,351]

Ethnic Minority and Low-Income Populations

Several factors are thought to contribute to the ethnic disparities in obesity in ways that potentially influence the nature of preventive interventions that will be effective.[352-354] Historical and current exposure to social inequities may lead to adverse eating and physical activity patterns through various mechanisms,[355] including the possibility that overeating is used as a mechanism to cope with stress or that children are overfed as "insurance" against hunger.[356] Studies have indicated ethnic differences in consumption of calories and fat,[357-359] which to some extent is associated with high levels of consumption of fast foods[360-362] and in levels of sedentary behaviors.[358,362] A number of studies have shown that African American women are more likely to accept a larger ideal body image[357,363-367] than are women from other ethnic groups, although the ways in which body image influences weight control are uncertain. Also, the nature and impact of body image variables for ethnic groups other than African Americans are unclear. The diversity of ethnic subgroups within the major categories of Hispanics/Latinos, American Indians, and Pacific Islanders makes it inappropriate to state generalities for these groups as a whole. The issue of body image is relevant, at least theoretically, to motivation for weight control and prevention of obesity. Survey data suggest that African American women who are overweight are less likely than Hispanic or non-Hispanic white women to try to lose weight[313] and may not perceive themselves to be overweight.[368] Ethnic minority populations in general are underrepresented in the weight-control literature, although this may reflect the access (both location and eligibility requirements) of minority populations to the studies that have been conducted. Studies comparing weight loss in African Americans and whites in the same program indicate lower average weight loss among African Americans than whites, within sex.[369-371]

This lesser level of success in weight-control programs could reflect social/environmental context issues, motivation, cultural appropriateness of the program, or other factors not yet identified. Again, whether this applies to other ethnic minority populations and also whether the results of treatment studies are informative for designing prevention strategies are unknown.

Recent attention has focused on aspects of the social contexts for obesity development that are less favorable for African Americans and other ethnic minority populations, including types of foods and retail food outlets available, range and accessibility of healthy food availability, opportunities for physical activity, and exposure to targeted marketing of less healthful foods.[352,372-375] Acculturation may play a significant role in the association of obesity with increased duration of US residence. In some studies conducted among Asian and Hispanic adolescents, acculturation to a US lifestyle was shown to be associated with adoption of unhealthy behaviors in those born outside of the United States, such as sedentary behavior and poor dietary habits.[376,377] However, culture of origin and circumstances after immigration are important variables to consider. There may also be instances in which less acculturation is associated with a higher occurrence of overweight, as suggested in a study of Chinese American children.[378]

Access to supermarkets, which increases access to healthy foods, has been associated with better dietary quality[379] (eg, greater consumption of fruits and vegetables). Supermarket access is relatively lower in census tracts with a high proportion of African American residents. For example, Morland and colleagues[380] reported that 4 times as many supermarkets were located in non-Hispanic white neighborhoods than in African American neighborhoods. In addition, the ratio of supermarkets:residents was substantially higher in predominantly non-Hispanic white neighborhoods (1:3816 residents) than in African American neighborhoods (1:23 582 residents). Zenk et al[381] found that the most impoverished neighborhoods in Detroit with high proportions of African Americans were farther away (1.1 miles on average) from the nearest supermarket than neighborhoods that were less impoverished and had low proportions of African American residents. In contrast, access to fast-food restaurants may be greater in black or low-SES neighborhoods. Block and colleagues[360] showed that the density of fast-food restaurants was greatest in neighborhoods in which residents were predominantly African American and low income. Neighborhoods in which 80% of the residents were African American had 2.4 fast-food restaurants per square mile, whereas neighborhoods in which 80% of the residents were non-Hispanic white had only 1.5 fast-food restaurants per square mile.

In addition to issues related to types of available food stores, the relative costs of low- versus high-calorie foods is another potentially critical influence on efforts to prevent obesity in low-SES communities. As reviewed by Drewnowski,[382] several lines of evidence converge to suggest that the likelihood of being able to consume a healthful diet with calories appropriate to energy needs decreases with decreasing income. Limited income means limited money to spend on food and less flexibility in food spending as a percentage of available funds. The current price structure of foods is such that products high in fat and sugar and low in other nutrients are the least expensive, whereas fruits, vegetables, and whole-grain products, which are both lower in calories per unit weight and higher in essential nutrients, are relatively more expensive. Therefore, even where supermarkets are available, people with low incomes may purchase a relatively higher-calorie diet of less expensive, higher-calorie foods. High-fat and high-sugar foods are "energy dense" (ie, have more calories per unit weight) and are often highly palatable, making them relatively easy to overconsume. The perception that people with low incomes can afford a healthful, calorically appropriate diet is perpetuated by federal policy—specifically the "Thrifty Food Plan" that is used to calculate the Food Stamp Program benefits—that assumes a base diet of raw foods that will be cooked "from scratch."[383] However, from a practical perspective, few people, including recipients of federal nutrition assistance or income support, are spending sufficient time in food preparation to consume such a diet.[383]

Studies that suggest that low-SES areas negatively influence physical activity include 1 study by Yen and Kaplan[384] based on data from the Alameda County Study, a population-based longitudinal cohort study that began in 1965. Overall physical activity decreased between 1965 and 1974 but decreased significantly more in areas of poverty than in nonpoverty areas. Even after adjustment for numerous potential confounds, including age, gender, baseline physical activity score, smoking, individual income, education, BMI, alcohol consumption, and perceived health status, living in an area of poverty was significantly associated with a greater decrease in physical activity. Observed interactions indicated differences in effects according to race/ethnicity and individual income. There were no racial/ethnic differences (comparing blacks with all others) in the pattern of changes within poverty areas but a greater decrease in physical activity among blacks versus others in the nonpoverty areas, adjusting for potential confounders. A similar interaction was seen with individual income (ie, similar patterns within poverty areas but greater decreases among those with inadequate incomes in nonpoverty areas). This reduction in physical activity in poorer areas may be owing to the possibility that physical activity-friendly environments (ie, safe, affordable, well maintained, and appealing) are less common in low-SES areas. For example, Powell et al[373] studied 409 communities and found high-poverty areas had significantly fewer sports areas, parks, greenways, and bike paths than areas characterized by higher median household income and lower poverty rates.

Considerations for Taking Action

The motivational and behavioral issues that people encounter in achieving and maintaining energy balance combined with the fact that the many environmental context factors that influence energy balance are beyond the individual's control provide a compelling rationale for taking a public health, or population-wide, approach to prevention of obesity. This type of approach is comprehensive, including educational and motivational messages aimed at the entire population, as well as societal, worksite, government, public health, and health-care organizations promoting health consciousness, providing opportunities for physical activity, and making healthy foods accessible.[19,20,236] Such efforts make healthy eating and physically active lifestyles easier to adopt and more socially acceptable and self-reinforcing. The pillar of the rationale for a public health approach to obesity prevention lies in the overall strategy for preventive medicine as outlined by the late Geoffrey Rose.[264]

Determining Where to Intervene: Targets for Action in an Ecological Framework

An Institute of Medicine[385] committee concluded that approaches informed by an ecological model are critical for effectively addressing major public health challenges generally, and a subsequent Institute of Medicine committee used an ecological framework as the basis for a comprehensive national action plan to address the epidemic of obesity in children and youth.[7] Ecological frameworks emphasize the importance of social, environment, and policy contexts as influences on individual behavior and the interactions and interdependence of influences across different levels extending from the individual to the society at large.

The need for a multilevel, multisectoral approach to population-based obesity prevention has been emphasized[8,19] and is illustrated in Figure 3. This "causal web" of societal-level influences on obesity provides a framework for conceptualizing the different sectors or processes from which they arise and act (eg, transportation, urbanization, commerce, social welfare, media and marketing, education, agriculture, food and nutrition, and health) and the different levels at which these factors operate to influence the contexts for food choices and activity patterns in the population at large (global, national, regional, and local, as well as immediate environments such as work, school, and home).[19] The arrows in Figure 3 indicate the complexity and interrelationships among processes and pathways emanating from different sectors.

Table [2.]3, which is complementary to Figure 3, was adapted from an ecological framework developed by the Partnership to Promote Healthy Eating and Active Living.[257] The listings in columns 1 to 3 give examples of specific categories of factors that might provide leverage points and settings for interventions in various sectors and contexts with a goal of shifting influences in a direction less conducive to chronic positive energy imbalance. Together with Figure 3, these listings illustrate that some influences that relate to obesity may require action through national and international channels (eg, those related to the food industry), whereas others can be influenced by policies and practices that are controlled by state or regional authorities, at the city or neighborhood level, or in schools and workplaces. The other 4 columns in Table [2.]3 reflect the societal and individual response variables that will affect the feasibility and effectiveness of obesity prevention initiatives. Many of these variables are reflected in the earlier described considerations for prevention in key risk sub-groups. A longitudinal analysis of patterns of weight gain among members of social networks, including unrelated individuals and spouses, as well as family members who were genetically related, underscores the potentially powerful influence of social relationships in transmission of environmental risks of obesity.[386]

Figure 3 illustrates the complexity of the social and environmental contexts that produce the greatest challenge for obesity prevention. Implicit in the causal web (Figure 3) are processes and pathways that are fundamental to the social fabric and to day-to-day lifestyles. The number and types of potential stakeholders and vested interests potentially affected by interventions in these sectors and channels are vast. Policy makers, industries, and consumers may not support making changes in these factors, even when they recognize the need for action on obesity, because of the structural nature of these factors and the perceived negative consequences for other outcomes, both commercial and personal. Also evident in this understanding of what is required for obesity prevention is that influences controlled by health professionals or health policy makers are only 1 type of influence and are not involved in many important pathways. Creating the multisectoral, multilevel, and interdisciplinary partnerships and initiatives that are needed to influence the many other sectors is one of the major challenges of obesity prevention.[20]

Increasing the emphasis on population approaches that go "upstream" to focus on environmental and policy change requires a shift in thinking for those trained in clinical or individually oriented interventions. It is difficult to know when one is being effective when taking action so far removed from the ultimate behavioral outcome of interest. Prevailing attitudes of health professionals and others may also argue against reducing the focus on individuals to change their behaviors. The "upstream-downstream" argument is often made by analogy to a situation in which a continuing number of people are struggling in the water downstream, about to drown. Going upstream to find out why people keep falling into the river (eg, a bridge might have collapsed) is as critical as working downstream to pull the people out of the river one at a time. This is not a dichotomy; the goal is both to save "those who are drowning" and to stop others from "falling in." The analogy is used to make the point that the clinical approaches in which we are so well trained and perhaps confident can never be sufficient to solve widespread population health problems unless broad-based population strategies are also applied. Moreover, upstream approaches are the most cost effective when problems are widespread because individualized screening and counseling are, by comparison, much more costly on a per capita basis. As noted previously, upstream approaches are also the most likely to level the playing field for socially disadvantaged populations whose options for healthy eating and physical

Table [2.]3

Influences on Physical Activity and Eating Behavior in Sectors and Settings: Ecological Layers From Macrosocietal to Individual Level

	Focal points and settings for interventions			Practical, social, and personal influences on intervention effectiveness			
Distal leverage points	Proximal leverage points	Behavioral settings	Enablers of choice	Social	Ethnic/Cultural	Individual
Architecture and building codes	Community	Community activity providers	Accessibility	Educational attainment	Beliefs	Genetics
Education system	Developers	Day care	Convenience	Interpersonal relationships	Ethnic identities	Hierarchy of needs
Entertainment industry	Employer	Food stores	Cost	Life stage	Habits	Physiology
Exercise, physical activity, and sports industry	Family	Health club	Knowledge	Social roles	Life experience	Pleasure
Food industry	Food stores	Home	Safety	Socioeconomic status	Values	Self identities
Government	Healthcare providers	Local school	Seasonality			
Healthcare industry	Local government	Neighborhood	Situation or context physical and social			
Information industry	Nongovernmental organizations	Parks, recreation centers, senior centers	Social trends			
Labor-saving device industry	Nonprofit providers	Religious, community, and nongovernmental	Source of information			
Political advocacy/lobbying	Property owners	Restaurants	Time			
Recreation industry	Recreation facilities	Shopping malls				
Transportation system	Restaurants and food outlets	Vehicle of transport				
School boards/districts	Workplace	Shopping mall				

Source: Reprinted from Booth et al., 257 with permission from Wiley-Blackwell.

activity patterns are the most limited, for a variety of reasons,[352,372] and who, because of limited resources and limited social capital or power, are more constrained by the available options than those with more advantages, who may be able to find ways to work around constraints and create new options for themselves.[387,388]

How to Intervene: Determining What to Do and Whether It Works

Figure 3 and Table [2.]3 describe potential targets for action—covering many different sectors, levels, and specific potential focal points. How to actually have an impact on these targets requires a more process-oriented perspective related to the design of specific intervention programs or community action initiatives. Useful insights for how to take action can be drawn from general public health and prevention models. For example, the "Spectrum of Prevention"[389] is useful for characterizing and differentiating interventions at all of the levels that may be needed to address obesity at the population level and how these levels interrelate. This framework, described in Table [2.]4 and discussed below in relation to obesity, has 7 bands or levels that indicate different types of strategies for environmental and policy changes, as well as community mobilization and individual education directed to selected combinations of the intervention targets outlined above. Consistent with an ecological model, the complementarity of these different strategies should be emphasized. In particular, the more upstream strategies at the upper levels of the spectrum (influencing policy and legislation, mobilizing communities and neighborhoods, changing organizational practices, and fostering coalitions and networks) are important for enabling the effectiveness of those oriented to individuals. Table [2.]4 also includes examples of activities at each level of the spectrum to promote increased physical activity, based on an initiative in California.[390] The following narrative, which is organized according to the 4 top bands in the spectrum (influencing policy and legislation, mobilizing neighborhoods and communities, changing organizational practices, and fostering coalitions and networks), provides further highlights of how obesity prevention might be approached at these more upstream levels. Guidance relevant to providers and individual education and counseling is referenced in Appendix 2.

Influencing Policy and Legislation

Initiatives to foster changes in policy and legislation may be undertaken at local, state, and federal levels with a focus on the relative availability or cost of high- versus low-calorie foods or on opportunities to be physically active. Formal or informal policy changes are core to upstream interventions in that they change behavioral options and can reach large numbers of people, regardless of individual health motivations. Food-related policy targets might include snack foods and sweetened beverages, for which the goal would be to decrease consumption, or fruits and vegetables or water, for which the goal would be increase consumption. Activity-related targets might include aspects of community design that are more

Table [2.]4

Components of the Comprehensive "Spectrum of Prevention" as Applied to Obesity Prevention

Prevention strategy	Rationale	Examples related to increasing physical activity*
Influencing policy and legislation	Both formal and informal policies have the ability to affect large numbers of people by improving the environments in which they live and work, encouraging people to lead healthy lifestyles, and providing for consumer protections	Land use policy established for community gardens Stable funding for Indian Health Service clinics to promote physical activity and nutrition
Mobilizing neighborhoods and communities	Particularly in low-income communities confronting more urgent concerns of violence, drug use, unemployment, and the struggle to keep families together, engaging community members in developing agendas and priorities is essential	Mapping community assets related to physical activity options Assisting community residents in setting priorities relevant to physical activity Providing technical assistance to help community residents implement action plans related to physical activity
Changing organizational practices	Modifying the internal policies and practices of agencies and institutions can result in improved health and safety for staff of the organization, better services for clients, and a healthier community environment; advocacy for such changes can result in a broad impact on community health	Protocols for physician assessment, sliding fees, counseling, and referral Bilingual staff at YMCA Work site policies Walking trail signage Improve safety in parks Provide fitness programs in public housing
Fostering coalitions and networks	Coalitions and networks, composed of community organizations, policy makers, businesses, health providers, and community residents working together, can be powerful advocates for legislation and organizational change and provide an opportunity for joint planning, system-wide problem solving, and collaborative policy development	Local project coalitions and advisory committees Local park and recreation departments Healthy Cities coalitions American College of Sports Medicine volunteers Local Governor's Council on Physical Fitness and Sports
Educating providers	Service providers within and outside the health system can encourage adoption of healthy behaviors, screen for health risks, contribute to community education, and advocate for policies and legislation	Training for physician screening and referrals Park and recreation staff training Community exercise leader training Curriculum at university

(continued)

Table 2.4 *(continued)*

Prevention strategy	Rationale	Examples related to increasing physical activity*
Promoting community education	Community education can reach the greatest number of individuals possible with health education messages and also build a critical mass of people who will become involved in improving community health. This includes the use of mass media to shape the public's understanding of health issues—termed "media advocacy"	Community walkathon Media campaign Work site programs Interdenominational sports leagues Community fitness event Community advocate training Community gardens Church and community bulletins
Strengthening individual knowledge and skills	This strategy involves working directly with clients in the home, community settings, or in clinics, providing health information to promote well-being among children, families, senior citizens, and other population groups. It also includes working with both youth and adults to build their capacity in areas such as media advocacy, community mobilizing, and working with policy makers to make positive changes in the health of their communities	Walking club orientation Exercise classes Education classes Field trips Handouts Outreach contacts Home visits/instructions Exercise demonstrations

Source: Adapted from Rattray et al,[389] with permission.

*Examples, except for those related to "mobilizing communities," were taken directly from Reference 390.

or less conducive to traveling on foot or by bicycle, availability and cost of recreational facilities, automobile use and availability of public transportation, and factors related to safety (eg, rates of street crime, condition of playgrounds, traffic-related measures to create safe routes for children to walk or bike to school).[7]

Options for types of policies include taxation of snack foods, subsidy of fruits and vegetables, regulations requiring foods served or sold in schools to meet specified nutritional standards, restrictions on advertising high-calorie foods to children, nutrition labeling regulations, financial incentives to industry (eg, to encourage siting of supermarkets in inner city areas with limited food access), or requiring school physical education classes and health education. Taxation mechanisms may be targeted to raising funds to support prevention programs directly. Worksite policies might include providing time off or facilities and equipment for exercise, providing bike racks and showers for people who cycle to work, providing weight-control programs or covering the cost of such programs or of gym memberships. Policies can also address monitoring and surveillance of weight levels (eg, of school children). Receptivity to various types of policy solutions varies among individuals and communities. There may be concerns that some policies will disadvantage commercial interests, limit individual freedom of choice, or create or aggravate social inequities. For example, taxation to raise the price of certain high-calorie foods could be problematic for people with very low incomes who depend on having cheap sources of calories.

The Institute of Medicine committee to evaluate progress to prevent childhood obesity[355] identified 717 bills (of which 123 were passed) and 134 resolutions (of which 53% were passed) relevant to childhood obesity that had been introduced in the United States between 2003 and 2005. Bills with a high rate of passage were related to farmers' markets, walking and biking paths, establishing task forces or study groups, and model school policies and safe routes to school. None of the 74 bills related to taxes on sodas and snacks passed. Policies to protect children specifically may garner more support than those directed to the general population because the potential vulnerability to environmental factors is relatively easier to argue with respect to children than for adults.

Mobilizing Communities and Neighborhoods

This level of the Spectrum of Prevention emphasizes the importance of community engagement, contrasting the traditional medical model, with the provider expert at the center (which also characterizes many public health activities), with the additional need to involve communities directly in assessing needs and planning and taking actions to address identified problems.[389] Such engagement with community members helps to align priorities as viewed by community members with those identified by public health workers and increases the likelihood that resulting initiatives will generate community interest and follow-through. Public health workers and academic research partners can support community-generated initiatives through technical assistance. Some obesity prevention research involves community-based participatory research.[391–393] There has been increasing recognition of the importance of community-based participatory research, particularly with respect to research to address health disparities. REACH 2010 (Racial and Ethnic Approaches to Community Health) projects funded by the CDC are examples of such efforts that have specifically mobilized community members through participatory research related to food access and broader issues related to obesity.[394] Resource inventories or assets mapping are useful tools in this approach.[395–397]

Changing Organizational Practices

Schools and child care facilities, workplaces, and primary care are important settings for implementation of policies and programmatic initiatives. Relevant policy or programs may involve specifying the nutrition composition or cost of foods served or sold in cafeterias, instituting requirements for physical education in schools, increasing the availability of physical activity options or the time available to take advantage of these options, implementing training programs to enable school teachers to provide nutrition or physical education, and providing financial support for programs and services related to weight control. The appeal of setting-based approaches of this type includes the ability to work with a "captive audience" and to also influence social norms within the setting, with possible transfer to behavior outside of the setting. For example, policies that foster integration of 10 minute physical activity breaks into the regular work day or school day appear to be feasible, well received, and associated with meaningful increases in physical activity and possibly improved performance. This approach may be sustainable given that the activity breaks can be led by regular staff or teachers.[398-400]

Of the possible setting-based interventions, the Task Force on Community Preventive Services has found sufficient evidence to recommend "multicomponent interventions aimed at diet, physical activity, and cognitive change" in worksite settings.[35] In this report, evidence was deemed insufficient to determine effectiveness of single component interventions in worksites or of school-based programs for children and adolescents, and reviews of evidence to support various types of healthcare system interventions and community-wide interventions were still pending. Key issues for intervening in specific settings relate to perceived or actual competition of the interventions with the mission or other priorities of the setting, fear of liability, resource issues, privacy issues, the potential for increasing discrimination against those with existing weight problems, or consumer dissatisfaction. For example, efforts to increase time spent in physical activity may compete with time needed for academic work. Efforts to change school food options may compete with the use of food sales to raise funds for other school activities, as well as be unpopular with students and parents, leading to other problems for school officials. Screening children for BMI levels is controversial owing to the potential for adverse psychosocial effects of identifying children as overweight or obese and also because it is meaningless without the ability to implement ameliorative interventions.[401] Workplace issues with respect to productivity, consumer acceptance, and the potential for discrimination are similar. Injuries associated with increased physical activity may be a liability concern. In workplaces, there is potential competition with time spent working, where productivity is at issue. Competition with time to address more pressing medical or social issues can be a deterrent to adding weight-related counseling to primary care settings. Although many primary care physicians and their patients may be very motivated to provide or receive such counseling, the length of typical visits is too short to allow this, and reimbursement for obesity-related counseling—if available at all—may be limited to people with established obesity-related comorbidities.

The Alliance for a Healthier Generation, a joint initiative of the American Heart Association and the William J. Clinton Foundation,[402] is an increasingly promi-

Table [2.]5

Components of the American Heart Association–Clinton Foundation Alliance for a Healthier Generation Initiatives to Foster Childhood Obesity Prevention

Founders	American Heart Association and William J. Clinton Foundation
Co-Leader	Governor Arnold Schwarzenegger of California
Mission	To eliminate childhood obesity and to inspire all young people in the United States to develop lifelong, healthy habits
Goals	To stop the nationwide increase in childhood obesity by 2010 and to empower kids nationwide to make healthy lifestyle choices The Alliance is positively affecting the places that make a difference to a child's health: homes, schools, restaurants, doctor's offices, and the community
Programs	Healthy Schools Program Industry Initiative Kids' Movement Healthcare Initiative

Source: Reference 402.

nent example of a comprehensive national-level obesity-prevention strategy that focuses on school settings. Components of this initiative are listed in Table [2.]5. Indicative of the importance of this program in the national obesity prevention effort, the Robert Wood Johnson Foundation, which has a major commitment to reversing the epidemic of child and adolescent obesity, initially awarded $8 million in 2006 to support the first phase of the Healthy Schools Program. A year later, it announced the award of an additional $20 million to support expansion of the program that will focus on states with the highest obesity rates, as well as expand on-line support for schools nationwide. As shown in Table [2.]5, the Alliance initiatives go beyond a school focus and address several other levels of the Spectrum of Prevention.

Fostering Coalitions and Networks

Community organizations or coalitions of community organizations or members who have a stake in obesity prevention may undertake community action to raise awareness of a problem, identify potential solutions, and seek to implement these solutions through changes in policy and practice. Some coalitions have a single focus, while others take on a broader set of community priorities. Community members may mobilize spontaneously (eg, in response to a perceived crisis or intolerable situation). Community mobilization may also be initiated as a health-promotion strategy (eg, through efforts of a state or local public health agency, other health services provider, or a community-based organization with a relevant mandate). Researchers who can provide technical assistance and advice are often partners in these efforts. Broadly based, multisectoral efforts may be particularly effective. For example, the Consortium to Lower Childhood Obesity in Chicago Children (CLOCC) provides a rubric for pooling the efforts of hundreds of organizations representing a variety of entities with relevant interests.[403] CLOCC activities include training public school teachers in strategies to improve student nutrition and physical activity, community-wide health-promotion events, website development, and an initiative to foster walk-to-school programs. A School Nutrition Task Force in Philadelphia mobilized a successful effort to create healthier vending options in schools.[404]

Evidence-Based Experience

In contrast to the extensive database available on obesity treatment, research to identify specific interventions to prevent obesity is still at a relatively early stage.[7,20,236,405] Elements of promising strategies for obesity prevention can be identified, and there are many relevant efforts under way. These efforts include programs generated spontaneously in communities, as well as formal research or demonstration projects undertaken based on program logic and combinations of strategies that appear to be effective. However, it is difficult to identify what set of interventions will be effective in shifting the BMI distribution for a whole community (also see Research Challenges). Effective interventions will, separately, improve dietary intake and the level of physical activity, but in combination, they must not only improve dietary quality and energy output or fitness but must also result in the avoidance of positive energy imbalance. Effects must also be sustainable over time in that the risk of excess weight gain is ever present. As explained previously, the applicability to obesity prevention of the literature on obesity treatment may be limited, because the challenges of achieving energy balance are different for prevention from those for treatment at the individual level. In addition, social and environmental changes, although relevant to both prevention and treatment, are fundamental to obesity prevention.

Numerous systematic reviews have assessed available scientific evidence on obesity prevention. Results of selected reviews published during the last decade are shown in Table [2.]6.[405-417] Two reviews focus on adults in primary care settings,[414,415] 2 focus on environmental and policy interventions,[412,413] and 2 cover all ages.[417,418] The remaining articles focus on children or school settings.[405-411] Almost all include studies both in the United States and abroad. Perhaps the most striking finding in Table [2.]6 is the relatively small numbers of eligible studies for these reviews of obesity prevention, although the number is increasing. Searches sometimes identify thousands of possible articles, but the number ultimately reviewed and included is relatively small. This is owing in part to the inclusion and exclusion criteria applicable to many reviews (not all of these criteria are included in the Table [2.]6 entries, for brevity; eg, requirements for controlled trials—either randomized or nonrandomized, inclusion of only completed trials, exclusions on the basis of a rating of poor quality, or exclusion of studies that did not provide a measurement of weight status or fatness). With respect to the findings on weight outcomes, the findings are encouraging in identifying many studies that were successful, although evidence of the ability of interventions to change average BMI levels is limited. The relatively limited breadth of studies identified, mainly school based and mainly individually oriented, indicates an urgent need to explore preventive interventions in other settings and at multiple levels upstream. Ongoing research may broaden the evidence base to some extent, but there is an overall impression that this critical area of research has far too little focus.

Research on how to implement effective environmental and policy change is a relatively new aspect to the field of obesity research, and appropriate measures and evaluation designs are still being developed. These measures and designs are needed not only for deliberate experimentation that involves environmental and policy changes, but also for the many spontaneous changes that are occurring in legislatures and communities on a day-to-day basis. Changes in school food and beverage vending policies are a prominent example of spontaneous changes that are being implemented with a limited empirical basis (ie, natural experiments). In addition, as noted above, evaluation of specific interventions is complicated by the fact that additive or synergistic effects of multiple interventions across different levels and sectors may be necessary to have an impact on behaviors related to energy balance and to see effects on weight.[411,418] This can be addressed in part by multilevel interventions or combinations of studies, but to date, these studies are few in number.[409,411] Another challenging and strongly debated issue is how study designs with the highest level of internal validity, randomized, controlled trials, apply in that they may impose limitations on both the feasibility and relevance of testing obesity prevention approaches in naturalistic settings.[418,419]

An example of a promising multilevel intervention, evaluated with a non-randomized, controlled trial design, is the "Shape Up Somerville" study.[420] This study compared the effects of a comprehensive intervention, conducted in partnership with entities in the study communities, on physical activity and food options during the child's entire day on BMI z-scores 1 year after the initiation of the interventions. Participants were 1178 elementary school-aged children in all 30 schools in 3 participating communities: 10 schools in the intervention community; 10 and 5 schools in the 2 control communities, which received no intervention. An extra control group was used to ensure against the spontaneous development of a nonstudy related intervention in 1 of the control communities. The numerous activities targeted the home, school, and community environments and included environmental changes and policy development related to food availability and physical activity options, newsletters, training of teachers and medical professionals, and implementation of a restaurant certification program. Children in the intervention community had a more favorable BMI trajectory than those in the comparison arm.

Table [2.]6

Highlights of Selected Systematic Reviews of Intervention Studies Related to Obesity Prevention (listed alphabetically by first author within year of publication, most recent first)

Reference	Focus, scope, and key inclusion criteria	Eligible studies identified	Main findings
Bluford et al[406]	**Preschool children** United States and international, published in 1966 through March 2005 Interventions to prevent or treat obesity in preschool children (ages 2 to <6 years) of at least 3 months' duration	7 studies Settings included schools, day care/Head Start programs, clinics, and home settings	Significant reductions in weight status or body fat were identified in 4 of the 7 studies, of which 3 sustained reductions 1 to 2 years after the program began 2 studies reported no change; the other study found no change in Latino or black children but an increase in weight status in white children
De Mattia et al[407]	**Children and adolescents** United States and international, published in 1966 to February 2005 Interventions to limit sedentary behaviors (recreational screen time but not homework or reading) in children or adolescents in natural settings (eg, at school or home or in a primary care setting	12 studies	All of the studies, including 6 that targeted clinic-based populations and 6 that were population-based, reduced sedentary behaviors (self-reported) and improved weight outcomes (measured)
Sharma[408]	**Children and adolescents** Only studies from countries outside of the United States, published in 1999–2005 School-based interventions for obesity prevention in children; not all studies included measured weight outcomes; and not all had been completed	21 interventions, of which 17 were from elementary schools	Most studies focused on individual level approaches; 16 of the 21 interventions were delivered by existing teachers, often with additional training Measured weight or fatness variables were available in 11 studies, of which 6 showed improvements; all 3 completed studies that included parents improved measured weight outcomes

Doak et al[409]	**Children and adolescents** United States and international, published through August 2005 Interventions and programs to prevent obesity in children and adolescents, with measured weight or fatness outcomes	25 interventions	17 of the 25 interventions reported statistically significant improvements in obesity measures; estimation of effectiveness differed according to whether skinfold or BMI measures were used 5 studies found gender differences in effects and 1 study found differences by ethnicity No ideal age for intervention could be identified from these studies Physical education and reduction of television viewing were highlighted as examples of effective approaches One of the effective interventions was also associated with an increase in underweight prevalence
Flodmark et al[410]	**Children and adolescents** United States and international, published until 2004 Setting or population-based interventions (ie, in groups of children not specifically selected for being overweight or obese) to prevent obesity of at least 12 months' duration; with measured weight or fatness outcomes Articles published until 2004 were added to a prior 2002 review; results of 5 other systematic reviews were also evaluated	24 studies in this review 39 total studies when including other reviews	8 studies reported significant positive results on measures of obesity, and 16 were neutral; none had negative results Considering these results together with those of 5 other systematic reviews yielded 39 studies of which 15 had positive results and the other 24 were neutral; no studies reported harmful effects on children Effective programs were relatively limited school-based programs that promoted a combination of healthful eating and increased physical activity

(continued)

Table [2.]6 *(continued)*

Reference	Focus, scope, and key inclusion criteria	Eligible studies identified	Main findings
Flynn et al[411]	**Children and adolescents** United States and international, including government reports and other published or unpublished sources identified apart from databases of published articles, 1982–2003 Accounts of programs that could shed light on best practices related to reduction of obesity and related chronic disease risk in children	147 programs were analyzed	No single program emerged as a model of best practice, although promising elements applicable to various populations and settings were identified More upstream and population-focused interventions are needed to balance the emphasis on individually oriented strategies There is a particular need for programs tailored to ethnic minority and new immigrant children and based in community or home settings
Health et al[412]	**Policy and environmental changes** United States and international, published through 2003 Studies of the effectiveness of urban design and land use and transport policies and practices for increasing physical activity; reviewed for the Guide to Community Preventive Services	12 studies on community-scale urban design, 6 studies on street-scale urban design, and 3 studies on transportation and travel policies and practices	Both community-scale and street-scale urban design and land use policies and practices were found effective in promoting physical activity, with evidence rated as "sufficient." The evidence to evaluate the effectiveness of travel and transport policies is insufficient Also reported are the following additional findings of the Guide to Community Preventive Services with respect to physical activity promotion, based on prior systematic reviews: strong evidence for community-wide campaigns, individually adapted health behavior change, school-based physical education, social support in community settings, and the enhancement of access to physical activity options combined with informational outreach activities There is sufficient evidence for point-of-decision prompts

Summerbell et al[405]	**Children and adolescents** United States and international, published in 1990 through February 2005 Interventions to prevent obesity, of at least 12 weeks' duration, in randomized controlled or controlled trials	10 long-term (at least 12 months) and 12 short-term (12 weeks to 12 months)	Of the long-term studies that focused on both diet and physical activity, 5 studies found improvements in weight or fatness outcomes for both boys and girls and 1 found improvements for girls only; a long-term study of a multimedia intervention to improve physical activity was effective; studies that focused on nutrition education only were not effective Two of the short-term studies were effective in improving weight or fatness outcomes; both focused on physical activity; 2 others that focused on physical activity and 10 that focused on both physical activity and diet were not effective
Matson-Koffman et al[413]	**Policy and environmental changes** United States and international, published in 1970–2003 Policy or environmental interventions to promote physical activity or good nutrition, excluding studies of the built environment and media-only campaigns; included studies in whole communities, schools, worksites and restaurants, and healthcare settings	65 studies before 1990 and 64 studies between 1990 and 2003	Strongest evidence was found for – Promoting stair use – Improving access to place and options for physical activity – Improving school physical education – Implementing comprehensive worksite approaches – Increasing availability of nutritious foods – Information at point of food purchase – Systems for reminding health-care providers to provide nutrition counseling
Pignone et al[414]	**Adults** United States and international, published in 1966–2001 Trials of counseling of adults in primary care settings to promote a healthy diet, of at least 3 months' duration, with behavioral outcomes reported, excluding trials in people selected on the basis of overweight or obesity or a chronic disease; reviewed for the US Preventive Services Task Force	21 trials	Relatively modest improvements in self-reported dietary intakes of saturated fat, fruits and vegetables, and possibly dietary fiber in response to brief interventions using a variety of modalities; greater intensity was associated with better results but had less potential feasibility in these settings

(continued)

Table [2.]6 (continued)

Reference	Focus, scope, and key inclusion criteria	Eligible studies identified	Main findings
Eden et al[415]	**Adults** United States and international, published in 1994 through March 2002 Trials in which counseling to improve physical activity was provided and some part of the intervention was performed by a primary care clinician (physician, nurse practitioner, nurse, or physician's assistant); reviewed for the US Preventive Services Task Force	8 trials; 5 other trials judged to be of poor quality were excluded	Limited support was found for the effectiveness of these interventions; 3 of the trials that included a usual care control group reported a significant improvement associated with the intervention; in 1 study, a written prescription was more effective than advice alone; another suggested that women may need more intensive counseling than men In the 1 study that reported harm, about 60% of all patients reported some type of musculoskeletal injury and some reported cardiovascular events that required hospitalization; however, no comparison data were available to estimate background rates
Hardeman et al[416]	**All ages** United States and International, published in 1966–1999 Published studies using any type of study design involving testing of an intervention to prevent weight gain among people not preselected on the basis of weight or age; studies in subpopulations such as those stopping smoking and studies of multifactorial interventions targeting specific diseases and studies targeting weight loss were not included	11 articles describing 9 distinct interventions 5 were in schools and 4 were in the community at large; 2 were in adults	Effectiveness seemed to be greater among older participants, men, nonsmokers, and those with high income Of 5 randomized, controlled trials, only 1 reported a significant effect on weight

Glenny et al[417]

All ages
US and international, published through 1995
Randomized trials of treatment and nonrandomized studies evaluating interventions for obesity prevention, at least 12 months' duration

Among 97 eligible trials of obesity treatment or prevention, only 4 were of prevention, 1 in children and 3 in adults

In the study in children, a 12-month family therapy intervention was initially successful compared with conventional treatment or no-treatment control, but effect was not present at 1-year follow-up
2 of the 2 studies involved comprehensive community-wide cardiovascular disease risk reduction programs; 1 reported a significantly smaller BMI increment over time in the intervention compared with control communities; the other study, based on mailed newsletters, optional group contact, and a financial incentive, reported a significant advantage for the intervention group after 1 year of follow-up

CONCLUSIONS

A main objective of this scientific statement is to provide an overview of the types of strategies needed to prevent obesity using a comprehensive, population-based approach rather than relying only on clinic-based or individually oriented strategies. Given that the ultimate determinants of obesity are individual eating and physical activity behaviors, the perception that one can solve the problem by refining the ability to help individuals to change their behaviors will persist. Central themes here are that what it will take for individuals on average to change their behaviors to the point of avoiding excess weight gain throughout the life course is affected by environmental factors that are not under their personal control. Research recommendations and programmatic initiatives for obesity prevention call for a broad range of strategies, many of which go beyond the knowledge, skill, and experience base of health professionals.

Investigators involved in pilot studies of obesity prevention identified a number of challenges to the design and conduct of research on obesity prevention in various organizational settings and study populations.[234,421] Foremost among these were the difficulty of motivating people to make the amount of effort needed for prevention of weight gain, the difficulty of measuring energy balance, the need to differentiate adverse weight gain from an increase in weight because of leaner body composition, and the large sample sizes needed to detect statistically significant differences when the primary outcome is no change in weight as opposed to the substantial weight losses obtained in treatment studies.[236] Perhaps partly for these reasons, the evidence to date includes many examples of obesity prevention interventions that have not shown significant differences in weight favoring the intervention group, making it especially important to identify examples of programs that might work.

Although the picture of how to intervene is far from complete, guidance and research recommendations developed by various expert panels,[7,355,422] working groups,[236] and systematic reviews (Table [2.]6) have led to an increase in obesity prevention research. One of these expert reports, developed by the Institute of Medicine, provides a national action plan for childhood obesity prevention and includes more than 50 recommendations for actions applicable to governments, industries, communities at large, schools, and homes.[7] A subsequent Institute of Medicine report provides a framework for evaluating progress and an update on progress in implementing elements of the plan.[355] Targeted funding from the National Institutes of Health,[423] from the CDC (www.cdc.gov), and, for childhood obesity prevention, from the Robert Wood Johnson Foundation (www.rwjf.org), for example, is a major incentive to conduct population-based obesity prevention research. This research includes community-partnered and community action research and research on the effectiveness of policies implemented in various sectors and at various levels. Unproven efforts will continue as an important part of the community response to this pressing health problem, but the mandate to ground these efforts with some type of mechanism for evaluation is increasingly emphasized and funded.[355]

Ongoing activities, such as the CDC Guide to Community Preventive Services[424] and Cochrane evidence reviews,[405] policy tracking, report cards,[425–428] and Web sites that serve as clearinghouses for sharing information about available resources and extant community programs,[429,430] are creating an increasingly strong platform for action. Several initiatives specifically designed to generate policy and environmental changes and identify effective approaches in this respect have been funded by the Robert Wood Johnson Foundation as part of its commitment to reversing the childhood obesity epidemic by 2015 (see www.rwjf.org). A study of 9 countries in Europe has set the precedent for comprehensive study of how various policy options for obesity prevention are viewed by a broad range of stakcholders.[431] With respect to direct physician involvement, a model of potential interest is the Physicians for Healthy Communities Initiative[432] developed by the California Medical Association Foundation in partnership with the California Nutrition Network for Healthy, Active Families and Kaiser Permanente. This initiative will promote policy and environmental changes in schools and communities and will also assist physicians with training in community collaboration, nutrition messages, and advocacy techniques to enable them to become champions to promote healthy eating and active living throughout California.

Finally, some aspects of the scenario with respect to obesity prevention should sound very familiar to those experienced with CVD prevention. Strategies across the spectrum have been applied to promotion of changes in food intake and physical activity and the needs for upstream interventions clearly articulated, both in the United States and globally.[433] The North Karelia project, in which policy-level interventions were implemented to generate population-wide reductions in intake of saturated fat, with benefits for reductions in CVD mortality, is perhaps the best known example of the success of policy changes for CVD risk reduction.[434] The concept of policy level interventions to change contexts for individual behavior is also well known from the experience with tobacco,[435] although the differences between food, which is essential to life and inherently good for health, and tobacco, which is nonessential and inherently bad for health, limit the direct transfer of some concepts and strategies. Many lessons from both tobacco and CVD prevention generally are applicable to obesity prevention. The most overarching lesson is that there is, indeed, the potential for success in combating such a far-reaching and deeply embedded societal pandemic.[435–437] Obesity treatment and prevention have always been a part of CVD prevention but, especially for prevention, have not been the primary focus. The rapid rise in obesity on a population level—associated with changes in the quantities of food available, marketed, and consumed, along with the very low level of obligatory physical activity for most people—makes obesity prevention efforts as a primary focus truly daunting. Furthermore, the inability to specify—at a population or individual level—the exact behaviors expected to result in energy balance considerably adds to the challenge. Avoiding unhealthy weight gain goes beyond the success of individual efforts to achieve good dietary quality and adequate physical fitness. It requires a broad range of strategies that include environmental and societal efforts.

Appendix [2.]1

AHA Statements and Workshop Proceedings Related to Obesity Etiology, Complications, Prevention, and Treatment, 2004–2006

Reference		Description
Williams et al[22]	Children and adolescents	Provides practical guidelines to clinicians to decrease CVD risk factors in youth, including low physical activity, obesity, insulin resistance and type 2 diabetes, high blood pressure, hypercholesterolemia, and cigarette smoking
Steinberger et al[23]	Children and adolescents	Summarizes evidence to provide a rationale for lifestyle modification and weight control in childhood to reduce risks of developing insulin resistance, type 2 diabetes, and CVD; oriented to clinical practitioners
Hayman et al[24]	Children and adolescents	Provides guidance about how to optimize school environments in population-based strategies to promote cardiovascular health for U.S. children and adolescents; intended for health and education professionals, child health advocates, policy makers, and community leaders; includes recommendations for school curricula, policies, and linkages to community resources and infrastructures
Mullis et al[25]	Adults, children, and families	Explains the complementarity of population-based and high-risk approaches to obesity prevention and treatment; describes important settings for instituting interventions to influence energy balance and the need for creative approaches to developing and evaluating broad policy approaches; makes research recommendations
Klein et al[26]	Adults	Reviews evidence on the clinical effects of weight loss on a variety of cardiovascular risk factors and outcomes and the clinical efficacy of treatments for obesity, including dietary and physical activity change, behavioral modification, pharmacotherapy, and surgery; summarizes guidelines for clinical evaluation and treatment of obese adults
Smith et al[21]	Adults in racial/ ethnic minority populations	Highlights the higher-than-average risk of some or all metabolic syndrome components in African Americans, Hispanic Americans, American Indians/Alaska Natives, Asian Americans and Pacific Islanders; makes recommendation to the AHA for initiatives to reduce the related health disparities through professional/lay programs, public policy/ advocacy, and research
Daniels et al[27]	Children and adolescents	Summarizes information on the pathophysiology and epidemiology of overweight in children and adolescents; provides an update on adverse health effects of childhood overweight and discusses approaches to prevention and treatment of overweight in children and adolescents

(continued)

Grundy et al[28]	Adults	Reviews and provides updated information in support of the AHA recommendations for clinical diagnosis, therapeutic goals and management of the metabolic syndrome; identifies related areas of needed research
Gidding et al[29]	Children and adolescents	Summarizes current available information on cardiovascular nutrition in children and makes recommendations for both primordial and primary prevention of cardiovascular disease beginning at a young age; emphasizes the importance of nutrition early in life, including the fetal milieu; includes brief overview of public health issues related to nutrition
Poirier et al[2]	Adults	Updates the evidence for the impact of obesity on CVD, including cardiac structure and function and summarizes the benefits of weight loss on the cardiopulmonary system; discusses potential CVD risks associated with certain clinical weight loss approaches
American Heart Association Nutrition Committee et al[30]	Adults primarily, although applicable to children	Updates the AHA public health and clinical recommendations for diet and other lifestyle behaviors to prevent and manage CVD, including the guideline to "aim for a healthy weight"; includes practical tips for individuals to achieve these guidelines; provides recommendations for practitioners, restaurants, the food industry, schools, and local governments to promote a more supportive environment for achieving goals
Pate et al[31]	Children and adolescents	Highlights physical activity to be a key determinant of weight status, summarizes the evidence supporting schools' potential for effectively improving and promoting physical activity, and recommends several key changes in school policy and practice
Kavey et al[32]	Children and adolescents	Provides guidelines for CVD prevention in children and adolescents who are at high risk for early coronary disease; these guidelines recommend more aggressive treatment of CVD risk factors, including obesity, than in the general population for children and adolescents with conditions such as familial hypercholesterolemia, diabetes, chronic kidney disease, heart transplantation, Kawasaki disease, systemic lupus erythematosus, rheumatoid arthritis, congenital heart disease, and past history of cancer treatment
Hayman et al[33]	Children and adolescents	Reviews rationale for primary prevention of CVD in youth and reports interventions at the population level and in high-risk individuals; provides guidelines with particular emphasis on nursing practice

Appendix [2.]2

Selected Evidence-Based Recommendations and Guidelines for Obesity Prevention and Treatment in Adults and Child/Adolescent Populations

Source	Relevance*
National Institutes of Health[34]	Adults
McTigue et al[17]	Adults
Katz et al[35]	Children/adolescents and adults
Koplan et al[7]	Children/adolescents
American Heart Association Nutrition Committee et al[30]	Children/adolescents and adults
Lau et al[36]	Children/adolescents and adults
National Initiative for Children's Healthcare Quality et al[37]	Children/adolescents

*Children under age 2 years are not targeted in any of the guidelines listed.

PART II

RESEARCH ON CONSUMER BIASES

CHAPTER 3

AN OUNCE OF PREVENTION, AN APPLE A DAY

Effects of Consumers' Lay Theories on Health-Related Behaviors

ANIRBAN MUKHOPADHYAY

Over 300 million people worldwide are obese (WHO 2010), including over 34 percent of the American adult population (Ogden et al. 2007). As these numbers grow ever faster every year and as people correspondingly succumb to health-related problems, the topic of health maintenance has become increasingly important and has begun to attract corresponding attention from consumer researchers (Agrawal, Menon, and Aaker 2007; Chandran and Menon 2004). A major focus of this scholarly attention has been on factors that lead individuals to overindulge in unhealthy behaviors instead of restraining themselves and making healthy choices. These include factors as disparate as social influence (McFerran et al. 2010), regulatory focus (Sengupta and Zhou 2007), and recollections of prior instances of indulgence or restraint (Mukhopadhyay, Sengupta, and Ramanathan 2008). Concomitant with this seemingly diverse set of factors, one area of investigation has demonstrated reliable and strong evidence of influence on health-related behaviors. This is the study of consumers' lay theories. Lay theories, also referred to as naive beliefs or implicit theories, have been shown to influence health-related goal setting and striving (Mukhopadhyay and Johar 2005), perceptions of taste versus healthiness (Raghunathan, Naylor and Hoyer 2006), and even parents' choices of foods for their children (Mukhopadhyay and Yeung 2010). The aim of this chapter is to detail these and other related advances in our understanding of how consumers' lay theories influence their health-related judgments and behaviors.

Lay theories are basic assumptions that ordinary people hold about themselves and their world (Dweck 1996; Wyer 2004). Consumer research has extensively studied lay theories as manifested in decision-making biases (Tversky and Kahneman 1974), expectancy disconfirmation–based product satisfaction (Oliver 1980), and beliefs regarding the association between price and quality (Rao and Monroe 1988). However, until recently, far less attention had been paid to lay theories in other, more general domains. Prominent among these are lay theories of personality, or "what ordinary men and women believe about the existence and power of individual differences in personality" (Ross and Nisbett 1991). Such lay theories pertain to human attributes such as intelligence or self-control. People acquire these lay theories from a variety of sources, including their everyday experiences (Ross and Nisbett 1991), folk wisdom (Briley, Morris, and Simonson 2000), their environments (Morris, Menon, and Ames 2001), or simply by observing themselves (Bem 1967). Importantly, once acquired, lay theories form an integral part of an individual's belief system (Wyer 2004) and therefore influence judgments and behavior across many if not most domains of human behavior (Butler 2000). As such, it is perhaps only to be expected that they should exert strong and systematic influences on health-related behaviors as well. The following discussion centers first on the health-related aspects of lay theories of self-control and then broadens to other key lay theories whose influence has been demonstrated in the literature.

LAY THEORIES OF SELF-CONTROL

Dweck's program of research (see Dweck 1999 for a comprehensive review) stands as the main body of research on the behavioral effects of lay theories. The key finding in this area is that the impact of failure on subsequent effort depends on children's lay theories regarding the nature of intelligence. Specifically, "incremental theorists," those who believe that intelligence and ability are malleable quantities that can be improved through effort, set themselves "learning goals" and treat failure as a challenge by increasing effort. On the other hand, "entity theorists" believe that intelligence and ability are fixed quantities and cannot be changed, set themselves "performance goals," and react to failure as an indictment of their ability (Dweck and Leggett 1988).

    While Dweck's research concerns itself largely with lay theories of intelligence, a growing body of research examines the behavioral effects of lay theories of self-control in particular. Kivetz and Simonson (2002) found that some people have a lay theory that people in general have "too much" self-control and, if gifted cash, would spend the money on "practical things." Hence they would prefer to give hedonic items as gifts. More specific to the context of health, Furnham and McDermott (1994) found that people believe that self-control can help overcome issues such as obesity, drug addiction, and marital problems. However, these researchers did not distinguish between people who differ in their beliefs about the nature of self-control itself.

    A more systematic analysis of the effect of lay theories of self-control on decisions and behavior was first provided by Mukhopadhyay and Johar (2005), who identified two distinct dimensions of lay theories of self-control. They established first that people might differ not only in terms of how much self-control they themselves have, but also on the amount of self-control they believe people in general have. Such beliefs can range across a continuum from very small (i.e., "limited theorists," who believe that reserves of self-control are inherently limited, as per Muraven and Baumeister 2000), to very large (i.e., "unlimited theorists," who believe that reserves of self-control are practically unlimited, as per much of Western philosophy, see Descartes 1649/1996). This lay theory therefore represents the quantum of self-control that a given individual believes that people have (with the labels "limited" and "unlimited" representing the two extreme ends of the continuum).

A second dimension relevant to such lay theories is whether, analogous to Dweck's entity versus incremental theorists, people vary on whether they believe that reserves of self-control can be changed over time or not. Those who tend to believe that people can increase (or decrease) their self-control over time are "malleable theorists," while those leaning toward the inclination that reserves of self-control are fixed for all time are "fixed theorists." These two conceptually orthogonal dimensions, beliefs regarding the quantum of self-control and its variability over time, lead in combination to four unique lay theories of self-control. Mukhopadhyay and Johar (2005) referred to these four combinations as the Limited-Fixed (small reserves that do not change over time), Limited-Malleable (small reserves that can be increased over time), Unlimited-Fixed (very large reserves that do not change over time), and Unlimited-Malleable (very large reserves that can be increased even further over time) lay theories of self-control.

Mukhopadhyay and Johar studied the effects of these four lay theories of self-control in the naturalistic but underexamined domain of New Year's resolutions. This popular annual practice closely mimics prototypical goal-directed behavior, offering a setting in which people attempt to choose and then work toward important outcomes that are often related to health. Indeed, the majority of resolutions that participants listed across experiments in this research were related to one of three categories: finances, diet, and exercise. Given this context, three experiments tested the effects of lay theories of self-control. The first two studies investigated the effects of lay theories that are manipulated or measured on setting resolutions, and the third study extended the investigation to assessing the extent of success at these resolutions.

In Study 1, participants in a 2 × 2 between-subjects design read passages from credible sources that either stated that self-control is a limited resource (Muraven and Baumeister 2000) or that it is an unlimited resource (Descartes, quoted in Elster 1979), which is also fixed (or malleable). Following this "Reading Comprehension" survey was a "Motivation Assessment Questionnaire," that looked completely different from the reading comprehension survey (e.g., a different font) to prevent participants from making any connections between the lay theory manipulation and this measure. Participants were presented with a blank table and asked to list all their current resolutions, in as much detail as possible. Results showed a significant interaction between the Limited-Unlimited and Fixed-Malleable lay theories, such that when lay theories were malleable, unlimited theorists set the highest number of resolutions. Fixed theorists did not show any effect of limited versus unlimited lay theory on their goal-setting. Moreover, the resolutions set were rated to be equally important across conditions. This finding, that everyone set equally important goals but there was systematic variation in the number of goals set, suggests that participants calibrated their goal setting based on their lay theories. As Mukhopadhyay and Johar 2005 or (2008) explain:

> The more individuals believe that they will be able to expend the effort required to achieve a desirable goal, the more likely they are to set themselves that goal. Since each additional goal requires additional effort at the margin, and hence decreasing expectations of success after a point, individuals tend to set only as many goals for the future as they expect to achieve. The belief that self-control is malleable or expandable to an unlimited extent (vs. limited or fixed) should therefore translate into increased expectancies of goal achievement and hence, the setting of more goals. Therefore, individuals who believe that people in general have malleable and unlimited self-control ("Unlimited-malleable theorists") are likely to set more goals than those who do not believe this to be the case ("Limited-malleable theorists" as well as "Fixed theorists").

Study 2 provided further evidence for the role of lay theories of self-control by showing that the effects replicate when lay theories are measured rather than manipulated. Moreover, results showed that these lay theories operate outside of awareness. Making them blatantly salient prior to setting goals can reverse the effect, but only for malleable theorists—fixed theorists continued to show no effect of lay theories on number of goals set. Importantly, self-reports of own self-control were assessed in both studies and did not have any effect in either case. This indicates that lay theories of self-control, which pertain to people in general, are distinct from perceptions of one's own self-control.

The final field experiment extended the investigation to success or failure at goal achievement, manipulating respondents' lay theories and assessing their impact on New Year's resolutions in real time. This study was conducted in two phases, with respondents listing their planned resolutions in November and then reporting on their success at keeping these resolutions the following March. Respondents' lay theories were again manipulated by making them read passages that either stated that self-control is a limited resource or an unlimited resource (but always malleable, since fixed lay theories had been seen to have no effect). Consistent with the previous studies, unlimited theorists (respondents who read the Descartes passage) set more resolutions than limited theorists. The effect of lay theories on success was moderated by respondents' self-efficacy (Bandura 1997), which, orthogonal to lay theories, is the extent to which one believes that one will be able to reach a given goal. Limited theorists who were also low in self-efficacy reported significantly less success at keeping their resolutions than those in other conditions—evidently goal achievement is jointly determined by the belief that reserves of self-control are low (i.e., the lay theory) in conjunction with the belief that one may be unable to reach a given goal (i.e., self-efficacy).

These studies demonstrated that people hold lay beliefs about the nature of self-control that can and do have direct and tangible impacts on their goal-setting and striving, even after controlling for important factors such as participants' ratings of own self-control, goal difficulty, and number of goals. In subsequent research, Mukhopadhyay and Johar (2008) investigated the additional effects of prior success or failure on subsequent goal-directed behavior and found that prior performance and lay theories jointly influence goal setting and striving by driving expectancies of subsequent capability. Compared to unlimited theorists, limited theorists are more likely to attribute success at time 1 to factors in their control, causing them to set more goals for time 2, persist longer and anticipate less doubt at achieving these goals, and strategize their goal pursuit more effectively.

From a pragmatic perspective, this research is important because it informs public policy by highlighting the utility of informing (or reminding) consumers about appropriate lay theories of self-control at appropriate points of time. For example, full disclosure about diets, nutritional contents of food, or side effects of medications may not work because they are not processed given motivational or cognitive limitations. However, a more general message about limited self-control, combined appropriately with interventions that boost domain-specific self-efficacy, could be a useful mechanism to prevent lapses of self-control such as overloading on cupcakes or succumbing to that next cigarette. More generally, it may be useful to sensitize consumers to the number of goals they set. Unlimited theorists may be prone to overextending themselves by setting too many goals—making them prioritize and focus their resources may lead to increased success. On the other hand, limited theorists may on occasion sell themselves short by setting too few goals, or goals that are too easy. Recall that goal difficulty was equal across conditions, yet limited theorists, who set fewer goals, were also more successful. It is conceivable that holding this lay theory, they may have left some "money on the table."

The finding that limited theorists set fewer goals than unlimited theorists is of use to marketers and salespeople who know that their targets are limited theorists (e.g., from a cultural perspective), in tailoring promotional messages accordingly (e.g., "If you only make one resolution this year let this be it" or "The only resolution you need to make"). Managers of health clubs (for instance) could construct inclusive targets rather than breaking each target down into constituent elements ("exercise for one hour" rather than "ten minutes on each of six machines"). Marketers whose customers are limited theorists might also consider increasing self-efficacy, either through supportive messages (e.g., at health clubs, or communications sent by healthful eating clubs) or through training programs or support systems that aid in consumption (e.g., dietary guides, reminder phone calls, and interventions).

Lay Theories and Choices of Products for Children

The above research investigates effects of lay theories of self-control on one's own goal-setting and striving. However, lay theories can also exert strong effects on interpersonal behaviors. (This is noteworthy, since lay theories often stem from observations of other people—this proposition implicates an influence in the reverse direction as well.) For instance, Dweck recounts an anecdote of a young child who described his parents' different reactions to his poor performance in class. The child's mother, evidently an incremental theorist, tried to console him by pointing out that he "tried his best." In contrast, his father scolded him for his underachievement and sent him to his room (Dweck 1999, 103). Not only are these two contrasting reactions excellent exemplars of the two lay theories as held by either parent, they are symptomatic of the types of reinforcements that over time lead children to become either incremental or entity theorists themselves.

In a similar vein, Mukhopadhyay and Yeung (2010) study how lay theories of self-control influence the products that people choose for young children, aged between four and six years old. Most parents consider self-control an important component of their children's development. However, when confronted by children's demand for indulgence—chips before dinner, toys advertised on television, candies on the supermarket shelf—parents allow indulgence more often than not. What makes adults give in to such demands? This research demonstrates that parents' lay theories of self-control, whether limited or unlimited and whether fixed or malleable, are key predictive factors in their decisions for children. Although these beliefs pertain to people in general rather than young children in particular, they are inappropriately projected onto children, leading to decisions that are inconsistent with the nurturing of children's self-control.

The basic premise of this research is that when limited-malleable theorists find themselves in situations where they can develop a child's self-control, they are inclined to act in ways that facilitate it. This includes restricting access to fast food and snacks, preferring educational television programs, and choosing gifts that help educate the child rather than give instant gratification. In contrast, unlimited-malleable theorists, who believe that people in general have large stores of self-control, and fixed theorists, who do not believe that the ability to self-control can be improved, do not take such actions to help build a child's self-control. Findings from experiments conducted in three countries (Hong Kong, the United States, and Singapore), across the domains of gift-giving, babysitting, television program preferences, and eating allowances, and in laboratory experiments as well as in the real world support these claims. Field experiments conducted with parents in Hong Kong and Singapore demonstrated that limited-malleable theorists take their children less frequently to fast-food restaurants (3.17 times per month, as opposed to 4.64 for unlimited malleable theorists and 3.52 times for fixed theorists) and give their children unhealthy snack foods less often (8.81 times per week, vs. 10.39 for unlimited-malleable theorists and 10.35 times for fixed theorists). Further, they are more inclined to restrict television viewing for their charges (television viewing being a natural correlate of unhealthy snacking, see Wansink 2007), and when they do allow the TV to be switched on, they prefer educational to entertaining television programs. Moreover, when choosing gifts for young children, limited-malleable theorists tend to prefer those offering greater value in the long term than the short term—for example, they prefer educational board games to entertaining video games. These effects are observed even after accounting for demographic characteristics such as family income, number of working hours for each parent, number of siblings, and domestic help, and relevant psychological characteristics of the parents. Again, accounting for self-reported self-control does not diminish the effects of lay theories.

These results demonstrate that lay theories of self-control have an influence not only on goal-directed behaviors undertaken by and for the self (i.e., self-regulation), but also on decisions made for others. Parents are gatekeepers for their children's consumption, and their decisions have lifelong implications for their children. It is therefore not unreasonable to assume that the problems of obesity and unfitness in the current day are in large part influenced by the intergenerational transfer of lay theories and associated behaviors. It would be an ambitious undertaking, but probably well justified from the public health perspective, to try to modify parents' lay theories in ways that would benefit their children's consumption. This may be attempted either via mass media or through point-of-sale communications at retail outlets of "vice" products such as fast-food restaurants. Such messages could, for instance, nudge parents toward limited-malleable lay theories by cueing the need to resist temptation, or perhaps sensitize them to their children's burgeoning self-control. Similarly, marketers of "virtue" products (such as healthy snack foods) may well be advised to subtly (but not blatantly) cue limited-malleable lay theories in communications and point of purchase materials.

Lay Theories and Temporal Perspectives

The above discussion has centered on health-related goal setting, striving, and product choice as reflective of such goal-setting and striving. A related question concerns how people plan toward their chosen goals. Mukhopadhyay and Agrawal (2006) studied the optimality of time frames for goal-directed behavior—does it matter whether people set their goals on a weekly basis or a yearly basis? New Year's resolutions are set every year, but should everyone use the same time frames? What time frame is best, for whom, and why? According to this research, individuals who believe that self-control is a small reserve (i.e., limited theorists) are likely to set goals, make plans, and pursue goals with due regard to this consideration of limited resources. Such individuals are more likely to focus on resources and constraints, and construe goals at lower levels. These lower-level construals should then lead to associations of temporal proximity. In contrast, unlimited theorists are less bound by considerations of constraints on their self-control and are hence likely to construe events as temporally distant. Therefore, Mukhopadhyay and Agrawal suggest that because limited theorists are more likely to think in terms of resources when setting goals, they should be more likely to set goals in proximal time frames. In contrast, unlimited theorists are likely to be more comfortable thinking of goals in distal frames and are more likely to set goals having distal time frames.

These propositions were tested in a study in which participants were presented with a one-page "Lifestyle Survey." The first question asked, "Looking ahead, how often do you plan to exercise?" with the response option given as "_____ sessions in the coming _____ {choose an appropriate time frame}." The choice of time frame was the dependent variable of interest. Lay theories of self-control were measured at the end of the questionnaire using two items, as in Mukhopadhyay and Johar (2005), which were averaged to form a composite measure. As expected, there was a significant relationship between lay theories and chosen time frame, such that those who held more limited theories of self-control were more likely to choose shorter time frames. Follow-up analysis demonstrated that limited theorists were significantly more likely than unlimited theorists to choose weekly horizons and correspondingly less likely to choose longer time frames; in contrast, some unlimited theorists scheduled their exercising frequency on an annual basis! These results demonstrate that lay theories of self-control co-occur with preferences for setting proximal versus distal goals.

What does this imply? Mukhopadhyay and Agrawal (2006) then demonstrate across multiple experiments that when a person's lay theory matches the temporal framing of a health-related goal, the time frame for the goal feels appropriate, and the pursuit of the goal feels efficacious. This compatibility translates into greater value associated with goal-relevant objects and tasks, better planning as evidenced by reduced conflicts in scheduled activities, greater persuasiveness of goal-related communications, and greater interest in and willingness to pay for goal-relevant activities and products. For instance, in one experiment, participants in a 2 × 2 between-subjects design had their lay theories manipulated by reading the same passages described earlier. Returning to the laboratory two months later, they were presented with a booklet titled "Health Focus Assessment Questionnaire," in which they were asked to list all the health-related activities they planned to take part in during the course of either "the next week" or "a week, one year from now"—a manipulation of temporal focus. They then saw a second booklet, purportedly a brochure for "The Iyengar Yoga Center of Hong Kong." This booklet contained a passage describing Iyengar Yoga and its benefits. Following the passage, participants responded to measures of attitude to Iyengar Yoga, willingness to pay for an Iyengar Yoga course, and how much the passage made them want to join any exercise program, Iyengar Yoga or otherwise.

Results revealed, as expected, that unlimited theorists valued the given Iyengar yoga program more when in a distant future mind-set rather than a near future mind-set, while limited theorists displayed the opposite pattern. Specifically, unlimited theorists had significantly more positive attitudes when in a distal (vs. proximal) mind-set, reported greater intentions to exercise, and were willing to pay nearly twice as much when in a compatible mindset (Ms = HK\$640.00 vs. HK\$334.81; approximately eight Hong Kong dollars equal one U.S. dollar). In contrast, limited theorists had significantly less positive attitudes when in a distal (vs. proximal) mind-set, were less likely to want to exercise, and were willing to pay only about half as much when in a distal mind-set (Ms = HK$374.40 vs. HK$601.43). This demonstrates an immediate detectable effect of lay theory–time frame compatibility and underscores the extent of the sway of lay theories on health-related behaviors, motivations, and cognitions.

LAY THEORIES IN OTHER DOMAINS

Until this point, the discussion has been limited to lay theories of self-control and their various effects. However, as mentioned, many other lay theories also exist and exert strong and systematic influences on health-related behaviors. The second part of this chapter discusses recent research on the health-related effects of other lay theories, under three heads: lay theories of experiences (specifically, emotions), lay theories that implicate the self (specifically, optimism), and lay theories that pertain to specific characteristics of food products (specifically, the relationship between healthiness and taste).

Experience-Centric Lay Theories: Emotion Transience

The first category of lay theories in this section involves experiences. Naive beliefs have been shown to affect predictions of dynamic hedonic experiences (Novemsky and Ratner 2003), predicted emotion (Xu and Schwarz 2009), and even how much one is willing to accept or pay in situations implicating the endowment effect (Van Boven, Dunning, and Loewenstein 2000). Loewenstein and Prelec (1993) famously demonstrated that people preferred to schedule unattractive dinners and meetings with unpleasant aunts ahead of fancy dinners and enjoyable afternoons, presumably driven by a belief that the experience of one would influence (or contaminate) the other, and Chan and Mukhopadhyay (2010) find evidence that such beliefs may vary nonlinearly with time and have ironic effects on postconsumption evaluations.

Among these various research domains, most relevant to the context of health are lay theories of emotion transience. Labroo and Mukhopadhyay (2009) demonstrate that these lay theories, the beliefs that emotions are stable versus transient, influence people's tendencies to choose hedonic options (for instance, a choice of a chocolate bar over an apple), depending on their current mood. The basic question in this research is: who is more likely to indulge in order to feel good in the moment even though exerting restraint is beneficial for the long term—a happy person or someone who is unhappy? Are happy or unhappy dieters more likely to indulge and eat a rich cake rather than exert restraint and choose a healthy apple?

Labroo and Mukhopadhyay argue that people strategically manage their actions both to accomplish their long-term interests and to attain immediate pleasures. If they believe they need to take actions to regulate their immediate feelings, they tend to indulge in immediate pleasures. In contrast, if they believe such actions are not required, they act in their long-term interests. The choice of actions between indulging to feel good or acting in one's long-term interest is determined interactively by people's current feelings and their chronic or situationally activated lay theories about the transience of emotion. People who feel good rather than bad are more likely to indulge *if they believe that emotion is fleeting*. This is because people who feel good infer that unless they take actions to feel better, their positive feelings will pass, but people who feel bad infer that actions to feel better are unnecessary because the negative feelings will pass on their own. In contrast, people who feel bad rather than good are more likely to indulge *if they believe that emotion is lasting*. This is because people who feel bad infer that unless they take actions to feel better, the negative feelings will persist, but people who feel good infer that they can act in their long-term interests because actions to preserve their mood are unnecessary.

Labroo and Mukhopadhyay (2009) observed these patterns across six studies featuring multiple manipulations and measurements of both mood and lay theories, and a variety of dependent variables. For instance, in one study, undergraduate students at the University of Chicago were recruited as they entered a local gym. All participants indicated that making healthy food choices was important to them, subsequent to which they were told that they were taking part in a short study on "time perception." The study involved a coloring task that simultaneously served as mood induction and theory manipulation. The cover story instructed participants that the experimenter was interested in peoples' estimates of duration of events and that their task was to color a line drawing presented to them as quickly and carefully as possible and then estimate how much time they took. Depending on the experimental condition, to manipulate mood, participants colored a line drawing of either a smiling face or a frowning face. In the positive-mood condition, participants colored a line drawing of a smiling face (☺), and in the negative-mood condition, participants colored a line drawing of a frowning face (☹). To manipulate transience, participants were provided with a thin-tipped pen or with a thick-tip Sharpie. Essentially, participants with a microtip pen should take longer to color the line drawing; thus, the task would seem less transient to them than participants who used the sharpie. This feeling of transience would be associated with the transience of emotion. As expected, if participants believed that emotion is fleeting, those exposed to positive (vs. negative) faces were more likely to indulge by choosing chocolate. In contrast, if they believed that emotion is lasting, participants exposed to positive (vs. negative) faces were less likely to indulge—they chose the apple. Hence dieters acted in their long-term interests and chose the apple unless they inferred a need to regulate their affect. Similar results were observed in another study, where individual differences in lay theories were measured, rather than situationally induced. Again, happy (vs. unhappy) participants were likely to prefer chocolate more strongly if they believed that emotion is fleeting, and they were less likely to prefer chocolate if they believed that emotion is lasting. These results suggest a different way of tempering indulgence if one knows the current mood of the target at the point when they are making their decision—remind them of stable reasons for their happiness if they are happy, and cue the transience of their feelings if not.

Self-Theories: Optimism

A second category of lay theory concerns beliefs that implicate the self. Particularly pertinent to the present context is the construct of optimism, which essentially functions as a lay belief that outcomes will be positive, good things will happen, and steps required to achieve these outcomes will be easy (Epstein and Meier 1989; Scheier and Carver 1985). For instance, consumers often purchase products that they are unable to use at the time of purchase, hoping that they may be able to do so in the future. Chan, Sengupta, and Mukhopadhyay (2010) demonstrate that under certain conditions, namely particular combinations of cognitive load, imagery, and a focus on process versus outcome, optimists are more likely than pessimists to buy clothes that are presently too small for them. The question then arises: how does the decision whether or not to purchase such smaller-sized clothes influence the subsequent decision to exercise or diet, so that one might wear these clothes? Chan, Mukhopadhyay, and Sengupta (2010) demonstrate the ways in which optimism influences the likelihood of subsequently behaving in ways that enable the usage of the purchase (e.g., exercising or dieting after having bought a pair of jeans that is one size too small).

The key premise here is that the purchase decision increases the salience of the health goal, to which optimists and pessimists respond differently depending on whether they are thinking of the outcome (looking good in the slim jeans) or the process required to achieve that outcome (exercising or dieting). When consumers focus on the outcome, the salience of the health goal leads optimists and pessimists to engage in different coping strategies. This is due to the difference in lay beliefs held by optimists and pessimists—optimists expect to attain the goal, so they are more likely to actively pursue it. As a result, optimists become more committed to the goal and therefore more likely to actively pursue it, leading them to be more likely to diet or exercise. In contrast, pessimists react in a nonadaptive manner by disengagement—they become less likely to engage in goal-congruent, healthy actions (Scheier, Weintraub, and Carver 1986).

A very different pattern emerges when the focus is on the process. Here, the purchase decision itself acts as a signal of progress toward the goal. For optimists, this sense of accomplishment provides a justification to move away from the focal goal (see Fishbach and Dhar 2005). Pessimists, because of their generally unfavorable beliefs, do not view the purchase decision as a measure of progress and hence are unaffected by it.

These propositions were supported in several experiments. For example, one experiment used a 2 (focus: outcome vs. process) × 2 (optimism: optimists vs. pessimists) × 2 (decision: buy vs. not buy) between-subjects design. Participants first took part in a survey, which included a question about the size of jeans that they could just fit into currently. After a filler task, they participated in a different survey about buying jeans. Thought focus was manipulated by asking participants to make their decisions by visualizing either the end benefits of wearing the jeans (outcome-focus) or the process they would have to go through in order to be able to fit into the jeans (process-focus). Next, they read the description of the jeans, which were always one size smaller than their current size. They then reported their likelihood of purchasing the jeans, after which they moved on to an ostensibly unrelated study, in which a type of exercise equipment was described. As the key dependent variable, participants were asked about their likelihood of trying out this equipment. Lastly, they filled out a standard optimism scale (Scheier and Carver 1985). As hypothesized, under outcome-focus, optimists were more likely to try the equipment as a consequence of buying (vs. not buying) the jeans, while the predicted negative effect was obtained for pessimists: buying (vs. not buying) the jeans reduced the likelihood of trying the exercise equipment. Under process-focus, on the other hand, optimists displayed a reduced likelihood of trying the exercise equipment after buying (vs. not buying) the jeans, while pessimists were unaffected by their purchase decision. Additional experiments replicate the results using manipulated (rather than measured) optimism and manipulated purchase decision, provide process measures of goal progress and commitment, and demonstrate the moderating effect of goal salience.

Optimism is a lay belief that things will go well. However, among scholars, there is disagreement regarding whether optimism itself is always beneficial or not. One perspective is that optimism helps in goal pursuit (Taylor and Brown 1988), while a counterargument is that it may lead to a false sense of security and accompanying lapses (Weinstein 1980). This research helps reconcile these differences by detailing when and how optimism helps and when it does not. Specifically, when the optimism functions as a belief that outcomes will be positive, prior goal-directed behavior spurs further goal-consistent behaviors. However, when the optimism functions as a belief that the steps taken to achieve a desired outcome will be easy, chances are that the optimist involved will slip up. These propositions have direct and actionable implications for policy-makers interested in ensuring that chosen health goals are indeed pursued with as few lapses as possible. Given a first healthy decision, such as signing up for a diet or buying an exercise cycle, subsequent goal-consistent behavior will be more likely for optimists if they had taken that first step while focused on the final goal, but for pessimists if they had instead been focused on the steps required to achieve that goal.

Product-Centric Lay Theories: The Unhealthy = Tasty Intuition

A final category of lay theories relevant to health implicates beliefs about associations between specific attributes of food products, namely, taste and healthiness. Raghunathan, Naylor, and Hoyer (2006) demonstrated that consumers have a lay theory that the less healthy the item is portrayed to be, the better is its taste. They showed that like many lay theories, this theory too is implicitly held and has strong effects on behavior. Specifically, the Unhealthy = Tasty Intuition leads to increased enjoyment of an item that is perceived to be unhealthy during consumption and increased preference for it in choice tasks when a hedonic goal is salient.

In an experiment conducted during a large dinner party, guests were requested to individually sample each of three food items, purportedly from a new Indian restaurant in town. One was unambiguously described as being healthy, and one correspondingly as unhealthy. The third, target item, was a mango lassi, a drink made by blending mango pulp with yogurt. Half the participants had this item described to them as being "generally considered very healthy," while the other half had it described as being "generally considered unhealthy." In line with the lay theory prediction, participants who were told that the mango lassi was unhealthy rated it as being significantly tastier than those who were told that it was healthy. Moreover, this main effect was stronger for those who explicitly believed that taste is inversely correlated with healthiness—further evidence of the power of this lay theory.

CONCLUSION

The study of the types and impact of lay theories is today at the cutting edge of psychology and consumer research. The research reviewed in this chapter details some important ways in which lay theories, of self-control and others, influence people's choices on diet and exercise. These findings are a subset of the growing body of work on lay theories, covering those lay theories that are most germane to obesity-related issues. Based on this evidence, it is inarguable that an understanding of lay theories is critical for an understanding of health-related behaviors and the design of interventions promoting healthfulness.

While each of the above studies has specific practical implications as discussed, are there any general principles that might prove useful in practice? One important lesson based on some of the above results is the substantiation of Wyer's (2004) observation that the effects of lay theories may be evidenced even when lay theories are situationally primed. Hence, while populations may vary in their distributions of any given lay theory, behavior may still be suitably directed if care is taken to institute appropriate priming procedures prior to the decision. The implementation of such procedures is naturally context-specific and may not always be straightforward, but the benefits reaped may be worth the cost incurred. Moreover, the data suggest that certain lay theories, such as limited-malleable theories of self-control, may lead to more healthful behaviors than others (for example, healthier choices for children and greater success in goal achievement when in concert with high self-efficacy). Therefore, coordinated public health campaigns that arise from disparate sources but carry the same message promoting limited-malleable theories may well prove to be superadditive in their effectiveness.

From a theoretical perspective, while the results reported in this chapter are all both robust and important, much still remains to be done. For instance, one limitation is that while the majority of these studies have looked at the incidence of healthy versus unhealthy choices, and some at the effects over time, an important area that remains underaddressed is the quantity of healthy versus unhealthy behavior—that is, the amounts of overindulgence or persistence at exercise. Moreover, a vast number of other possible lay theories could also conceivably have had concurrent effects. For instance, a possible corollary of a lay theory of self-control is a lay theory of effort— people may be more likely to restrain at one time if they believe it is relatively easy to exert self-control, but they may also be more likely to indulge because the same belief leads them to view future occasions of restraint as no big problem. Clearly, many such lay theories may be at play, and their interrelationships, antecedents, mechanisms, consequences, and superstructure all remain to be explored.

It is important to keep sight of two key points that unify this seeming smorgasbord of lay theories. The first is that lay theories are, in general, beliefs. The fact that beliefs influence behaviors is not new (Ajzen 1985); what the study of lay theories adds is a much more general and inclusive perspective. As Wyer (2004) avers, implicit theories play a very large part both in explaining past events and guiding future behaviors, and a given implicit theory can be applied in many different circumstances. Some of the research reviewed in this chapter bears this point out strongly—for example, lay theories of self-control are seen to influence goal setting, planning, achievement, and even the choices of products for children. From this generalized perspective stems a second key point, one that bears reiteration. This is that lay theories of personality, specifically, are beliefs about how people may vary on a given personality trait. Hence lay theories of personality are conceptually distinct from their referent personality traits and, as found in several of the studies discussed here, have effects that are observable over and above these traits. Indeed, at times their influence on behavior is palpable even when the referent trait itself has no observable effect. In essence, what people believe about other people in the world they inhabit appears to influence their own behaviors even more than how they view themselves. Our personalities are reflected in the choices we make, and the study of lay theories suggests that we are more what we believe than who we think we are.

ACKNOWLEDGMENTS

I am grateful to Elaine Chan, Iris Hung, and Jaideep Sengupta for their insightful and constructive comments on earlier versions of this article. Much of the research described here was made possible by the Hong Kong RGC Grant CERG 6463/05H. All errors are mine.

REFERENCES

Agrawal, Nidhi, Geeta Menon, and Jennifer L. Aaker. 2007. "Getting Emotional About Health." *Journal of Marketing Research*, 44 (February), 100–113.
Ajzen, Icek. 1985. "From Intentions to Actions: A Theory of Planned Behavior." In *Action Control: From Cognition to Behavior*, ed. Julius Kuhl and Jurgen Beckmann, 11–39. Berlin and New York: Springer-Verlag.

Bandura, Albert. 1997. *Self-Efficacy: The Exercise of Control.* New York: W.H. Freeman.

Bem, Daryl J. 1967. "Self-Perception: An Alternative Interpretation of Cognitive Dissonance Phenomena." *Psychological Review*, 74 (May), 183–120.

Briley, Donnel A., Michael Morris, and Itamar Simonson. 2000. "Reasons as Carriers of Culture: Dynamic vs. Dispositional Models of Cultural Influence on Decision Making." *Journal of Consumer Research*, 27 (September), 157–178.

Butler, Ruth. 2000. "Making Judgments About Ability: The Role of Implicit Theories of Ability in Moderating Inferences from Temporal and Social Comparison Information." *Journal of Personality and Social Psychology*, 78 (May), 965–978.

Chan, Elaine, and Anirban Mukhopadhyay. 2010. "When Choosing Makes a Good Thing Better: Temporal Variations in the Valuation of Hedonic Consumption." *Journal of Marketing Research*, 47 (June), 497–507.

Chan, Elaine, Anirban Mukhopadhyay, and Jaideep Sengupta. 2010. "Understanding Optimism: The Consequences of Anticipatory Purchase." Working paper, Hong Kong University of Science and Technology.

Chan, Elaine, Jaideep Sengupta, and Anirban Mukhopadhyay. 2010. "Means and Ends: The Two Routes to Understanding Optimism." Working paper, Hong Kong University of Science and Technology.

Chandran, Sucharita, and Geeta Menon. 2004. "When a Day Means More Than a Year: Effects of Temporal Framing on Judgments of Health Risk." *Journal of Consumer Research*, 31 (September), 375–389.

Descartes, Rene. 1649/1996. "Les Passions de L'Ame." In *Ouevres de Descartes*, ed. Charles Adam and Paul Tannery, 368–369. Paris: Vrin/CNRS.

Dweck, Carol S. 1996. "Implicit Theories as Organizers of Goals and Behavior." In *The Psychology of Action: Linking Cognition and Motivation to Behavior*, ed. Peter M. Gollwitzer and John A. Bargh, 69–90. New York: Guildford Press.

———. 1999. *Self Theories: Their Role in Motivation, Personality and Development.* Philadelphia: Taylor and Francis.

Dweck, Carol S., and Ellen L. Leggett. 1988. "A Social-Cognitive Approach to Motivation and Personality." *Psychological Review*, 95 (April), 256–273.

Elster, Jon. 1979. *Ulysses and the Sirens: Studies in Rationality and Irrationality.* New York: Cambridge University Press.

Epstein, Seymour, and Petra Meier. 1989. "Constructive Thinking: A Broad Coping Variable with Specific Components." *Journal of Personality and Social Psychology*, 57 (2), 332–359.

Fishbach, Ayelet, and Ravi Dhar. 2005. "Goals as Excuses or Guides: The Liberating Effect of Perceived Goal Progress on Choice." *Journal of Consumer Research*, 32 (3), 370–377.

Furnham, Adrian, and Mark R. McDermott. 1994. "Lay Beliefs About the Efficacy of Self-Reliance, Seeking Help and External Control as Strategies for Overcoming Obesity, Drug Addiction, Marital Problems, Stuttering and Insomnia." *Psychology and Health*, 9 (October), 397–406.

Kivetz, Ran, and Itamar Simonson. 2002. "Self-Control for the Righteous: Towards a Theory of Pre-Commitment to Indulgence." *Journal of Consumer Research*, 29 (September), 199–217.

Labroo, Aparna A., and Anirban Mukhopadhyay. 2009. "Lay Theories of Emotion Transience and the Search for Happiness: A Fresh Perspective on Affect Regulation." *Journal of Consumer Research*, 36 (August), 242–254.

Loewenstein, George, and Drazen Prelec. 1993. "Preferences for Sequences of Outcomes." *Psychological Review*, 100 (January), 91–108.

McFerran, Brent, Darren W. Dahl, Gavan J. Fitzsimons, and Andrea C. Morales. 2010. "I'll Have What She Is Having: Effect of Social Influence and Body Type on the Food Choices of Others." *Journal of Consumer Research*, 36 (April), 915–929.

Morris, Michael W., Tanya Menon, and Daniel R. Ames. 2001. "Culturally Conferred Conception of Agency: A Key to Social Perception of Persona, Groups, and Other Actors." *Personality and Social Psychology Review*, 5 (April), 169–182.

Mukhopadhyay, Anirban, and Nidhi Agrawal. 2006. "Planning for Which Future? Lay Theories of Self-Control and the Temporal Framing of Goal-Directed Behavior." Annual Conference of the Association for Consumer Research, Orlando, Florida.

Mukhopadhyay, Anirban, and Gita V. Johar. 2005. "Where There Is a Will, Is There a Way? Effects of Lay Theories of Self-Control on Setting and Keeping Resolutions." *Journal of Consumer Research*, 31 (March), 779–786.

———. 2008. "Never Give Up Givin' It Up: How Lay Theories of Self-Control and Recent Success or Failure Affect Goal-Directed Behavior." Annual Conference of the Society for Consumer Psychology, New Orleans, Louisiana.

Mukhopadhyay, Anirban, Jaideep Sengupta, and Suresh Ramanathan. 2008. "Recalling Past Temptations: An Information-Processing Perspective on the Dynamics of Self-Control," *Journal of Consumer Research*, 35 (4) (December), 586–599.

Mukhopadhyay, Anirban, and Catherine W.M. Yeung. 2010. "Building Character: Effects of Lay Theories of Self-Control on the Selection of Products for Children." *Journal of Marketing Research*, 47 (April), 240–250.

Muraven, Mark, and Roy F. Baumeister. 2000. "Self-Regulation of Limited Resources: Does Self-Control Resemble a Muscle?" *Psychological Bulletin*, 126 (March), 247–259.

Novemsky, Nathan, and Rebecca K. Ratner. 2003. "The Time Course and Impact of Consumers' Erroneous Beliefs About Hedonic Contrast Effects." *Journal of Consumer Research*, 29 (March), 507–516.

Ogden, Cynthia L., Margaret D. Carroll, Margaret A. McDowell, and Katherine M. Flegal. 2007. "Obesity among Adults in the United States: No Change since 2003–2004." NCHS data brief (1). Hyattsville, MD: National Center for Health Statistics.

Oliver, Richard L. 1980. "A Cognitive Model of the Antecedents and Consequences of Satisfaction Decisions." *Journal of Marketing Research*, 17 (November), 460–469.

Raghunathan, Rajagopal, Rebecca W. Naylor, and Wayne D. Hoyer. 2006. "The Unhealthy = Tasty Intuition and Its Effects on Taste Inferences, Enjoyment, and Choice of Food Products." *Journal of Marketing*, 70 (October), 170–184.

Rao, Akshay R., and Kent B. Monroe. 1988. "The Moderating Effect of Prior Knowledge on Cue Utilization in Product Evaluations." *Journal of Consumer Research*, 15 (September), 253–264.

Ross, Lee, and Richard E. Nisbett. 1991. *The Person and the Situation: Perspectives of Social Psychology*. New York: McGraw-Hill.

Scheier, Michael F., and Charles S. Carver. 1985. "Optimism, Coping and Health: Assessment and Implications of Generalized Outcome Expectancies." *Health Psychology*, 4 (3), 219–247.

Scheier, Michael F., Jagdish K. Weintraub, and Charles S. Carver. 1986. "Coping with Stress: Divergent Strategies of Optimists and Pessimists." *Journal of Personality and Social Psychology*, 51 (6), 1257–1264.

Sengupta, Jaideep, and Rongrong Zhou. 2007. "Understanding Impulsive Choice Behaviors: The Motivational Influences of Regulatory Focus." *Journal of Marketing Research*, 24 (May), 297–308.

Taylor, Shelley E., and Jonathon D. Brown. 1988. "Illusion and Well-Being: A Social-Psychological Perspective on Mental Health." *Psychological Bulletin*, 103 (2), 193–210.

Tversky, Amos, and Daniel Kahneman. 1974. "Judgment under Uncertainty: Heuristics and Biases." *Science*, 185, 1124–1131.

Van Boven, Leaf, David Dunning, and George F. Loewenstein. 2000. "Egocentric Empathy Gaps Between Owners and Buyers: Misperceptions of the Endowment Effect." *Journal of Personality and Social Psychology*, 79 (July), 66–76.
Wansink, Brian. 2007. *Mindless Eating: Why We Eat More Than We Think*. New York: Bantam-Dell.
Weinstein, Neal D. 1980. "Unrealistic Optimism About Future Life Events." *Journal of Personality and Social Psychology*, 39 (5), 806–820.
World Health Organization. 2010. Obesity and Overweight. www.who.int/dietphysicalactivity/publications/facts/obesity/en.
Wyer, Robert S., Jr. 2004. *Social Comprehension and Judgment: The Role of Situation Models, Narratives and Implicit Theories*. Mahwah, NJ: Erlbaum.
Xu, Jing, and Norbert Schwarz. 2009. "Do We Really Need a Reason to Indulge?" *Journal of Marketing Research*, 46 (February), 25–36.

CHAPTER 4

CALORIE ESTIMATION BIASES IN CONSUMER CHOICE

ALEXANDER CHERNEV AND PIERRE CHANDON

Despite the increase in the number of healthy options available to consumers, the proportion of overweight individuals has increased as well (Chandon 2009; Heini and Weinsier 1997; Wansink 2006). Calorie overconsumption has been identified as one of the primary sources contributing to this obesity epidemic (CDC 2007; Olshansky et al. 2005). Reduced-calorie diets result in clinically meaningful weight loss regardless of which macronutrients (fat or carbohydrates) they emphasize (Sacks et al. 2009). Managing calorie intake has been singled out by the U.S. Department of Health and Human Services as the primary method to maintain optimal body weight (Thompson and Veneman 2005). Assessment of calorie intake has also been documented as playing a central role in the prevention and treatment of many diseases, including diabetes, coronary heart disease, and some forms of cancer (Allison et al. 1999; Goodhart and Shils 1980; Keys 1997; Must et al. 1999; USDA 2008).

To encourage individuals to consume fewer calories, the majority of nutritional programs recommend specific daily calorie intakes. Most packaged goods are now required by the Food and Drug Administration to display their calorie content, a measure designed to regulate calorie intake. Despite the availability of nutritional information for many products, however, calculating one's actual calorie intake is not a trivial task. Indeed, while the calorie content of packaged goods is usually readily available, restaurants are not required by the FDA to provide nutrition information. Although many chains—including McDonald's, Burger King, Dunkin' Donuts, and Starbucks—already provide calorie information on their websites, posters, or tray liners, this information is rarely available to consumers at the time of food selection and food intake.

Even when nutritional information is readily available, it typically describes the calorie content per serving of one item, rather than the content of the entire meal consumed by individuals. This further complicates estimation of the total calorie intake since the packaging of most foods and drinks involves multiple servings, and consumers are typically unaware of or unable to determine the recommended serving size. Furthermore, the overall calorie count is often not available for meals comprising multiple items. The unavailability of meal-specific nutritional information at the time of food selection raises the question of how consumers evaluate the calorie content of individual food items and how they integrate these estimates into an overall estimate of the calories contained in a particular meal.

Given that consumers make food-related decisions every day, one could argue that they should be able to estimate more or less accurately the calorie content of popular meal options, such as fast-food meals, snacks, and soft drinks. Recent evidence, however, has questioned the accuracy of consumers' estimates of calorie intake. It has been shown that people—even trained dieticians—tend to make large errors in estimating both calories and the quantity of food consumed (Chandon and Wansink 2007b; Lansky and Brownell 1982; Lichtman et al. 1992). Multiple studies have further documented people's tendency to underestimate their calorie intake (see Livingstone and Black 2003 for a review). Despite the overwhelming evidence for this underestimation bias in evaluating calorie intake, little is known about its antecedents.

This chapter offers an overview of recent consumer research that sheds light on categorization-based factors biasing estimation of the calorie content of food-related items.[1] It reviews research showing that calorie underestimation can be attributed to two types of categorization-driven decision biases: the halo bias and the averaging bias. The halo bias refers to the tendency of a particular feature of the food, such as nutrition labels or marketing claims that it is healthy, to influence the overall estimation of the calorie content of the food item or of an entire meal. The averaging bias refers to people's tendency to average the calorie content of combinations of healthy and unhealthy items. Although driven by different psychological processes, both biases stem from people's tendency to categorize food-related items according to a healthy/unhealthy dichotomy.

The notion that people tend to categorize food-related information according to a good/bad dichotomy of healthy and unhealthy has been advanced by researchers in different domains, including psychology (Chernev 2011b; Rozin, Ashmore, and Markwith 1996), marketing (Raghunathan, Naylor, and Hoyer 2006; Wertenbroch 1998), and nutrition (Oakes 2005; Oakes and Slotterback 2001). These studies show that asking consumers to rate the health benefits of different foods leads to a bimodal distribution, indicating the use of good/bad categorization. Thus, foods such as fruits and vegetables tend to be classified as inherently healthy, whereas candy, bacon, and popcorn are considered to be inherently indulgent and unhealthy.

The healthy/unhealthy categorization is influenced not just by the nature of the food, but by nutrition-related information communicated by the name of the brand or by the specific claims or qualifiers used to describe the food. Foods described as organic, light, fat-free, and low-fat tend to be classified as healthy, whereas options described by qualifiers such as regular, rich, creamy, and decadent are more likely to be classified as unhealthy. Similarly, people tend to classify restaurants according to the degree of their perceived healthiness, whereby outlets such as Jamba Juice and Subway are perceived to be healthier than Burger King and McDonald's.

The remainder of this chapter is organized as follows. We first examine calorie estimation biases in cases when people evaluate meals comprising either healthy or unhealthy items. In this context, we show that nutrition labels or marketing claims lead to a halo bias categorization of food-related items as healthy and unhealthy such that people tend to overweight categorization-consistent features but discount the categorization-inconsistent ones. We then show that combining both healthy and unhealthy items leads to an averaging bias in which people underestimate the calorie content of the combined meal. The chapter concludes with a discussion of the public policy implications of calorie estimation biases, focusing on ways to correct these biases and improve food-related decision-making.

HALO BIAS IN ESTIMATING THE CALORIE CONTENT OF EITHER HEALTHY OR UNHEALTHY FOOD AND MEALS

In the absence of salient, unambiguous calorie information, people infer calorie content from other cues. A plethora of research (e.g., Kardes, Posavac, and Cronley 2004) has shown that consumers frequently draw inferences about missing attributes from other attributes (e.g., "What is the fat content?"), from the brand's overall positioning (e.g., "Does it claim to be healthy or not?"), or from the attributes of comparable products (e.g., "What else is on this restaurant's menu?"). According to selective accessibility models of information processing, unless consumers are specifically asked to do the opposite, these cues increase the accessibility of category-consistent information on the target food or meal, leading to the assimilation of calorie estimations toward the cue (for a review, see Mussweiler 2003). The result is a halo bias, which leads to lower calorie estimates when people rely on cues suggesting that an item is healthy than when cues suggest that the item is unhealthy.

Prior research on health halos has shown that people tend to generalize specific health claims inappropriately—for example, believing that foods low in cholesterol are also low in fat (Andrews, Netemeyer, and Burton 1996). The results of some of these studies, however, are inconclusive because they did not control for differences in the calorie content of healthy and unhealthy food (e.g., studies 1 and 3 in Wansink and Chandon 2006). For example, Burton et al. (2006) found that people underestimated the calorie content of a number of relatively healthy foods (including chicken breasts and turkey sandwiches) by 9 percent but underestimated the calorie content of relatively unhealthy foods (including fettuccine Alfredo, hamburgers, and fries) by 93 percent. A potential problem with these findings is that the unhealthy food used in the study contained significantly more calories than the healthy food (1336 vs. 543, on average). This is problematic because Chandon and Wansink (2007b) have established that calorie underestimation increases with actual calorie content, which implies that the above findings could be attributable to the higher calorie content of unhealthy food rather than to health halos.

To control for the potential confound between health halos and calorie content,

Figure 4.1 **Health Halo Effects in Food Portion Estimations**

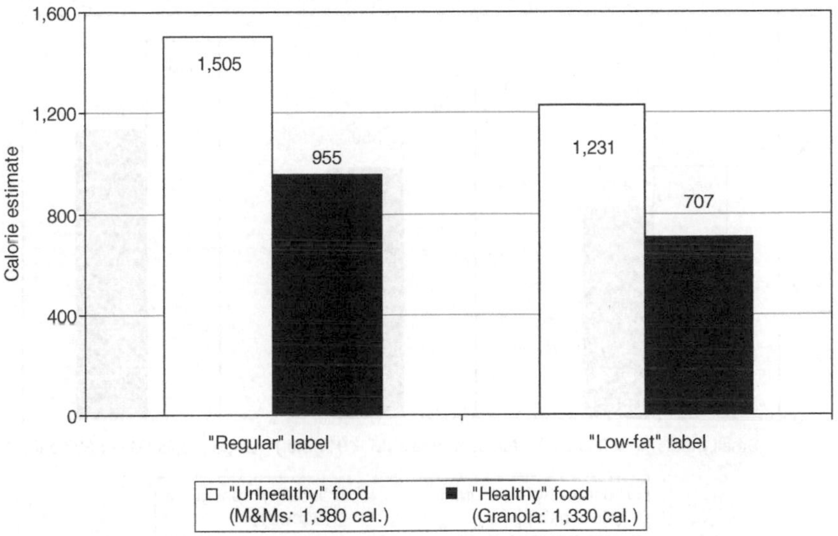

Note: Calorie estimates are lower for foods perceived as healthy and labeled as "low-fat."

Wansink and Chandon (2006) asked consumers to estimate the number of calories contained in two ten-ounce cups, one containing M&Ms (1,380 calories) and the other containing granola (1,330 calories). The two snacks were chosen based on pretests indicating that although both foods have similar calorie density, granola is perceived as healthier and less indulgent than M&Ms. Consistent with the halo hypothesis, participants underestimated the calorie content of the relatively healthy granola by 28 percent but overestimated the calorie content of the relatively un-healthy M&Ms by 9 percent (Figure 4.1).

Wansink and Chandon (2006) further examined the effects of another health halo source: "low-fat" nutrition claims.[2] They found that health halos created by "low-fat" labels reduced calorie estimation by a similar amount for both products (18 percent for M&Ms and 26 percent for granola). They also observed that the health halo effects caused by food stereotyping (M&Ms vs. granola) and by nutri-tion claims ("low-fat" vs. "regular" labels) equally affected both overweight and normal-weight participants. This suggests that health halos are not driven by the individual differences typically observed between these two groups (e.g., restrained eating, gender, socioeconomic level, and appearance self-esteem).

In a related series of studies, Chandon and Wansink (2007a) examined the effects of the health claims of fast-food restaurant brands on the perceived caloric content of entire meals, not just of single food portions. To illustrate, in one experiment, the authors asked people who had just finished eating a meal at either Subway (a fast-food chain that claims to serve healthy meals) or McDonald's (a fast-food

Figure 4.2   **Health Halo Effects in Fast-Food Meal Estimations**

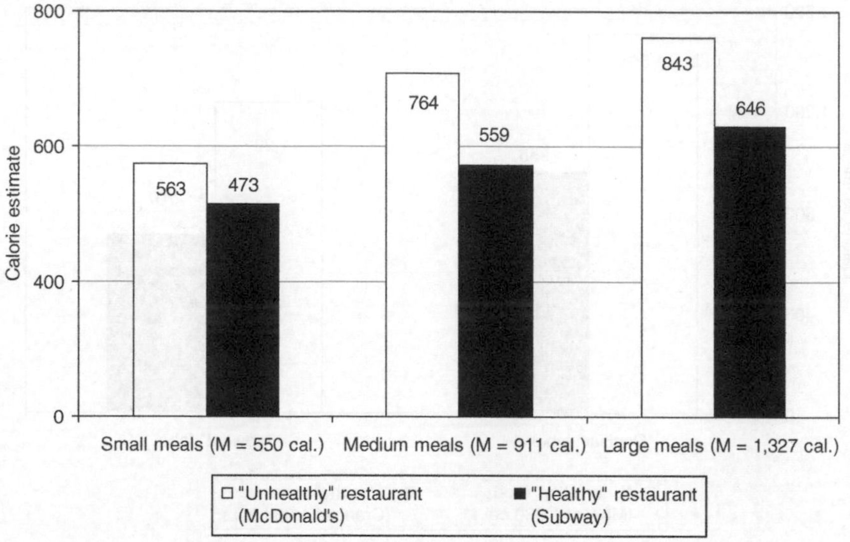

Note: People eating at Subway, a restaurant claiming to serve healthy meals, underestimate the caloric content of their meals more than people eating at McDonald's, a restaurant not making health claims, regardless of the size of their meal.

chain that does not make that claim) to estimate the caloric content of their meal. The researchers then recorded the type and size of the foods and drinks from the wrappings left on the trays and obtained information about the actual number of calories in the foods and beverages from the restaurant's website. To increase the comparability of McDonald's and Subway meals, they only analyzed meals consisting of a sandwich, a soft drink, and a side order. The data summarized in Figure 4.2 show the mean calorie estimate of people eating small, medium, or large meals (categorized on the basis of actual number of calories) at either Subway or McDonald's. On average, Subway meals were perceived to contain 21.3 percent fewer calories than same-calorie McDonald's meals. These results were replicated in a scenario in which the health positioning of the fast-food restaurant was empirically manipulated, rather than measured.

AVERAGING BIAS IN ESTIMATING THE CALORIE CONTENT OF MEALS COMBINING HEALTHY AND UNHEALTHY ITEMS

Conventional wisdom suggests that deriving calorie estimates of combinations of food items should be fairly trivial: The calorie content of a meal comprising several individual items should be equal to the sum of the individual estimates of these items. Recent research has shown, however, that this is not always the case and that individuals display systematic biases in evaluating the calorie content of combinations of items (Chernev 2011b, Chernev and Gal 2010). In particular, when evaluating combinations of items representing indulgence and health goals, consumers tend to underestimate their calorie content.

Consider a calorie-conscious person who is choosing between two meals: a lone hamburger or the same hamburger with a green salad on the side. After some deliberation, the consumer chooses the second meal even though, objectively, the two-item meal contains more calories and is, therefore, inconsistent with the primary goal of consuming fewer calories. Despite its inconsistency with a consumer's weight-management goals, the preference for combinations of healthy and indulgent items is not unusual and has been documented in multiple studies.

What motivates consumers to act in a way that is inconsistent with their goals? Building on the notion that people tend to automatically classify food items into healthy and unhealthy (Chandon and Wansink 2007b; Krider, Raghubir, and Krishna 2001), Chernev and Gal (2010) argue that when evaluating combinations of healthy and unhealthy food items, people tend to average their benefits, which leads them to believe that the combination of a healthy and an unhealthy item is healthier than the unhealthy item alone. To illustrate, people tend to think that a hamburger and a salad is healthier than the hamburger alone.

Furthermore, in the absence of readily available calorie information, people are inclined to rely on their impressions of a meal's overall healthiness to infer its calorie content. Because health halos lead people to believe that healthier meals have fewer calories than unhealthy meals, adding healthier items can make the overall meal seem healthier, which in turn can lower its perceived calorie content. This line of reasoning leads to the erroneous conclusion that because the combination of a healthy and an unhealthy item seems healthier than the unhealthy item alone, the combined meal is likely to have fewer calories.

The paradox here is that adding a healthy option can lower the perceived calorie content of the combined meal even in cases when the actual number of calories has not changed or even has increased. For example, people might think that a meal comprising a cheeseburger and a green salad has 500 calories even though they believe the cheeseburger alone to have 600 calories when they evaluate it separately. This, in turn, might lead to the erroneous belief that by consuming a healthy item (e.g., salad) in addition to an unhealthy one (e.g., cheeseburger), a person can actually decrease rather than increase the amount of calories consumed.

Consumers' tendency to perceive that a meal containing both a healthy and an unhealthy item has fewer calories than the unhealthy item by itself has been documented in numerous experiments. In one study (Chernev and Gal 2010), respondents were randomly assigned to estimate the calorie content of a hamburger alone, a broccoli salad alone, or a meal containing both. Respondents estimated that the hamburger by itself had 761 calories and that the broccoli salad by itself had 67 calories. Logically, one would expect that the combined meal would, therefore, have approximately 830 calories. In contrast, respondents estimated that the

Figure 4.3   **Averaging Bias in Combining Healthy and Indulgent Items**

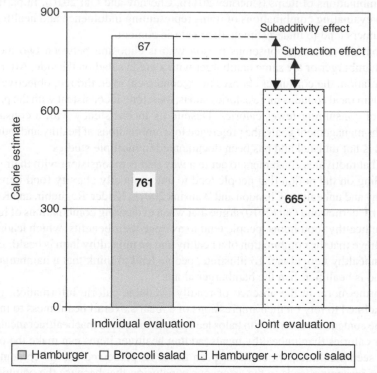

Note: Adding a healthy item to an unhealthy one decreases the perceived calorie content of the combined meal.

hamburger-and-broccoli meal would have 583 calories, which was not only lower than the combined estimates of both dishes but also lower than the perceived calorie content of the hamburger by itself (Figure 4.3). Thus, adding a broccoli salad to the hamburger lowered the estimated calorie content of the entire meal by an average of 96 calories, or 12.6 percent. The fact that respondents evaluated the broccoli salad separately as having positive calories indicates that these data cannot be attributed to the popular belief that broccoli has "negative" calories because the energy used to digest it exceeds its caloric content.

Chernev and Gal (2010) further showed that the observed averaging bias is particular to combinations of healthy and indulgent items and does not hold for a combination of two indulgent items. They asked a separate set of respondents from the same population to estimate the caloric content of a meal comprising the same burger paired with a chocolate chip cookie. The data show that adding a cookie instead of the broccoli salad had the opposite effect of increasing rather than decreasing the perceived calorie content of the combined meal. In particular, respondents perceived the burger/cookie combination to have 859 calories, significantly more than the burger alone. Thus, adding a cookie to the hamburger increased the perceived calorie content of the entire meal by 98 calories, or 12.9 percent.

These data indicate that the averaging bias is conceptually different from a simple psychophysical summation bias, whereby a meal is perceived to have fewer calories than the sum of the estimates of its individual components (Chandon and Wansink 2007b; Krider, Raghubir, and Krishna 2001). Indeed, whereas summation bias can predict the subadditivity of the estimates of the individual components of a meal, it cannot account for the subtraction effect in which the perceived calorie content of the combined meal is estimated to be less than the unhealthy item alone (Figure 4.3). Moreover, summation bias cannot account for the fact that the subtraction effect occurs only when combining healthy and indulgent items but not when combining two indulgent items. These findings suggest that averaging bias is conceptually independent from a simple summation bias.

The averaging bias is a function of the degree to which people classify options as healthy or indulgent: combining options that are perceived to be more extreme in their healthiness or indulgence should produce a greater averaging bias. To illustrate, in one experiment (Chernev and Gal 2010) respondents were randomly assigned to estimate the calorie content of a cheeseburger alone, a Caesar salad alone, or a meal containing both. The degree of the perceived healthiness of the Caesar salad was manipulated by giving respondents an evaluation task in which they were asked to compare the healthiness of the Caesar salad to a reference meal. Some of the respondents were asked to evaluate the healthiness of the Caesar salad relative to a broccoli salad, whereas others were asked to evaluate the healthiness of the Caesar salad relative to a black bean chili salad. The rationale for this manipulation was that comparing the Caesar salad to a chili salad would highlight its healthiness, whereas comparing it to a broccoli salad would make the Caesar salad appear less healthy.

The data summarized in Figure 4.4 show that respondents perceived a meal comprising a cheeseburger and a "healthier" (compared to a black bean chili salad) Caesar salad to have fewer calories than the cheeseburger alone (583 vs. 698 calories). In contrast, combining the cheeseburger with the "less healthy" (compared to a broccoli salad) Caesar salad resulted in a directionally opposite effect (779 vs. 721 calories).

Note that even though the subtraction bias (estimating the calorie content of the combined meal as lower than one of its components) was observed only in the presence of the healthier option (Caesar salad compared to chili salad), both conditions produced an averaging bias whereby the combined meal was perceived to have fewer calories than the sum of its individual components (583 < [698 + 102] and 779 < [721 + 164]). This finding lends further support to the proposition that people tend to underestimate the calorie content of combinations of healthy and unhealthy items.

Figure 4.4   **Averaging Bias as a Function of the Perceived Healthiness of the Combined Items**

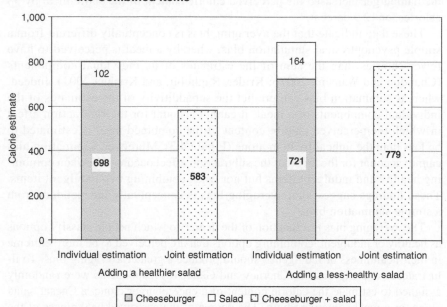

Note: The underestimation bias resulting from combining a healthy and an unhealthy item is a function of the degree of perceived healthiness of the items.

POLICY IMPLICATIONS

The reported decision biases have important public policy implications stemming from the fact that people's beliefs about the calorie content of food items influence their purchase and consumption behavior. Below, we review some of the key public policy implications following from the calorie-estimation biases.

Studies have shown that health halos increase consumption and lead people to choose high-calorie beverages, side dishes, and desserts. Wansink and Chandon (2006) found that labeling food as "low-fat" strongly increases intake during a single consumption occasion, especially if the food is categorized as healthy. For example, they found that moviegoers who were given granola labeled as "low-fat" consumed 50.1 percent more granola than moviegoers who were given granola labeled as "regular." Chandon and Wansink (2007a) found that consumers chose beverages, side dishes, and desserts containing up to 131 percent more calories when the main course was a supposedly healthy twelve-inch Italian BLT Subway sandwich compared to when it was a supposedly unhealthy McDonald's Big Mac (even though the Subway sandwich already contained 50 percent more calories than the Big Mac). As a result, they found that meals ordered from "healthy" restaurants frequently contain more calories than meals ordered from "unhealthy" restaurants.

The averaging bias associated with combining healthy and unhealthy options also influences people's choice of a meal. To illustrate, in one experiment respondents were given a choice between two meals—a lone hamburger or a hamburger with an apple. The choice task involved two different hamburgers, labeled as Hamburger A and Hamburger B. Some respondents saw the apple paired with Hamburger A, while others saw the apple paired with Hamburger B. Among respondents who saw the Hamburger A by itself, 32 percent indicated that a calorie-conscious person would choose it. When Hamburger A was paired with the apple, however, the percentage of participants who chose the Hamburger A-and-apple meal over the lone hamburger increased to 62 percent. The paradox here is that even though the apple alone was estimated to contain a positive number of calories, adding it to a hamburger increased rather than decreased the preference for this burger among consumers concerned with minimizing their calorie intake.

The ubiquity of the halo and averaging biases in calorie estimation and their strong impact on people's consumption decisions raise the question of identifying strategies that will attenuate, if not eliminate, these biases. Below we discuss five such strategies:

1. motivating consumers to pay more attention to nutrition information,

2. mandating the disclosure of calorie information in away-from-home consumption,

3. counterfactual thinking,

4. piecemeal evaluation of meals comprised of multiple items, and

5. de-emphasizing categorical thinking by focusing on quantitative estimates such as meal size.

We then review the existing evidence on the effectiveness of the first three strategies for reducing health halos and of the last two strategies for reducing averaging halos.

Nutrition Involvement

Encouraging consumers to pay more attention to nutrition information is a widespread goal of government intervention. Unfortunately, existing research has cast doubt on its effectiveness. In one study, Chandon and Wansink (2007a) measured consumers' nutrition involvement using a five-item scale that included statements such as "I pay close attention to nutrition information." They then asked consumers with high or low levels of nutrition involvement to estimate the caloric content of typical calorie-equivalent foods from supposedly healthy (Subway) or unhealthy (McDonald's) restaurants. They found that although nutrition involvement improved the quality of calorie estimations, it did not reduce the halo effects of the restaurant brand's health positioning. Similarly, Provencher, Polivy, and Herman (2008) found that neither dietary restraint nor weight salience moderated health halos. In their study, cookies were perceived to contain fewer calories and were consumed in larger quantities when they were described as "healthy snacks" than when they were described as "gourmet cookies," regardless of whether people were weighed before or after the calorie estimation task and whether or not they were trying to restrict their food consumption.

Mandatory Calorie Disclosure

One obvious solution to reduce health halos would be to mandate the disclosure of calorie information not just for packaged goods but also in away-from-home consumption situations. Although opposed by the restaurant industry on the grounds that it is impractical and anticommercial, legislation to that effect is being put in place.[3] The question of whether this legislation will prove effective, however, is still open. Thus, one study (Howlett et al. 2009) showed that providing calorie information about a sandwich unexpectedly high in calories reduced consumers' intention to purchase it and reduced their subsequent intake of cookies and candies. On the other hand, prior research conducted for packaged goods suggests that mandatory calorie disclosure alone is unlikely to be sufficient to eliminate health halos simply because not enough consumers pay attention to nutrition information. For example, although some studies found that the Nutrition Labeling and Education Act increased consumer search for and comprehension of nutrition information for packaged goods (Moorman 1996), other studies found no effect on search, recall, or choice (Balasubramanian and Cole 2002).

Counterfactual Thinking

If health halos are caused by priming and selective activation, one solution is to encourage consumers to question the validity of the health claims. The effectiveness of this debiasing strategy is enhanced if people are asked to consider evidence inconsistent with the prime because it increases the accessibility of claim-inconsistent knowledge (Mussweiler, Strack, and Pfeiffer 2000). In one study, Chandon and Wansink (2007a) asked people to estimate the number of calories in a meal consisting of a ham sandwich and a soda (660 calories). They asked another group of people whether they would like to have chips with this meal. They manipulated health halos by way of the restaurant name ("Good Karma Healthy Foods" vs. "Jim's Hearty Sandwiches") and the food available on its menu (e.g., carrot soup vs. a sausage sandwich). Participants in the "consider the opposite" condition were also asked to find arguments supporting the idea that the ham sandwich was a generic meal and not typical of the restaurant serving it. Participants in the control condi-

Figure 4.5 **Counterfactual Thinking Reduces the Effects of Health Halos on Calorie Estimations**

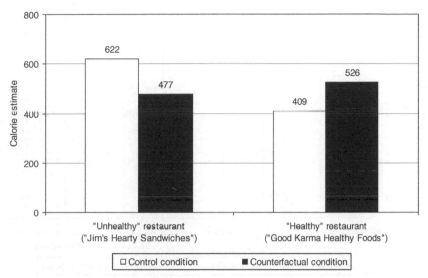

Note: Prompting people to question the health claims of the restaurant eliminates the effects of health halos on calorie estimation.

tion more deeply underestimated the calorie content of the target meal and were more likely to order chips with this meal when it came from the supposedly healthy restaurant than when it came from the supposedly unhealthy restaurant (see Figure 4.5). However, the effects of health halos disappeared in the "consider the opposite" condition in which calorie estimations and side-order consumption intentions were essentially the same regardless of the health claims. Prompting people to question the validity of health primes therefore eliminated halo-based biases.

Piecemeal Evaluation

Prior research indicates that piecemeal estimation tends to improve people's calorie estimations of a meal (Chandon and Wansink 2007b). Piecemeal evaluation is especially effective in attenuating the averaging bias. Indeed, because the averaging bias is caused by individuals forming an overall evaluation of the healthiness of a meal comprising both healthy and unhealthy items, this bias is less pronounced, or even eliminated, in cases when individuals form separate evaluations of the items. To illustrate, in one experiment (Chernev and Gal 2010) one group of respondents was shown a meal comprising a cheeseburger and a green salad, and another group was shown a meal comprising the same cheeseburger and a piece of cheesecake instead of a salad. In addition, some of the respondents in each group were asked to estimate the calorie content of the entire meal, whereas others were asked to

Figure 4.6   **Piecemeal Evaluations Tend to Reduce the Averaging Bias**

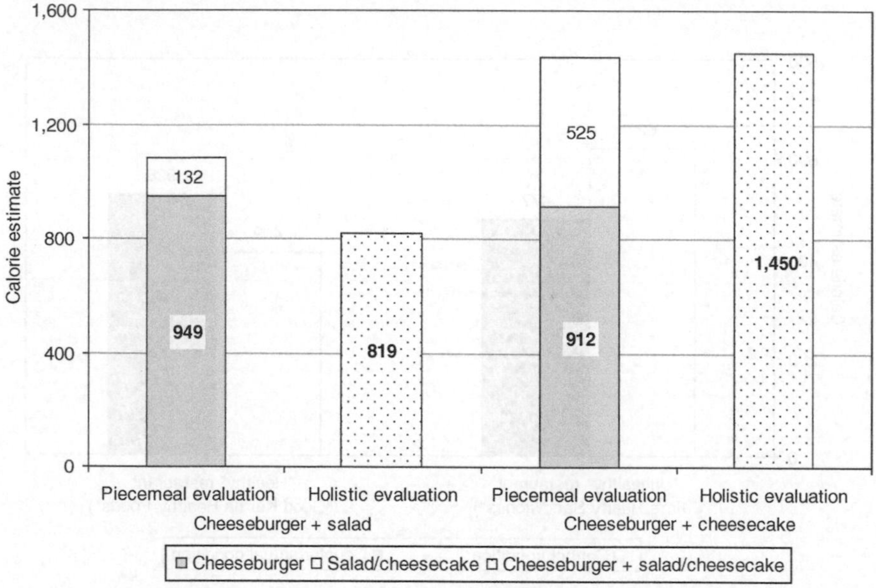

Note: The averaging bias is greater for a meal combining a healthy and an unhealthy item when consumers form an overall evaluation of the items than when the items are evaluated in a piecemeal fashion.

estimate the calorie content of the individual components. In both cases, the meal viewed by respondents was exactly the same; only the manner of estimating (overall vs. piecemeal) differed. The data summarized in Figure 4.6 show that respondents asked to evaluate the calorie content of the cheeseburger-and-salad combination perceived it to have fewer calories than respondents asked to estimate the calorie content of the meal's individual components (819 vs. 1,082). In contrast, respondents asked to evaluate the calorie content of the cheeseburger-and-cake combination perceived it to have virtually the same amount of calories, regardless of whether they estimated its calorie content in an overall or a piecemeal fashion (1,450 vs. 1,437). Thus, when evaluated in a piecemeal fashion, the calorie content of the cheeseburger was essentially the same regardless of whether it was paired with a healthy or unhealthy option (949 vs. 912 calories); however, when evaluated in a holistic fashion, adding a healthy option was perceived to detract calories from the indulgent option.[4] Piecemeal evaluation therefore improved the accuracy of calorie estimation and attenuated the averaging bias (see also Chernev 2011a).

Size-Based Evaluation

Because the averaging bias is a function of individuals' categorical beliefs about a meal's overall healthiness, eliminating this bias might be accomplished by de-

Figure 4.7   **Focusing on Meal Size Tends to Reduce the Averaging Bias**

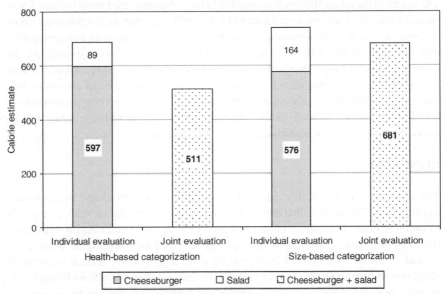

Note: The averaging bias is greater when consumers focus on the healthiness of a meal rather than its size.

emphasizing people's attention on the healthiness of the available food items. One approach to shifting people's attention away from healthiness-based categorization is to emphasize other aspects of the available meals such as meal size. Because larger meals are perceived to have more calories (Chandon and Wansink 2007b; Scott et al. 2008), size-based inferences are likely to work in a direction opposite to health-based inferences, leading to an increase, rather than a decrease, in the perceived calorie content of the combined meal vis-à-vis its individual components. Therefore, when people use alternative means, such as size, to infer a meal's calorie content, the underestimation effect associated with people's evaluations of a meal's healthiness should be attenuated or even disappear.

The impact of evaluating a meal's size is illustrated by the following experiment (Chernev and Gal 2010). Respondents were divided into three groups: some were shown a meal comprising a cheeseburger, others were shown a meal comprising a carrot-and-celery salad, and the rest were shown a meal comprising the cheeseburger and the carrot-and-celery salad. In addition, all respondents were initially presented with three pairs of items: a cake and an apple, a tomato and a burger, and a chocolate chip cookie and a kiwi. To manipulate consumers' focus on either the health-related or on the size-related aspect of the meal, some of the respondents were asked to indicate which item in each of the three pairs was healthier, while the others were asked to indicate which item in each pair was bigger. The data summarized in Figure 4.7 show that the latter type of categorization led to a reversal of the averaging bias. Respondents asked to compare the initially presented items according to their healthiness perceived the cheeseburger/salad meal to have fewer calories than the cheeseburger alone (511 vs. 597). In contrast, respondents asked to compare the initially presented meals by size did not display an averaging bias, and their estimates of the cheeseburger/salad combination were essentially the same as the sum of the individual components (681 vs. [576 + 164]). Thus, whereas health-based evaluations were more likely to promote the use of an averaging rule and an underestimation of the calorie content of healthy/unhealthy combinations, size-based evaluations were likely to promote the use of an additive rather than an averaging rule, thus attenuating calorie underestimation.

CONCLUSION

The research outlined in this chapter has important managerial and public policy implications. The finding that adding healthy options to the menu leads consumers to underestimate the calorie content of all foods on the menu (health halo), par-ticularly of meals combining healthy and unhealthy foods (averaging bias), casts a shadow on the potential of healthy options to significantly reduce overeating. While providing an alternative for individuals interested in a healthier lifestyle, the introduction of healthier options ironically can lead to overconsumption stemming from underestimation of the calorie content of the considered meals. Therefore, an important implication of the findings reported in this research is that providing calorie information in a user-friendly format at the time of food selection could help minimize the overconsumption resulting from the reported averaging bias.

Our findings also raise important questions regarding the implications of people's reliance on a healthy/unhealthy classification to make their food consump-tion decisions. Categorizing foods according to their healthiness is rooted in the actions of many government and private institutions, which use such categoriza-tions to help consumers regulate their food intake. Yet our findings suggest that this approach can sometimes yield exactly the opposite results when it comes to monitoring calorie intake since health-based categorization can lead to underes-timating the calorie content of healthy foods and combinations of healthy and indulgent items. This, in turn, can lead to counterproductive behaviors because people think they are eating a healthier and less caloric meal when they actually are consuming more calories.

NOTES

1. Prior research has shown that errors of calorie estimation partly stem from psy-chophysical biases in quantity estimation, which lead people to slightly overestimate the calorie content of small portions, to strongly underestimate the calorie content of large portions, and to underestimate the magnitude of portion size changes. For a review of this research, see Chandon (2009).
2. Foods can claim to be low-fat as long as they contain less than three grams of fat per serving, regardless of their caloric content. On average, foods labeled as low-fat do

not contain significantly fewer calories per serving than foods without this label (National Institutes of Health 2004).

3. In 2008, California was the first U.S. state to pass a law stating that restaurant chains with twenty or more locations will be required to post caloric information on menus and indoor menu boards and to provide brochures with nutritional content upon request by January 1, 2011.

4. In addition to providing a remedy for the averaging bias, this experiment illustrates the conceptual distinction between the averaging and halo biases. Indeed, if the observed underestimation was a result of a healthiness "spillover" from the healthy to the unhealthy item, then the underestimation effect should have persisted regardless of the nature of the decision task (overall vs. piecemeal), since respondents in both conditions saw the healthy and unhealthy items next to each other. In contrast, the data show that the observed underestimation effect has its own antecedents that go beyond the halo effect.

REFERENCES

Allison, David B., Kevin R. Fontaine, JoAnn E. Manson, June Stevens, and Theodore B. VanItallie. 1999. "Annual Deaths Attributable to Obesity in the United States." *Journal of American Medical Association*, 282 (16), 1530–1538.

Andrews, J. Craig, Richard G. Netemeyer, and Scot Burton. 1996. "Consumer Generalization of Nutrient Content Claims in Advertising." *Journal of Marketing*, 62 (4), 62–75.

Balasubramanian, Siva K., and Catherine Cole. 2002. "Consumers' Search and Use of Nutrition Information: The Challenge and Promise of the Nutrition Labeling and Education Act." *Journal of Marketing*, 66 (3), 112–127.

Burton, Scot, Elizabeth H. Creyer, Jeremy Kees, and Kyle Huggins. 2006. "Attacking the Obesity Epidemic: The Potential Health Benefits of Providing Nutrition Information in Restaurants." *American Journal of Public Health*, 96 (9), 1669–1675.

Centers for Disease Control and Prevention (CDC). 2007. "Overweight and Obesity: Contributing Factors." www.cdc.gov/nccdphp/dnpa/obesity/contributing_factors.htm.

Chandon, Pierre. 2009. "Estimating Food Quantity: Biases and Remedies." In *Sensory Marketing: Psychological Research for Consumers*, ed. Aradhna Krishna, 323–342. New York: Taylor and Francis.

Chandon, Pierre, and Brian Wansink. 2007a. "The Biasing Health Halos of Fast-Food Restaurant Health Claims: Lower Calorie Estimates and Higher Side-Dish Consumption Intentions." *Journal of Consumer Research*, 34 (3), 301–314.

———. 2007b. "Is Obesity Caused by Calorie Underestimation? A Psychophysical Model of Meal Size Estimation." *Journal of Marketing Research*, 44 (1), 84–99.

———. 2011. "Semantic Anchoring in Sequential Evaluations of Vices and Virtues." *Journal of Consumer Research,* 37 (February).

Chernev, Alexander, and David Gal. 2011a. "Categorization Effects in Value Judgments: Averaging Bias in Evaluating Combinations of Vices and Virtues." *Journal of Marketing Research*, 47 (August), 738–747.

Chernev, Alexander. 2011b. "The Dieter's Paradox." *Journey of Consumer Psychology*, 21 (April).

Goodhart, Robert S., and Maurice E. Shils. 1980. *Modern Nutrition in Health and Disease.* 6th ed. Philadelphia: Lea and Febiger.

Heini, Adrian F., and Roland L. Weinsier. 1997. "Divergent Trends in Obesity and Fat Intake Patterns: The American Paradox." *American Journal of Medicine*, 102 (3), 259–264.

Howlett, Elizabeth A., Scot Burton, Kenneth Bates, and Kyle Huggins. 2009. "Coming to a Restaurant Near You? Potential Consumer Responses to Nutrition Information Disclosure on Menus." *Journal of Consumer Research*, 36 (3), 494–503.

Kardes, Frank R., Steven S. Posavac, and Maria L. Cronley. 2004. "Consumer Inference: A Review of Processes, Bases, and Judgment Contexts." *Journal of Consumer Psychology*, 14 (3), 230–256.

Keys, Ancel. 1997. "Coronary Heart Disease in Seven Countries." *Nutrition*, 13 (3), 249.

Krider, Robert E., Priya Raghubir, and Aradhna Krishna. 2001. "Pizzas: Pi or Square? Psychophysical Biases in Area Comparisons." *Marketing Science*, 20 (4), 405–425.

Lansky, David, and Kelly D. Brownell. 1982. "Estimates of Food Quantity and Calories: Errors in Self-Report Among Obese Patients." *American Journal of Clinical Nutrition*, 35 (4), 727–732.

Lichtman, Steven W., Krystyna Pisarska, Ellen Raynes Berman, Michele Pestone, Hillary Dowling, Esther Offenbacher, Hope Weisel, Stanley Heshka, Dwight E. Matthews, and Steven B. Heymsfield. 1992. "Discrepancy Between Self-Reported and Actual Caloric Intake and Exercise in Obese Subjects." *New England Journal of Medicine*, 327 (27), 1893–1898.

Livingstone, M. Barbara, and Alison E. Black. 2003. "Markers of the Validity of Reported Energy Intake." *Journal of Nutrition*, 133 (3), 895S–920S.

Moorman, Christine. 1996. "A Quasi Experiment to Assess the Consumer and Informational Determinants of Nutrition Information." *Journal of Public Policy and Marketing*, 15 (1), 28–44.

Mussweiler, Thomas. 2003. "Comparison Processes in Social Judgment: Mechanisms and Consequences." *Psychological Review*, 110 (3), 472–489.

Mussweiler, Thomas, Fritz Strack, and Tim Pfeiffer. 2000. "Overcoming the Inevitable Anchoring Effect: Considering the Opposite Compensates for Selective Accessibility." *Personality and Social Psychology Bulletin*, 26 (9), 1142–1150.

Must, Aviva, Jennifer Spadano, Eugenie H. Coakley, Alison E. Field, Graham Colditz, and William H. Dietz. 1999. "The Disease Burden Associated with Overweight and Obesity." *Journal of American Medical Association*, 282 (16), 1523–1529.

National Institutes of Health. 2004. Diet Myths. Bethesda, MD: NIH Publication No. 04–4561. http://win.niddk.nih.gov/publications/myths.htm.

Oakes, Michael E. 2005. "Stereotypical Thinking About Foods and Perceived Capacity to Promote Weight Gain." *Appetite*, 44 (3), 317–324.

Oakes, Michael E., and Carole S. Slotterback. 2001. "What's in a Name? A Comparison of Men's and Women's Judgments About Food Names and Their Nutrient Contents." *Appetite*, 36 (1), 29–40.

Olshansky, S. Jay, Douglas J. Passaro, Ronald C. Hershow, Jennifer Layden, Bruce A. Carnes, Jacob Brody, Leonard Hayflick, Robert N. Butler, David B. Allison, and David S. Ludwig. 2005. "A Potential Decline in Life Expectancy in the United States in the 21st Century." *New England Journal of Medicine*, 352 (11), 1138–1145.

Provencher, Veronique, Janet Polivy, and C. Peter Herman. 2008. "Perceived Healthiness of Food: If It's Healthy, You Can Eat More!" *Appetite*, 52 (2), 340–344.

Raghunathan, Rajagopal, Rebecca W. Naylor, and Wayne D. Hoyer. 2006. "The Unhealthy = Tasty Intuition and Its Effects on Taste Inferences, Enjoyment, and Choice of Food Products." *Journal of Marketing*, 70 (4), 170–184.

Rozin, Paul, Michele Ashmore, and Maureen Markwith. 1996. "Lay American Conceptions of Nutrition: Dose Insensitivity, Categorical Thinking, Contagion, and the Monotonic Mind." *Health Psychology*, 15 (6), 438–447.

Sacks, Frank M., George A. Bray, Vincent J. Carey, Steven R. Smith, Donna H. Ryan, Stephen D. Anton, Katherine McManus, Catherine M. Champagne, Louise M. Bishop, Nancy Laranjo, Meryl S. Leboff, Jennifer C. Rood, Lilian de Jonge, Frank L. Greenway, Catherine M. Loria, Eva Obarzanek, and Donald A. Williamson. 2009. "Comparison of Weight-Loss Diets with Different Compositions of Fat, Protein, and Carbohydrates." *New England Journal of Medicine*, 360 (9), 859–873.

Scott, Maura L., Stephen M. Nowlis, Naomi Mandel, and Andrea C. Morales. 2008. "The Effects of Reduced Food Size and Package Size on the Consumption Behavior of Restrained and Unrestrained Eaters." *Journal of Consumer Research*, 35 (3), 391–405.

Thompson, Tommy G., and Ann M. Veneman. 2005. *Dietary Guidelines for Americans*. 6th ed. Washington, DC: U.S. Government Printing Office.

USDA. 2008. Steps to a Healthier You. www.mypyramid.gov.

Wansink, Brian. 2006. *Mindless Eating: Why We Eat More Than We Think*. New York: Bantam Books.

Wansink, Brian, and Pierre Chandon. 2006. "Can 'Low-Fat' Nutrition Labels Lead to Obesity?" *Journal of Marketing Research*, 43 (4), 605–617.

Wertenbroch, Klaus. 1998. "Consumption Self Control by Rationing Purchase Quantities of Virtue and Vice." *Marketing Science*, 17 (4), 317–337.

CHAPTER 5

FOOD TEMPTATIONS VERSUS SELF-CONTROL

Friends or Enemies?

KELLY GEYSKENS

Consumers today live in an "obesogenic environment" characterized by a multitude of unhealthy and easily accessible temptations. Besides genetic determinants (Aitman 2003; Dietz 1991) and shifts toward less physically demanding work, consumers today encounter convenience-oriented foods with a higher proportion of fats and sugars (Cutler, Glaeser, and Shapiro 2003; Mitka 2003) and market forces such as decreased prices, greater availability, and increased flavor variety (Raynor and Epstein 2001; Tardoff 2002). Foods today come in larger serving sizes (Nielsen and Popkin 2003; Wansink 1996) and via more convenient eating opportunities (e.g., ready-to-eat meals and eating in restaurants). All these have led, over the past decades, to an enormous increase in the consumption of fattening snacks and have often been cited as driving the obesity epidemic (Critser 2003; Nestle 2002). The remedies that are put forward by health organizations, such as stimulation of the market penetration of low-fat products, increasing the price of high energy products and beverages, and reducing the price of fruit and vegetables (WHO 2006), typically aim at reducing the strength of and exposure to unhealthy food temptations.

In addition, consumers themselves have come to believe that the more "vice" products they store at home, the more "vice" products they will consume. (Vice products are those that satisfy a short-term goal but hurt long-term goals, e.g., chocolate, cake, and candy.) Therefore consumers ration the purchase quantities of vice products, for example by forgoing quantity price discounts (Wertenbroch 1998). In other words, consumers prefer to pay higher unit costs for one candy bar than for a twelve-pack of the same candy bar, presumably to keep control over the amount eaten. Prior research and observations from everyday life support this common intuition that food temptations constitute a permanent threat to the accomplishment of consumers' long-term food intake regulation goals. Indeed, larger package sizes increase consumption (Wansink 1996), and stockpiling accelerates the consumption rate of convenience goods due to a higher salience of the food products (Chandon and Wansink 2002). Other research has shown that external cues such as visual prominence (e.g., seeing half a cake on a counter) or aromatic prominence of food (e.g., the scent of cookies in a room) can make it salient (Painter, Wansink, and Hieggelke 2002; Schachter 1971; Wansink 1994). The increase in food salience following appetizing olfactory food cues has been shown to activate a craving for food and stimulate eating behavior (Fedoroff, Polivy, and Herman 2003; Lambert and Neal 1992). Shiv and Fedorikhin (2002) found that increasing the salience of the food options in a choice task, by placing the options in front of consumers rather than showing pictures of the food, causes a relative vice food option (e.g., pizza) to be preferred over a relative virtue food option (e.g., tomato soup).

However, recent research suggests that these strategies, designed to prevent self-control failure, can often backfire, because people react differently to these cues compared to what people intuitively would expect (e.g., Coelho do Vale, Pieters, and Zeelenberg 2008; Geyskens et al. 2008; Scott et al. 2008; Wansink and Chandon 2006). We argue here that exposure to strongly tempting food cues, resistance to which requires self-control, might actually be better in helping consumers resist subsequent food temptations.

RESEARCH SUGGESTING SELF-CONTROL–ENHANCING EFFECTS OF FOOD TEMPTATIONS

Some recent findings suggest that control might be initiated by the mere exposure to tempting food stimuli (Fishbach, Friedman, and Kruglanski 2003). The model of asymmetric associations between temptations and higher priority goals (Fishbach, Friedman, and Kruglanski 2003) states that automatic associations can develop between goals that are active at the same time. These connections between goals result in mutual facilitation or mutual inhibition, depending on whether the goals are related or opposing. For example, the goal of leading a healthy life can be facilitated by the goal of wanting to go swimming but it can be opposed by the goal of wanting to eat at McDonald's. In other words, temptations that threaten the achievement of important long-term goals could activate these opposing long-term goals and in this way facilitate self-regulation. Repeated attempts at self-control lead to frequent co-occurrence of a temptation (a dessert) and a goal (having a slim body). For example, if a person does not eat dessert because of the long-term goal of having a nice and thin body, which implies dieting, the link between the dessert (the temptation) and dieting (the goal) is made. This results in an asymmetric link, implying that temptations activate inhibitory goals but the goals inhibit the temptations. Because of many activations of this link, it can become overlearned, which implies that the activation of the goals by (opposing) temptations could be relatively independent of cognitive resources and that even subliminal activation of the temptation could be sufficient to activate the goal. Moreover, Fishbach, Friedman, and Kruglanski (2003) state that the direct priming of the goal increases the awareness of the goal but does not enhance self-control attempts, while the priming of temptations activates a narrower set of self-control intentions, which does enhances self-control.

Recently Fishbach and Shah (2006) also found that, in addition to the activation of the overriding goal, the automatic response to food stimuli is a tendency to approach these stimuli. However, at the same time, especially for dieters, there is an automatic tendency to avoid these food stimuli. This suggests that the self-control conflict caused by exposure to food cues emerges by the simultaneous approach and avoidance tendencies that they induce. Self-control is successful when the original tendency to approach these stimuli is overridden by the tendency to avoid the stimuli.

The prediction that food temptations might help resistance against subsequent food offers may also be derived from the finding of Gilbert et al. (2004) that active attempts to solve a problem arise only when the problem becomes serious enough. People's problem-solving strategies seem to be triggered only by critical levels of hedonic states because they expect intense states (e.g., pain from a bruised leg) to last longer than mild states (e.g., pain from a numb leg). Intense hedonic states are overestimated (Gilbert et al. 1998) and trigger self-control strategies, whereas mild states are underestimated and therefore linger unsolved (Snell, Gibbs, and Varey 1995). In the case of food temptations, a similar nonlinear relationship might apply. A large number of candies may trigger concerns about health and diet objectives whereas small numbers might not. This implies that people might paradoxically consume more candies when there are only a few candies in the kitchen cabinet than when a lot of candies are present (Gilbert et al. 2004), although consumers seem to believe the opposite (Wertenbroch 1998). The application of Gilbert et al.'s (2004) theory to the food consumption domain implies that consumers might be wrong when they buy smaller amounts of vice foods as a strategy to keep their consumption under control. According to the critical level perspective, exposure to food temptations that exceed the critical level beyond which self-control strategies are triggered might help to control food intake on a subsequent consumption occasion.

THE PIVOTAL ROLE OF FOOD TEMPTATION ACTIONABILITY OF PRIOR FOOD TEMPTATIONS ON GOAL ACTIVATION AND CONSUMPTION

We investigated when prior exposure to food temptations hurts or helps consumers' capability to control their subsequent food intake (Geyskens et al. 2008). Since little is known about the specific circumstances that determine whether food temptations lead to increased food intake through the activation of eating goals or decreased food intake through the activation of inhibition goals, we investigated the pivotal role of the actionability of the food temptation. We compared prior food temptations that do not offer the opportunity to consume the food temptation, and prior food temptations that do offer the opportunity to consume the tempting food, with respect to their effects on current consumption. We compared those effects with a control condition without prior temptation. The food temptation that is not actionable (e.g., pictures of food) does not create a self-control conflict. In other words, we assumed that nonactionable food temptations do not exceed the critical level beyond which self-control strategies are triggered, because there is no self-control conflict present. In contrast, a food temptation that is actionable (e.g., a basket full of delicious cookies), while consumption is not appropriate, implies the self-control conflict induced by the opportunity of immediate consumption. We assumed that actionable food temptations push the consumer beyond the critical level at which self-control strategies are triggered. So our main prediction was that, as compared to exposure to nonactionable temptations, exposure to actionable temptations will reduce subsequent consumption.

In a first study, we replicated the findings of Fishbach, Friedman, and Kruglanski (2003), showing that nonactionable as well as actionable food temptations activate the goal to restrict food intake. In other words, exposure to food temptations activates the opposing goal (i.e., dieting), independent of the level of actionability of the food temptation. Considering our claim that exposure to nonactionable food temptations does not trigger self-control strategies whereas actionable food temptations do, this finding raised the question by which other process self-control enhancement (i.e., food intake control) is obtained. Activation of a food restriction goal is theoretically only one, albeit the literature's favorite route to successful self-control (e.g., Metcalfe and Mischel 1999; Shiv and Fedorikhin 2002). Following that account, a temptation, upon activating an eating goal, triggers the activation of the food restriction goal, which is believed to reduce consumption. Assuming, however, that the choice in a self-control conflict follows from the balance between desire and willpower (Hoch and Loewenstein 1991), another route to successful consumption control may be through the down-regulation of the desire for food, as reflected in a decreased activation of the eating goal. Fishbach and Shah (2006) recently found that, in addition to the activation of a food restriction goal, the automatic response to food stimuli is a tendency to approach these stimuli (see also Shiv and Fedorikhin 2002).

In a second study, we tested the role of actionability in the activation of the eating goal in tempting situations, by measuring the activation of the eating goal resulting from the exposure to food temptations differing in actionability and the presence (yes or no) of a subsequent temptation. We found that exposure to nonactionable as well as actionable food temptations activated the eating goal, as compared to the no-temptation condition when no subsequent temptation opportunity was present. However, when a subsequent temptation was present, prior exposure to the actionable food temptations down-regulated the desire to eat. That is, when consumers are exposed to an actionable temptation that cannot be consumed ad libitum, they adapt by down-regulating their desire to eat. This self-control strategy used to deal with the tempting situation during preexposure is easily reactivated in a subsequent tempting situation and is reflected in a reduction of the eating goal, despite the presence of a temptation. Only actionable food temptations that exceed a critical level (Gilbert et al. 2004) will trigger self-control strategies that result in down-regulating the desire to eat upon exposure to a subsequent temptation.

In a third and final study, we investigated whether the goal activation findings can be confirmed in behavioral findings. In this study, we tested whether the inhibitory effect of prior exposure to actionable food temptations, on the desire to eat, also results in the elimination of the effect of rendering food more salient on subsequent consumption. We relied on the well-documented effects that appetizing food cues, such as scent (Fedoroff et al. 2003; Lambert and Neal 1992) and the convenience of the food offered (Wansink 2004), increase consumption. We used a food cue external to the subsequent consumption situation and one internal to the subsequent consumption situation to generalize the scope of the effect. Based on prior literature (Fedoroff et al. 2003; Wansink 2004), we expected these cues (scent and convenience) to increase consumption in the control condition because they increase the salience of the cued food. The typical effect of these food cues should be suppressed after preexposure to actionable food temptations, as it reduces the eating goal activation, but not after preexposure to nonactionable food temptations or no temptations. The consumption increasing effect of scent and convenience was validated. The consumed amount of M&Ms in the taste test was higher when participants smelled the scent of freshly baked brownies or when they could grab the M&Ms from a larger and more convenient surface. Moreover, the findings show that the preexposure to an actionable food temptation suppressed this consumption-increasing effect of scent and convenience.

In sum, these findings imply that the exposure to food temptations needs to exceed a certain critical level (Gilbert et al. 2004) that makes the food temptations threatening for the achievement of the long-term goal, in order to eventuate in self-control enhancement. Self-control actually takes place through the prevention of the activation of an eating goal, which leads to actual control of real consumption behavior in a subsequent taste test. In other words, as suggested by Fishbach, Friedman, and Kruglanski (2003), it might be better to expose consumers to real actionable food cues (i.e., hot nodes) instead of exposing consumers to concepts related to food inhibition (i.e., cool nodes) in order to enhance food intake control. Food cues are threatening to the long-term goal of being slim and healthy. When the critical level of this threat to the long-term goal is exceeded, the activation of the food restriction goal that resulted from exposure to these food cues will result in self-control-enhancing strategies by preventing the activation of the goal to eat. Nonactionable food temptations (e.g., pictures of foods as in ads) are not threatening and thus cannot exceed the critical level of threat. This might explain why the activation of hot nodes is more efficient in triggering self-control strategies, in comparison to the direct activation of cool nodes, as already suggested by Fishbach, Friedman, and Kruglanski (2003). Indeed, exposure to goal-related stimuli is not threatening. Therefore, the critical level is not exceeded and thus self-control strategies are not triggered.

SUBSEQUENT SELF-REGULATION IN CONSUMER DECISIONS IS ENHANCED FOR SIMILAR RESPONSE CONFLICTS

At first sight, these findings seem to conflict with the ego-depletion literature. This literature states that exerting self-control taxes a limited resource that is akin to energy or strength, thus reducing people's capacity to exert self-control in the next phase (Muraven and Baumeister 2000). According to this theory, the initial self-control exertion through resistance of the actionable food temptation should lead to self-control failure in a subsequent task that requires self-control (i.e., overconsumption in a taste test). We explored this apparent inconsistency with the ego-depletion literature (Dewitte, Bruyneel, and Geyskens 2009).

In this study, participants were, in a first phase, either tempted with attractive chocolates but asked not to eat any; exposed to an actionable food temptation (e.g., Baumeister et al. 1998); or asked to engage in a nondemanding task. In the second phase, half of the participants were asked to engage in a difficult anagram in which we measured their persistence in seconds (Baumeister et al. 1998). The other half of the participants was asked to engage in a taste test. Controlling food intake in a taste test of attractive sweets requires self-control (e.g., Baumeister et al. 1998, study 1; Shiv and Fedorikhin 1999; Vohs and Heatherton 2000). Backed by almost a decade of consistent findings, the self-control strength model unequivocally predicts that persistence on the anagram task as well as food intake control in the taste test will reduce in the group that was previously tempted and had to exert self-control to resist their urge to take a sweet, as compared to the control group. We found that the initial food intake restriction task was depleting and thus decreased self-control performance in a different domain, in this case reduced persistence on a subsequent anagram task, in line with predictions from the ego-depletion literature. For the taste test, however, we again found that the resistance to actionable food temptations resulted in self-control enhancement in a subsequent taste test. These results and the contradiction with ego-depletion can be explained by the cognitive control theory (Botvinick et al. 2001). This theory states that performance on tasks involving conflict improves through temporal adaptation of one's behavior to highly demanding situations. This adaptation temporarily results in a more focused, conservative approach and thus an increase in task performance, which spills over to a subsequent task with a similar response conflict. At the same time, this temporary sustained activation of the rules necessary to perform the task deteriorates task performance when the subsequent task involves a different response conflict. These results suggest that self-control strength theory (Muraven and Baumeister 2000) seems to apply only when the consecutive self-control tasks involve different response conflicts. When two similar self-control tasks follow each other, adjustment to the response conflict in the first task seems to enhance self-control performance in a subsequent similar self-control task. This implies that the exertion of self-control is not always detrimental to subsequent self-control performance.

In contrast, self-control exertion in one conflict situation enhances self-control performance in a subsequent self-control-requiring situation if these consecutive self-control tasks involve a similar response conflict.

SUMMARY AND LIMITATIONS OF FINDINGS

Taken together, the findings of our research (Dewitte, Bruyneel, and Geyskens 2009; Geyskens et al. 2008) suggest that when consumers are confronted with a self-control threat that exceeds the critical level of threat, such as exposure to actionable food temptations, the consumer's focus will be on successfully performing this self-control-demanding task. The results of our studies show that consumers adapt to this self-control conflict by down-regulating their desire to eat. When a subsequent task involves a similar response conflict, the previously initiated adaptation to that response conflict will enable performance on the second task. Indeed, when a subsequent taste test arises, the down-regulation of the desire to eat helps in preventing consumption from the effects of food cues that make the food more salient, like the scent of freshly baked brownies. Exerting self-control in a situation that involves a certain response conflict appears to facilitate self-control in a subsequent situation that involves a highly similar response conflict. More specifically, inhibiting food intake in a first phase enhances food intake control in a subsequent taste test.

It has been shown that consumers do ration the purchase quantities of vice products in order to solve their self-control problem (Wertenbroch 1998). They do so because they believe that limiting the stock of vice products reduces the temptation to overconsume vices. Together with our findings, this suggests that people might paradoxically end up consuming more vice products when they ration the purchased quantity of these vice products. In other words, buying less and thus having fewer vices at home might not activate the self-control strategies needed to deal with these vices, whereas buying and having a lot of vices might do so.

We note that we do not claim that food temptations never lead to loss of self-control. Numerous researchers (Chandon and Wansink 2002; Fedoroff, Polivy, and Herman 2003; Lambert and Neal 1992; Painter, Wansink, and Hieggelke 2002; Schachter 1971; Shiv and Fedorikhin 2002; Wansink 1994, 1996) have showed that consumers lose their self-control when food is made more salient. Our contribution consists of providing evidence that salient actionable food cues can lead to self-control enhancement when the self-control conflict that these cues create exceeds the critical level of threat. When the threat exceeds this critical level, the conflict will be detected and self-control strategies to deal with this conflict will be recruited (Botvinick et al. 2001). In other words, this suggests that prior exposure to actionable food cues that exceed the critical level activates control strategies that prepare the consumer to deal with subsequent temptations. At this point, however, it is not clear how this critical level is determined, which brings us to the discussion of future research opportunities.

IMPLICATIONS AND FUTURE RESEARCH

The findings suggest some interesting ideas for future research. For example, it might be interesting to find out how and when the critical level is reached. How threatening should the temptation be in order to trigger self-control strategies? Or is it necessary to have two consecutive food temptations and thus two consecutive self-control conflicts to achieve the effects? In this view, it could also be interesting to compare the effects of food temptations differing in salience, namely a few candies versus a lot of candies. Such a study might reveal the required amount of food that is required to exceed the critical level.

We also showed that the exposure to actionable food temptations prevents consumers from increasing consumption when they are exposed to convenient food cues or an appetizing scent. In the same vein, prior research showed that larger package size could increase consumption (Wansink 1996), as can the increasing size of portion servings in kitchens and in restaurants (Rolls, Morris, and Roe 2002). Indeed, portions and package sizes have grown larger over the past thirty years (Nielsen and Popkin 2003; Young and Nestle 2002). Moreover, people rely on visual cues or rules of thumb (such as eating until a bowl is empty) to determine the appropriate amount to eat. As a result of this rule of thumb, the amount of food on a plate or in a bowl implicitly suggests the "normal" or "appropriate" amount to consume (Fisher, Rolls, and Birch 2003; Kahn and Wansink 2004). Consequently, we often eat a lot without realizing it, thereby doing our part to promote the current obesity epidemic. The consumption-increasing effect of the portion sizes should not be underestimated, as Wansink, Painter, and North (2005) show that people use their eyes to count calories and not their stomachs. People consumed dramatically more from refilling soup bowls than from normal soup bowls, implying that the amount of food on a plate or bowl influences the consumption norm independent of people's monitoring process that keeps track of how much they are eating. These visual cues increase the amount eventually consumed. It seems interesting to explore whether a certain portion size can exceed the critical level and in this way curb the consumed amount.

In addition, it might be possible that the self-control conflict caused by the threat of exposure to actionable food cues helps to control food intake on a subsequent consumption occasion, even when big portions are offered. Recent research by Coelho do Vale, Pieters, and Zeelenberg (2008) supports this possibility by showing that consumers' belief that smaller packages, which are becoming more prevalent very recently (e.g., Ben and Jerry's ice cream and Pringles and Lay's chips are now being offered in small, single-serve packages), help them in regulating consumption leads them to misjudge small packages as not threatening. As a consequence, the small package does not elicit a self-control conflict between the desire to indulge and overarching goals like losing weight, and thus the strategies to deal with self-control conflicts are not activated. The small package formats fly under the critical level of threat, whereas large package formats are more readily detected as a threat to self-control.

Another opportunity that deserves further investigation is the question whether the exposure to unhealthy food cues activates a general goal to eat or whether this craving is limited to the food cue itself. In other words, what is the role of the similarity between the food in the two phases, and the effect of the two types of temptations (actionable and nonactionable)? In our studies, similarity between the food of phase 1 and phase 2 was high but not perfect. However, the slight difference between the temptation and the consumption domain testifies to the relevance and strength of our effects. Indeed, exposure to a food temptation, actionable or nonactionable, influences the consumed amount of any tempting (unhealthy) food, even if it is dissimilar from the initial temptation, offered at a later point in time. The fact that the effects were obtained for slightly differing domains implies that our findings would in all probability also be obtained if the domains were identical. However, we are less certain when dissimilarity would be higher (e.g., chocolate and cake, chocolate and pizza, or even chocolate and Coke). We know from previous research (Fedoroff, Polivy, and Herman 2003; Lambert and Neal 1992) that exposure to the appetizing scent of food induces craving, liking, and consumption of the cued food. However, if the offered food (i.e., pizza or cookies) differed more strongly from the cued food (i.e., cookies or pizza), the effects were not found. These findings imply that exposing consumers to a nonactionable pizza temptation would lead them to consume more pizza-related food, but not more pizza-unrelated food, because the initial nonactionable pizza temptation induces a desire to eat pizza. For nonactionable temptations, then, high similarity seems to be a requirement. However, for actionable temptations, prior literature is less clear about the role of similarity between the food items in the two phases. Exposure to an actionable pizza temptation might help consumers to control the consumption of pizza-related, as well as pizza-unrelated, food because of the general initial activation of strategies to solve the self-control conflict. This initial activation pushes consumers beyond the critical level of threat by the second self-control conflict, even if this concerns a food cue unrelated to the first food cue.

Another opportunity for future research is to explore to what extent the effect of the actionable temptation depends on the success of the food restriction. Some research suggests that tasting a little bit of a food temptation could successfully inhibit the urge to eat for binge eaters (Jansen 1998). As a result, small transgressions against the personal norm of rational food intake may push the consumer across the critical level and in this way lead to the enhancement of food intake control. However, the disinhibition effect suggests that small transgressions may break down inhibition and hence food intake control. When people exceed the caloric limit they set for themselves for any given day, they tend to stop restraining their food intake for that specific day and overindulge because the day is already lost—also called the "what-the-hell" effect (Cochran and Tesser 1996; Polivy and Herman 1985). If consumers succumb to the actionable food temptation, they might overconsume the food offered at a later point in time because they already lost control by consuming the food temptation.

Related to the effect of the success of the food restriction, it would be worthwhile to explore the role of the awareness of an earlier successful self-control attempt. In other words, is it necessary that consumers are aware that they acquired self-control in the first phase and in this way might be motivated to continue this route to success? It is for example possible that making consumers mindful or conscious of ongoing events (Deikman 1982) by explicitly giving them feedback that they were successful might be enough in triggering self-control strategies in a subsequent self-control conflict.

We suggest that tasting a small amount of the actionable food temptation does not lead to self-control loss in a subsequent consumption opportunity. We assume that the consumption of a small amount of the food temptation should at least be as threatening as having the opportunity to consume the food. This is also consistent with cognitive control theory, which states that whenever a response is successful in a certain situation, reinforcement signals increase the corresponding pattern of activity by strengthening connections between the control strategy that is activated by that response (Botvinick et al. 2001; Miller and Cohen 2001). Because of this strengthened pathway, task-relevant responses and thus control of the conflict situation may gradually become automatic (e.g., riding a bike; Norman and Shallice 1986). This would imply that training in successfully resisting strongly tempting food stimuli might be a very effective strategy to untangle the obesity epidemic.

It is of high importance for public policy-makers and marketers to know under which conditions food temptations (dis)enhance self-control. This information could be used for the development of more efficient strategies to combat the obesity epidemic. For example, the results show that exposure to strongly tempting food cues whose resistance requires self-control might help consumers resist them more effectively than safeguarding consumers from these threatening temptations (e.g., by offering low-fat snack products). This implies that the increased consumption of low-fat snacks (Wansink and Chandon 2006) could be explained by the fact that they fly under the radar of self-regulatory surveillance and are consumed immediately without major thought. Moreover, because consumers believe that the more vice products they store at home, the more vice products they will consume (Wertenbroch 1998), they therefore ration the purchase quantities of vice. However, they might not ration snack products that are not perceived as a threat to their self-control, such as low-fat snacks. This implies that low-fat versions of unhealthy snacks may be more readily stockpiled at home, thus possibly encouraging overconsumption of these low-fat snacks. Taken together, public policy should consider strategies that increase, instead of decrease, the strength of and exposure to unhealthy food temptations. However, as suggested in the ideas for future research, the exact boundary conditions of these effects need further exploration before concrete guidelines for public policy can be formulated.

In sum, the findings of our studies suggest that exposure to strongly tempting food cues whose resistance requires self-control might help consumers resist them more effectively than safeguarding consumers from these threatening temptations.

REFERENCES

Aitman, Timothy J. 2003. "Genetic Medicine and Obesity." *New England Journal of Medicine*, 348 (21), 2138–2140.

Baumeister, Roy F., Ellen Bratslavsky, Mark Muraven, and Dianne M. Tice. 1998. "Ego Depletion: Is the Active Self a Limited Resource?" *Journal of Personality and Social Psychology*, 74, 1252–1265.

Botvinick, Matthew M., Todd S. Braver, Deanna M. Barch, Cameron S. Carter, and Jonathan D. Cohen. 2001. "Conflict Monitoring and Cognitive Control." *Psychological Review*, 108, 624–652.

Chandon, Pierre, and Brian Wansink. 2002. "When Are Stockpiled Products Consumed Faster? A Convenience-Salience Framework of Postpurchase Consumption Incidence and Quantity." *Journal of Marketing Research*, 39, 321–335.

Cochran, Winona, and Abraham Tesser. 1996. "The 'What the Hell' Effect: Some Effects of Goal Proximity and Goal Framing on Performance." In *Striving and Feeling: Interactions among Goals, Affect, and Self-Regulation*, ed. Leonard. L. Martin and Abraham Tesser, 99–120. Mahwah, NJ: Erlbaum.

Coelho do Vale, Rita, Rik Pieters, and Marcel Zeelenberg. 2008. "Flying Under the Radar: Perverse Package Size Effects on Consumption Self-Regulation." *Journal of Consumer Research*, 35, 380–390.

Critser, Greg. 2003. *Fat Land: How Americans Became the Fattest People in the World.* New York: Mariner/Houghton Mifflin.

Cutler, David M., Edward L. Glaeser, and Jess M. Shapiro. 2003. "Why Have Americans Become More Obese?" *Journal of Economic Perspectives*, 17 (3), 93–118.

Deikman, Arthur J. 1982. *The Observing Self.* Boston: Beacon Press.

Dewitte, Siegfried, Sabrina Bruyneel, and Kelly Geyskens. 2009. "Self-Regulating Enhances Self-Regulation in Subsequent Consumer Decisions Involving Similar Response Conflicts." *Journal of Consumer Research*, 36 (3) (October).

Dietz, William. 1991. "Factors Associated with Childhood Obesity." *Nutrition*, 7 (4), 290–291.

Fedoroff, Ingrid, Janet Polivy, and Peter C. Herman. 2003. "The Specificity of Restrained versus Unrestrained Eaters' Responses to Food Cues: General Desire to Eat, or Craving for the Cued Food?" *Appetite*, 41 (1), 7–13.

Fishbach, Ayelet, Rohn S. Friedman, and Arie W. Kruglanski. 2003. "Leading Us Not Unto Temptation: Momentary Allurements Elicit Overriding Goal Activation." *Journal of Personality and Social Psychology*, 84: 296–309.

Fishbach, Ayelet, and James Y. Shah. 2006. "Self-Control in Action: Implicit Dispositions Toward Goals and Away from Temptations." *Journal of Personality and Social Psychology*, 90 (5), 820–832.

Fisher, Jennifer Orlet, Barbara J. Rolls, and Leann L. Birch. 2003. "Children's Bite Size and Intake of an Entree Are Greater with Large Portions than with Age-Appropriate or Self-Selected Portions." *American Journal of Clinical Nutrition*, 77, 1164–1170.

Geyskens, Kelly, Siegfried Dewitte, Mario Pandelaere, and Luk Warlop. 2008. "Tempt Me Just a Little Bit More: The Effect of Prior Food Temptation Actionability on Goal Activation and Consumption." *Journal of Consumer Research*, 35, 600–610.

Gilbert, Daniel T., Matthew D. Lieberman, Carey K. Morewedge, and Timothy D. Wilson. 2004. "The Peculiar Longevity of Things Not So Bad." *Psychological Science*, 15 (1), 14–19.

Gilbert, Daniel T., Elizabeth C. Pinel, Timothy D. Wilson, Stephen J. Blumberg, and Thalia P. Wheatley. 1998. "Immune Neglect: A Source of Durability Bias in Affective Forecasting." *Journal of Personality and Social Psychology*, 75, 617–638.

Hoch, Stephen J., and George F. Loewenstein. 1991. "Time-Inconsistent Preferences and Consumer Self-Control." *Journal of Consumer Research*, 17 (4), 492–507.

Jansen, Anita. 1998. "A Learning Model of Binge Eating: Cue Reactivity and Cue Exposure." *Behavior Research and Therapy*, 36, 257–272.
Kahn, Barbara E., and Brian Wansink. 2004. "The Influence of Assortment Structure on Perceived Variety and Consumption Quantities." *Journal of Consumer Research*, 30, 581–596.
Lambert, Kelly G., and Tara Neal. 1992. "Food-Related Stimuli Increase Desire to Eat in Hungry and Satiated Human Subjects." *Current Psychology*, 10 (4), 297–304.
Metcalfe, Janet, and Walter Mischel. 1999. "A Hot/Cool-System Analysis of Delay of Gratification: Dynamics and Willpower." *Psychological Review*, 106, 3–19.
Miller, Earl K., and Jonathan D. Cohen. 2001. "An Integrative Theory of Prefrontal Cortex Function." *Annual Review of Neuroscience*, 24, 167–202.
Mitka, Mike. 2003. "Economist Takes Aim at 'Big Fat' U.S. Lifestyle." *Journal of the American Medical Association*, 289 (1), 33–34.
Muraven, Mark, and Roy F. Baumeister. 2000. "Self-Regulation and Depletion of Limited Resources: Does Self-Control Resemble a Muscle?" *Psychological Bulletin*, 12, 247–259.
Nestle, Marion. 2002. *Food Politics: How the Food Industry Influences Nutrition and Health.* Berkeley: University of California Press.
Nielsen, Samara Joy, and Barry M. Popkin. 2003. "Patterns and Trends in Food Portion Sizes, 1977–1998." *Journal of the American Medical Association*, 289 (4), 450–453.
Norman, Donald A., and Tim Shallice. 1986. "Attention to Action. Willed and Automatic Control of Behavior." In *Consciousness and Self-regulation*, ed. Richard J. Davidson, Gary E. Schwartz, and David Shapiro, 1–18. New York: Plenum Press.
Painter, James E., Brian Wansink, and Julie Hieggelke. 2002. "How Visibility and Convenience Influence Candy Consumption." *Appetite*, 38 (3), 237–238.
Polivy, Janet, and Peter C. Herman. 1985. "Dieting as a Problem in Behavioral Medicine." In *Advances in Behavioral Medicine*, ed. Edward Katkin and Stephen Manuck, 1–37. New York: JAI.
Raynor, Hollie A., and Leonard H. Epstein. 2001. "Dietary Variety, Energy Regulation, and Obesity." *Psychological Bulletin*, 127, 325–341.
Rolls, Barbara J., Erin L. Morris, and Liane S. Roe. 2002. "Portion Size of Food Affects Energy Intake in Normal-Weight and Overweight Men and Women." *American Journal of Clinical Nutrition*, 76, 1207–1213.
Schachter, Stanley. 1971. "Some Extraordinary Facts about Obese Humans and Rats." *American Psychologist*, 26, 129–144.
Scott, Maura L., Stephen M. Nowlis, Naomi Mandel, and Andrea C. Morales. 2008. "The Effect of Reduced Food Sizes and Packages on the Consumption Behavior of Restrained Eaters and Unrestrained Eaters." *Journal of Consumer Research*, 35 (October), 391–405.
Shiv, Baba, and Alexander Fedorikhin. 1999. "Heart and Mind in Conflict: The Interplay of Affect and Cognition in Consumer Decision Making." *Journal of Consumer Research*, 26, 278–292.
———. 2002. "Spontaneous Versus Controlled Influences of Stimulus-Based Affect on Choice Behavior." *Organizational Behavior and Human Decision Processes*, 87 (2), 342–370.
Snell, Jason, Brian J. Gibbs, and Carol Varey. 1995. "Intuitive Hedonics: Consumer Beliefs about the Dynamics of Liking." *Journal of Consumer Psychology*, 4, 33–60.
Tardoff, Michael G. 2002. "Obesity by Choice: The Powerful Influence of Nutrient Availability on Nutrient Intake." *American Journal of Physiology* 51 (5), 1536–1539.
Vohs, Kathleen D., and Todd F. Heatherton. 2000. "Self-Regulatory Failure: A Resource-Depletion Approach." *Psychological Science*, 11 (3), 249–254.
Wansink, Brian. 1994. "Antecedents and Mediators of Eating Bouts." *Family and Consumer Sciences Research Journal*, 23 (2), 166–182.

———. 1996. "Can Package Size Accelerate Usage Volume?" *Journal of Marketing*, 60 (3), 1–14.

———. 2004. "Environmental Factors That Increase The Food Intake and Consumption Volume of Unknowing Consumers." *Annual Review of Nutrition*, 24, 455–79.

Wansink, Brian, and Pierre Chandon. 2006. "Can 'Low-Fat' Nutrition Labels Lead to Obesity?" *Journal of Marketing Research*, 43, 605–617.

Wansink, Brian, James E. Painter, and Jill North. 2005. "Bottomless Bowls: Why Visual Cues of Portion Size May Influence Food Intake." *Obesity Research*, 13, 93–100.

Wertenbroch, Klaus. 1998. "Consumption Self-Control by Rationing Purchase Quantities of Virtue and Vice." *Marketing Science*, 17, 317–337.

World Health Organization. 2006. Obesity and Overweight. www.who.int/mediacentre/factsheets/fs311/en/index.html.

Young, Lisa R., and Marion Nestle. 2002. "The Contribution of Expanding Portion Sizes to the U.S. Obesity Epidemic." *American Journal of Public Health*, 92, 246–249.

CHAPTER 6

THINKING ABOUT HEALTH AND OBESITY

How Consumers' Mental Experiences Influence Health Judgments

IAN SKURNIK, CAROLYN YOON, AND NORBERT SCHWARZ

Obesity is a global public health problem that cuts across age, race, social class, and culture. The causes of the international trend toward obesity are complex, and combating the condition requires changing public policy, the consumer's social environment, and the health behavior of individual consumers. In this chapter, we focus on a particular kind of influence on consumer health: consumers' own subjective mental experience while thinking about health-related issues. Because consumers cannot acquire, retain, and process all the information that they see, they often turn to their own subjective mental experiences as a source of information. For example, a statement can "feel" familiar or unfamiliar, a memory can come to mind easily or with effort, and printed messages can seem easy or hard to read (for a review, see Schwarz et al. 2007). We review how mental experiences such as these systematically influence consumers' assessments of their own health behavior and risk status, and their judgments about whether information is true or false. Throughout this chapter we suggest ways for health communicators to improve their message design and execution, and to avoid or minimize some systematic consumer biases.

OBESITY, HEALTH, AND CONSUMER DECISION-MAKING

By recent estimates, 300 million people across the world are obese, and over 1 billion people are overweight (Edwards and Roberts 2009). A worldwide trend toward obesity continues, and population weight has been shifting toward the heavier end of the distribution (Bell, Ge, and Popkin 2001). According to the U.S. Centers for Disease Control and Prevention (CDC), nearly one-third of adults and one-sixth of children in the United States are classified as obese, tripling the rate of obesity in the United States since 1980. The effects and consequences of obesity are serious and wide-ranging. Obese individuals and their families experience diminished health and fitness, and increased risk of related disease (especially cardiovascular diseases and type 2 diabetes). Care for obese people is also expensive: obese people are much more costly to treat than people of normal weight, and over the five years ending in 2001, obesity-related diseases accounted for over one-quarter of the increase in U.S. medical costs (CDC 2009). The obesity trend has even been linked to global warming, through increased greenhouse gas emissions from heightened consumption, production, and transportation of food (Edwards and Roberts 2009).

Combating obesity, like other social marketing and public health efforts, is difficult. The "product" being promoted is not a traditional good or service, but a change in behavior, environment, or policy. Public health messages that target individual consumers usually try to convince consumers to give up a current behavior, to replace a current behavior with an alternative, or to refrain from a behavior in the future. Even if consumers embrace the advocated behavior in the abstract, they may consider it unimportant or intrusive, and it may oppose a long-established behavior that they value. In response to these impediments to behavior change, many public health campaigns aim to reinforce healthy behaviors positively through education or reminders, in the hope that providing comprehensive and accurate information will lead consumers to change their unhealthy behaviors. Of course, it is critical that consumers base their health choices on correct data. But merely conveying detailed health facts and advice to consumers ignores the way they acquire and use that information. As we review in more detail below, consumers' judgments and decisions are not only a function of *what* is on their minds—that is, the declarative information they attend to; instead, the subjective experiences that accompany thinking are informative in their own right and influence the conclusions consumers draw and the decisions they make.

For many consumers, the underlying causes of obesity are linked to mundane daily behaviors and choices. No one consciously makes a plan to adopt a diet that will be unhealthy over the long run. Instead, an unhealthy diet often results from small, repeated choices in consumption whose effects accumulate over time, such as deciding what to eat in what portion size, choosing what leisure activities to engage in or abstain from, and assessing one's own risk of unwanted consequences from any particular behavior. In addition, for any given decision, consumers often have access to a wide range of health information from a variety of sources, such as health professionals, websites, advertisements, friends, and television dramas. To make optimal decisions, consumers face several daunting challenges: sorting through the information, remembering it later on, and putting it to use. During the course of their daily lives, we argue, consumers often make these small choices rapidly and without detailed reflection or reliance on background research and records, conditions that give considerable weight to momentary gut reactions and intuitive decision-making at the expense of more analytic considerations.

Next, we address how mental experiences influence consumers' health-related judgments and decisions when they ask themselves certain questions: Am I at risk?

Is the remedy realistic and feasible? Am I confident that changing my behavior will help? Subsequently we turn to the implications of mental experiences for the design of information campaigns and review how mental experiences influence recipients' assessment of the truth-value of the information presented to them.

IS THIS RISKY?

Assessing the Implications of One's Own Behavior

Suppose that two men are considering the extent to which they are personally at risk for heart disease, a potential consequence of long-term obesity. One man recalls three risk-increasing behaviors, and the other recalls eight similar behaviors. Which of the two is likely to feel more at risk for heart disease? No one has perfect and instant recall of all their past behaviors, so the logical answer seems to be that the man who listed eight reasons will feel more at risk; after all, he has more evidence to support the conclusion. In fact, the answer is often the opposite: the man who recalled three behaviors will feel most at risk. The reason for this counterintuitive judgment has to do with the mental experiences that accompany retrieving information from memory. When the information comes to mind relatively easily, as it does when listing just three behaviors, the experience of ease is taken to imply that the recalled behaviors are relatively frequent, recent, or representative (a bias known as the availability heuristic; Schwarz et al. 1991; Tversky and Kahneman 1973). In other words, the risk judgment did not depend solely on what information came to mind, but also on the mental experience that accompanied its coming to mind.

To illustrate this process, Rothman and Schwarz (1998) asked young men to remember either three or eight behaviors that they had engaged in that either increased or decreased their risk for heart disease. (A pretesting procedure had already established that most people found recalling three such behaviors easy and eight hard.) After this memory task, the men reported their personal perceived risk of heart disease and their intentions to change their behavior. If the amount of behavior that the men could recall was the main driver of their risk assessment, then they should feel more at risk the more risk-increasing behaviors they recalled, and less at risk the more risk-decreasing behaviors they recalled. However, the opposite pattern would be expected if the men based their judgments on the relative ease of recalling their behaviors: the men should feel more at risk when they recall fewer risk-increasing behaviors, and less at risk when recalling fewer risk-decreasing behaviors.

An operative assumption is that risk assessments of this type are constructed in a somewhat ad hoc fashion. That is, individuals may not have a stable and chronically accessible assessment of their own risk for heart disease, so they construct a risk assessment in response to a request for one; their assessment is likely to be influenced by information that is available at the moment and seems relevant. Following this assumption, Rothman and Schwarz separated the responses of men

Figure 6.1   **Ease of Retrieval and Perceived Risk Vulnerability**

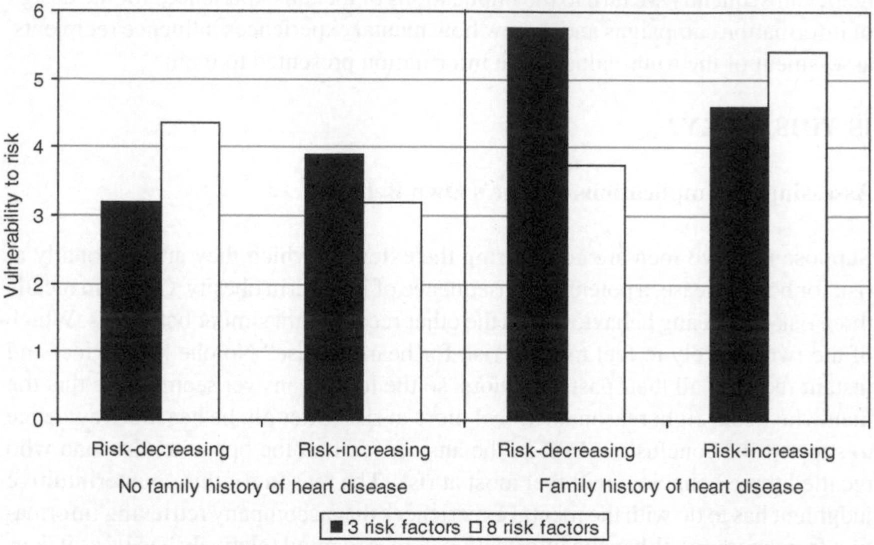

Source: Adapted from Rothman and Schwarz (1998).

who had a family history of heart disease from those who did not. Men without a family history of heart disease may be less motivated to think carefully about their responses and the implications of their behaviors. If so, these men would tend to rely on the more heuristic strategy of drawing inferences based on ease of recall. In contrast, men with a family history of the disease may think more carefully about the implications of the behaviors they recall; these men would be likely to rely on the content of what they recalled and place less weight on the ease of its retrieval.

Figure 6.1 shows the findings for risk assessments, which conform to the predictions outlined above. The left panel shows risk assessments for men with no family history of heart disease. These respondents concluded that they were at *less* risk after listing three risk-decreasing behaviors than after listing eight such behaviors. Similarly, they felt they were *more* at risk after listing three than eight risk-increasing behaviors. These findings are consistent with the explanation that the men were relying on the ease of recalling their behaviors, over and above the implications of the amount of recalled behavior. The right panel shows results for men who had a family history of heart disease. These men inferred that they were at a lower risk after listing eight risk-decreasing behaviors than after listing three of these behaviors, and at a higher risk after listing eight rather than three risk-increasing behaviors. This pattern of findings for men with a family history of heart disease matches the notion that they relied on the content of what was recalled over and above the ease of its retrieval.

Figure 6.2 shows results for the behavior change measure. Men with no family

Figure 6.2 **Ease of Retrieval and Perceived Need to Change Behavior**

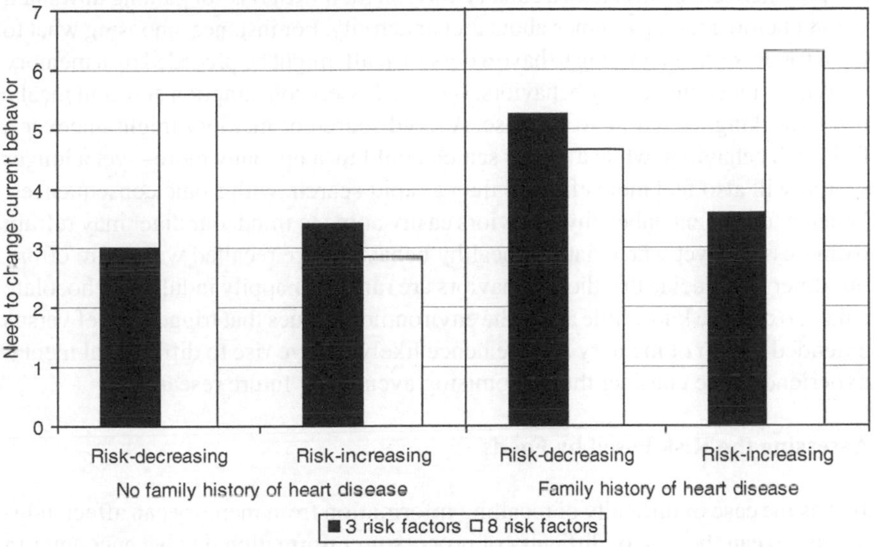

Source: Adapted from Rothman and Schwarz (1998).

history were *less* concerned about changing their own behavior after listing fewer (3 vs. 8) risk-decreasing behaviors, and reported *greater* intentions to change after listing fewer (3 vs. 8) risk-increasing behaviors. As with the risk assessments, men who had a family history showed the opposite pattern: their perceived need for behavior change was reduced when they listed more risk-decreasing behaviors, or when they listed more risk-increasing behaviors.

The overall pattern of results illustrates the impact of ease of recall on judgments, and highlights the circumstances where mental experiences such as ease of retrieval are likely to play a role. Men *with* a family history of heart disease, which is a major risk factor for the disease, made judgments in line with the implications of the content and amount of behavior that they recalled. In contrast, men *without* a family history of heart disease, who were less motivated to reflect extensively on the implications of their behaviors, seemed to rely on their mental experiences as a source of information that qualified the implications of what they recalled. In general, research on mental experiences suggests that people are more likely to rely on mental experiences in judgment as a heuristic strategy: that is, when their motivation is low, they are under time pressure, or they are otherwise unable or unwilling to process information extensively. When people are highly motivated and able to process information extensively and make choices in a compensatory fashion, the role of mental experiences is minimized or eliminated. The impact of mental experiences can also be eliminated when the relevance or source of the experience is called into question (Schwarz et al. 2007).

Ease of recall can play a role in many behavioral choices relating to obesity. People often reflect, in at least a cursory way, on their own risk for gaining unwanted weight before making a choice about diet or activity. For instance, choosing what to have for dessert, or choosing to have a dessert at all, might be preceded by a memory search for recent unhealthy behaviors, such as dessert consumption at recent meals, prior snacking, or failing to exercise. A rapid search of memory might uncover a few such behaviors, while a longer search could turn up many more—yet a longer search will also feel more effortful than a rapid search, with ironic consequences. When a few recent unhealthy behaviors easily come to mind, our diner may refrain from dessert—yet when many unhealthy behaviors are recalled with more effort, our diner may decide that those behaviors are rare and happily indulge in chocolate cake. To date we know little about the environmental cues that trigger a brief versus extended search of memory and are hence likely to give rise to differential mental experiences. We consider this a promising avenue for future research.

Assessing the Risk Posed by Foods

Just as the ease or difficulty of recalling information from memory can affect judgments, so can the ease or difficulty of processing information that we encounter in the environment. In general, familiar information that we have seen many times before is easier to perceive, recognize, learn, and remember than novel information that we encounter for the first time. This (correct) observation often gives rise to the reverse (and often erroneous) inference: if it is easy to process, it must be familiar. Accordingly, people perceive information that is easy to process as more familiar than information that is difficult to process—even when the mental experience results merely from an easy- or difficult-to-read print font or the ease with which a word can be pronounced (for a review see Schwarz 2004). This impression of familiarity has important implications for risk perception. As many researchers have observed, familiar hazards are perceived as less dangerous than unfamiliar ones, and consumers' concern about a given hazard decreases as its familiarity increases (for a review see Breakwell 2007).

Studies by Song and Schwarz (2009) illustrate this relationship. They asked consumers to estimate the health risk posed by various (fictitious) food additives. To manipulate how easily consumers could process information about the food additives, the researchers gave them easy-to-pronounce (e.g., Magnalroxate) or hard-to-pronounce names (e.g., Hnegripitrom). Additives that were hard to pronounce were rated as more novel and more hazardous than easy-to-pronounce additives. Such findings suggest that easy-to-pronounce names have a familiar ring to them that makes it less likely that a product is considered hazardous.

Other research (e.g., Song and Schwarz 2008a) further showed that familiar information is less likely to be critically scrutinized than unfamiliar information— and an easy- versus difficult-to-read print font is sufficient to trigger different perceptions of familiarity, resulting in differential levels of scrutiny. In combination with the risk findings, this observation suggests that mental experiences of ease or difficulty may influence how people think about their food. When background knowledge about a food item is low and new information about the food is easy to process, the food item may not only seem more familiar and less hazardous, but also be less likely to become the topic of extensive scrutiny to begin with. From this perspective, familiar foods, ingredients, or additives may pose a higher health risk than unfamiliar foods because they are less likely to become the subject of thoughtful attention. Moreover, contextual variables that make food seem less familiar may encourage more thoughtful eating.

On the other hand, when background knowledge about a food item is high, the effect of ease of processing is harder to predict. In some cases, people may ignore ease of processing in favor of the more extensive processing or recall that arises when rendering a judgment. If so, then ease of recall or processing would have relatively little influence on judgments (see the men with family history of heart disease in Rothman and Schwarz 1998). However, if people interpret ease of processing as familiarity due to their established subject-area expertise, they may feel more confident in an ease-based impression and may feel less need for a more thorough search of memory. Under such circumstances, ease of processing or recall would play a relatively larger role in judgment. These possibilities await empirical testing.

HOW HARD WILL IT BE TO DO THE RIGHT THING?

Prior research suggests that self-efficacy and motivation are generally predictive of health-promoting behaviors (e.g., Bandura 2004; Kelly, Zyzanski, and Alemagno 1991; Strecher et al. 1986), as are appropriate goal-setting (e.g., Cullen, Baranowski, and Smith 2001; Strecher et al. 1995) and self-regulatory processes (e.g., Carver and Scheier 1998; Schwarzer 1999). These lines of research reflect the view that in order for consumers to be successful in changing their health-related behaviors, the behaviors must be planned, initiated, and maintained. Unfortunately, strict adherence to health-promoting behaviors is difficult, which often leads to disengagement and failure.

Thus common sense suggests that people may be more likely to adopt healthy behaviors when the required change is easy rather than difficult to implement. Supporting this everyday experience, numerous studies show that high perceived effort is a major impediment to behavior change, from adopting an exercise routine (e.g., DuCharme and Brawley 1995) to changing one's diet (e.g., Sparks, Guthrie, and Shepherd 1997). At present, it is poorly understood how people estimate the effort involved in novel and unfamiliar behavior. It seems likely, however, that one strategy of effort estimation involves mental simulation: when we want to know how effortful something is, we may run a mental simulation to see how it feels. If so, we may conclude that the behavior change requires tremendous effort when the new behavior is difficult to imagine, but much less effort when it is easy

Figure 6.3   **Exercise Instructions**

Easy to Read

> Tuck your chin into your chest, and then lift your chin upward as far as possible. 6–10 reps.

Hard to Read

> *Tuck your chin into your chest, and then lift your chin upward as far as possible. 6–10 reps.*

Source: From Song and Schwarz (2008b).

to imagine. Studies by Song and Schwarz (2008b) provide empirical support for this possibility and highlight, once again, how minor incidental influences can profoundly affect people's judgments.

In one study, Song and Schwarz (2008b) asked people to read instructions for a new exercise routine. The instructions were printed in a font that was either easy or hard to read (see Figure 6.3 for an example). People who read the exercise instructions in an easy-to-read font estimated that the exercise would take less time to complete, would flow more naturally, and would be more enjoyable than people who read the same instructions in a difficult-to-read font. Not surprisingly, the former participants were also more willing than the latter to make the exercise part of their daily routine.

These and related findings (Song and Schwarz 2008b) illustrate that people misread the difficulty of reading as indicative of the difficulty of doing: the harder instructions are to read and the harder a behavior is to imagine, the more effortful it seems and the lower is the motivation to engage in it. Accordingly, variables that facilitate easy processing of health information—such as print fonts, layouts, and color contrast—may have a profound influence on recipients' willingness to adopt a behavioral recommendation. Future research may fruitfully explore the power of these variables in naturalistic settings.

CAN I TRUST THE INFORMATION OFFERED?

As seen in our discussion of risk judgments, information that is easy to process is perceived as less novel and more familiar (e.g., Song and Schwarz 2009). This gives rise to the impression that one must have heard or seen it before, or why else would it seem familiar? This association between ease of processing and perceived familiarity has many important consequences, from perceptions of risk

(Song and Schwarz 2009) to perceptions of social consensus and truth, to which we turn next.

Perceptions of Truth

As Festinger (1954) noted, when the objective truth is difficult to assess, we often rely on social consensus as a heuristic cue: when many people believe it, there is probably something to it. If so, any variable that makes a statement seem more familiar should also increase the likelihood that the statement is accepted as true. Empirically, this is the case.

For example, Skurnik and Monin (2010) had people read a series of rhyming and nonrhyming novel ad slogans (e.g., for a brand of olive oil, people saw either "The cooking aid that nature made" or "The cooking aid that nature crafted"). Rhyming slogans, compared to their nonrhyming counterparts, were rated as more familiar, despite the fact that all brands and slogans had been created for the research study. More important, the rhyming slogans were also rated as more believable than their nonrhyming counterparts. That is, people inferred from the ease of processing that resulted from rhyme structure that the statement was familiar as well as true. Similarly, Reber and Schwarz (1999) observed that a given statement was more likely to be accepted as true when the color contrast of its print font made it easy rather than difficult to read.

A particularly powerful variable that increases ease of processing and perceived familiarity and truth is actual repetition: the more often we hear a statement, the more familiar it becomes, the more we assume that others agree (e.g., Weaver et al. 2007) and the more likely we are to accept it as true (e.g., Festinger 1954). This is the case even when all repetitions are simply due to a single repetitive voice. For example, Weaver et al. (2007) had people read information from a single communicator, who repeated some statements many times. Later, people were asked to estimate how widely the conveyed beliefs were shared. The more often a statement was presented, the higher the consensus was perceived for the statement, even though the only source of the statement was a single communicator. Numerous other studies (for a review see Schwarz et al. 2007) found that repeating the same statement reliably increases its perceived truth (e.g., Begg, Anas, and Farinacci 1992; Hasher, Goldstein, and Toppino 1977) unless the specific context suggests that familiar statements are probably not credible (Skurnik, Schwarz, and Winkielman 2000; Unkelbach 2007).

In addition, people may rely on ease of processing to infer the credibility of the communicator: when the message sounds familiar and true, the communicator appears more credible. This inference reverses the usual connection between credible sources and the information they convey. For example, Fragale and Heath (2004) had people read statements such as "The wax used to line Cup-o-Noodles cups has been shown to cause cancer in rats" either two or five times. Next, people tried to guess whether each statement had been taken from the *National Enquirer* (a low-credibility source) or *Consumer Reports* (a high-credibility source). The more often a statement had been presented, the more it was attributed to *Consumer Reports* rather than to the *National Enquirer*, an attribution that is well suited to further enhance the credibility of the statement.

Implications for Information Campaigns and Warnings

As the preceding findings indicate, the old saying that if you repeat something often enough, it will seem true has considerable empirical support. This observation has important implications for information campaigns that are designed to correct false beliefs and to dispel rumors. In a comprehensive study of World War II rumor transmission, Allport and Lepkin (1945) found that the biggest predictor of belief in a rumor was frequency of exposure to the rumor—this factor had a bigger impact on belief than education, political affiliation, age, and so on. This repetition-based enhancement of truth for rumors is especially relevant for social marketers, who are often in the position of trying to refute rumors about a treatment or behavior change that they are promoting.

An intuitive strategy to fight the influence of rumors is to counter the rumors by publicizing them as false information. However, the foregoing theorizing argues against this approach. Although such an anti-rumor campaign may have the desired impact immediately by convincing people about the false nature of a rumor, it may fail by ignoring how people will remember the information after a delay. Specifically, recall of specific information such as the source of a communication fades from memory, while processing fluency for previously seen information remains fairly intact (e.g., Johnson, Hashtroudi, and Lindsay 1993). Remembering a joke but forgetting who told it, or recalling a news story but forgetting its source, are everyday examples of this dissociation in memory. The implication is that warning people about false information could backfire over time: when people hear the rumor again, it seems more familiar and they are more likely to perceive it as true—having forgotten that the only reason why it seems familiar is that they had been told several times that it is false.

Skurnik et al. (2005) tested this possibility with claims about health behaviors and diet. They exposed people either once or three times to statements such as "Corn chips have twice as much fat as potato chips"; each statement was explicitly identified as "true" or "false" as it was presented. The people participating in the research were either younger adults (around age twenty) or older adults (over age seventy-two). The pattern of memory for statements suggests that older adults may be particularly vulnerable to the backfire effects of information campaigns. Numerous studies show that explicit memory—for example, recall of detailed source information—declines with age, whereas implicit memory—for instance, feelings of fluency and familiarity—stays largely intact (Park 2000). If so, older adults may be less likely to remember the details of previously seen information, which would be required to identify the information as false, but they may still

Figure 6.4 **Truth Judgments for True and False Statements**

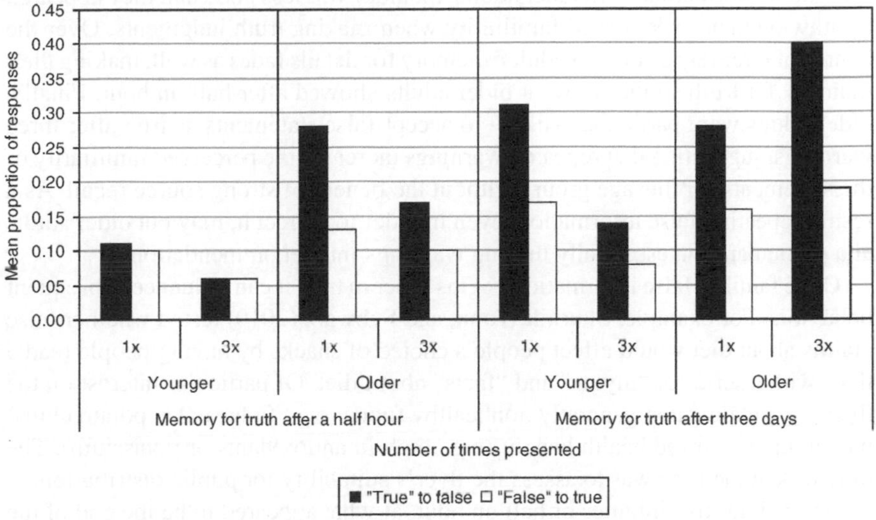

Source: Adapted from Skurnik et al. (2005).
Note: Bars indicate the proportion of false statements misremembered as true ("true" to false) and true statements misremembered as false ("false" to true) after no delay (*top panel*) and a delay of three days (*bottom panel*).

find previously seen statements easy to process and familiar, making the statements seem true.

Either immediately after reading the statements or after a three-day delay, people read the statements again and were asked to identify each one as true or false. Figure 6.4 shows the results. After a short delay (Figure 6.4, *top panel*), the younger adults were equally likely to misidentify a true statement as false and a false statement as true, indicating overall good memory for truth with a few random errors. The older adults, on the other hand, were more likely to misremember a false statement as true than a true statement as false. This "illusion of truth" effect shown in the older adults was more pronounced for information seen only once than three times, indicating that three exposures resulted in more accurate memory for truth.

After a three-day delay (Figure 6.4, *bottom panel*), memories of the younger adults mirrored those of the older adults after half an hour almost exactly. For statements seen once, younger adults showed an illusion of truth effect and misidentified 24 percent of the false statements as true; this effect was less pronounced for statements seen three times. The benefits of repetition to source recall were still with the younger adults. Finally, older adults misidentified 29 percent of the once-presented false statements as true. For statements shown three times, older adults thought that a full 40 percent of the false statements were true.

The overall pattern of results suggests an increasing reliance on experienced familiarity as source memory fades. Without a delay, younger adults remembered the presented information well; older adults' memory was less good and they appeared to draw on their experienced familiarity when making truth judgments. Over the course of three days, younger adults' memory for details fades as well, making their memory for truth similar to what older adults showed after half an hour. Finally, older adults were particularly likely to accept false statements as true after three warnings, suggesting that repeated warnings increases the perceived familiarity of the statements for this age group, without the benefit of strong source recall. As a result, repeating false information, even in order to correct it, may put older adults at a particular risk, essentially turning warnings into recommendations.

Once familiar false information begins to seem true, it can influence subsequent behaviors. For example, Skurnik, Yoon, and Schwarz (2010) tested whether false claims about diet would affect people's choice of snacks by having people read a flyer with a series of "myths" and "facts" about diet. Of particular interest on the flyer were claims that generally nonhealthy foods (e.g., fudge cake, potato chips) had an unrecognized health benefit (e.g., high in antioxidants or potassium). The only task at the time was to assess the flyer's suitability for public distribution.

After either five minutes or half an hour, at what appeared to be the end of the research session, people were asked to rate various statements about health and diet, including the statements from the earlier flyer. Then, ostensibly as part of a separate activity, people chose snacks for themselves from a set of alternatives, some of which were mentioned among the diet facts and myths on the flyer. If people were swayed by the flyer's claims, then in the short term they may be willing to choose the unhealthy foods when their benefits were described as factual, but reject the same foods when the benefits were described as myths. However, if the fact and myth designations fade from memory more quickly than the core claim, then as time passes people may embrace the unhealthy foods they initially rejected.

Figure 6.5 shows mean truth ratings of statements from the flyer and new statements that did not appear on the flyer. True claims are consistently rated truer than new claims, and false claims are consistently rated more false than new claims. However, the truth rating of false claims changes between the five-minute and half-hour delays. Specifically, false claims are rated as less false after half an hour has passed, in line with predictions. Figure 6.6 shows the likelihood of selecting a nonhealthy snack that was mentioned as having a health benefit in the flyer. As expected, when the benefit was described as a fact, people chose the food consistently across the delay. In contrast, when the benefit was described as a myth, people avoided the food immediately, but chose it more frequently after half an hour had passed.

The overall picture is that warnings about false information can be effective at first, evoking the desired behavior from people. But as time passes, the details of the warning's context fade from mind, leaving a core proposition that feels familiar; this familiarity makes the now-vague information seem true. In the end, the warning, which was initially effective, can have the opposite effect of what was intended.

Figure 6.5 **Truth Ratings of Claims About Snack Foods**

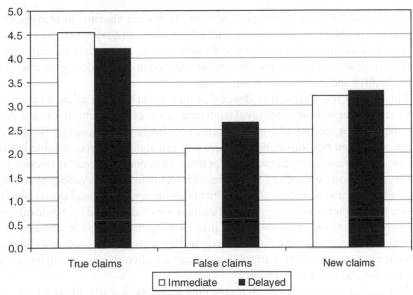

Source: From Skurnik, Yoon, and Schwarz (2010).
Note: Higher numbers indicate greater rated truth.

Figure 6.6 **Likelihood of Choosing an Unhealthy Snack Food**

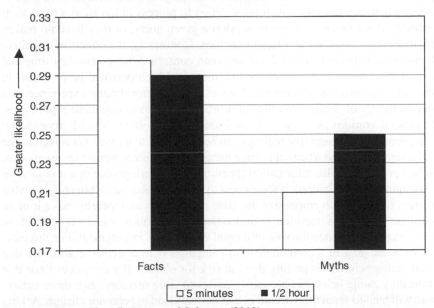

Source: From Skurnik, Yoon, and Schwarz (2010).

CONCLUSION

As this review illustrates, experiential information that accompanies thinking plays a crucial role in judgment. This experiential information can qualify and even reverse the conclusions implied by declarative thought content alone. Understanding how consumers draw conclusions and form judgments requires considering the interplay of declarative and experiential information.

This chapter has reviewed evidence that mental experiences affect a variety of specific judgments: ease of retrieval from memory is often interpreted as a sign of the frequency or recency of what was retrieved, fluency of processing is taken as a sign of reduced risk, difficulty in processing can signify harm or trouble in performance, and familiarity can stand in for truth. In domains relevant to obesity and health, people are exposed to a great deal of information from a variety of sources (e.g., news reports, websites, advertisements, contact with medical professionals, advice from friends and family). Not all sources are credible, and even information from credible sources can change over time. Sorting through this information is a critical but difficult task. The difficulties of dealing with this abundant and complex dynamic array of information mean that consumers often process health messages in a passive and heuristic manner.

It is during such situations that consumers are particularly likely to rely on their subjective mental experiences to assess health information and behaviors. What seem like mundane, low-stakes decisions, with no import for long-term health and happiness, can thus build through their repetition into a public health problem. Consumers are most likely to base their judgments on cognitive experiences when they have too much information to process in too short a time, their memory is not precise enough to support a given query, or they have no reason to doubt their intuitions and rapid reactions. Conversely, the effects of cognitive feelings on judgment should decrease when consumers have abundant time and expertise to consider the bases for judgment and high personal involvement in the judgment process or outcome. Factors such as prior dieting experience or a family history of obesity may thus minimize the effects of cognitive experiences. In general, consumers should be more immune to the effects of subjective mental experiences when cognitive feelings can be attributed to a cause not linked to the judgment at hand and when supporting materials can replace incomplete memories. When presenting false information (presumably to warn people that it is false or to debunk the information), it seems best to focus the audience's attention on what is true, rather than to emphasize the false information and thereby make it more familiar. Finally, it is important to understand circumstances when it is desirable to encourage or minimize the role of mental experiences in judgment. For instance, suppose the goal of a communication campaign is to convince consumers that their eating behavior is putting them at risk for obesity. If a consumer finds that unhealthy eating behaviors are easily retrieved from memory, then those behaviors will tend to seem more frequent and perhaps lead to behavior change. Asking these consumers to reflect on all their unhealthy behaviors may have the opposite effect; if the examples are so hard to recall, consumers may reason, then there are probably not too many of them. Exploring the links between mental experiences and message strategies is a fruitful area for future research.

REFERENCES

Allport, Floyd H., and Milton Lepkin. 1945. "Wartime Rumors of Waste and Special Privilege: Why Some People Believe Them." *Journal of Abnormal and Social Psychology*, 40 (1), 3–36.

Bandura, Albert. 2004. "Health Promotion by Social Cognitive Means." *Health Education and Behavior*, 31 (2), 143–164.

Begg, Ian M., Ann Anas, and Suzanne Farinacci. 1992. "Dissociation of Processes in Belief: Source Recollection, Statement Familiarity, and the Illusion of Truth." *Journal of Experimental Psychology: General*, 121 (4), 446–458.

Bell, A.Collin, Keyou Ge, and Barry M. Popkin. 2001. "Weight Gain and its Predictors in Chinese Adults." *International Journal of Obesity Related Metabolic Disorders*, 25 (7), 1079–1086.

Breakwell, Glynis M. 2007. *The Psychology of Risk*. New York: Cambridge University Press.

Carver, Charles S., and Michael F. Scheier. 1998. *On the Self-Regulation of Behavior*. New York: Cambridge University Press.

Centers for Disease Control and Prevention (CDC). 2009. *Obesity. Halting the Epidemic by Making Health Easier. At a Glance 2009*. www.cdc.gov/nccdphp/publications/AAG/obesity.htm.

Cullen, Karen Weber, Tom Baranowski, and Stella P. Smith. 2001. "Using Goal Setting as a Strategy for Dietary Behavior Change." *Journal of the American Dietetic Association*, 101 (5), 562–566.

DuCharme, Kimberley A., and Lawrence R. Brawley. 1995. "Predicting the Intentions and Behavior of Exercise Initiates Using Two Forms of Self-Efficacy." *Journal of Behavioral Medicine*, 18 (5), 479–497.

Edwards, Phil, and Ian Roberts. 2009. "Population Adiposity and Climate Change." *International Journal of Epidemiology*, 38 (4), 1137–1140.

Festinger, Leon 1954. "A Theory of Social Comparison Processes." *Human Relations*, 7 (May), 123–146.

Fragale, Alison R., and Chip Heath. 2004. "Evolving Information Credentials: The (Mis) Attribution of Believable Facts to Credible Sources." *Personality and Social Psychology Bulletin*, 30 (2), 225–236.

Hasher, Lynn, David Goldstein, and Thomas Toppino. 1977. "Frequency and the Conference of Referential Validity." *Journal of Verbal Learning and Verbal Behavior*, 16 (1), 107–112.

Johnson, Marcia K., Shahin Hashtroudi, and D. Stephen Lindsay. 1993. "Source Monitoring." *Psychological Bulletin*, 114 (1), 3–28.

Kelly, Robert B., Stephen J. Zyzanski, and Sonia A. Alemagno. 1991. "Prediction of Motivation and Behavior Change Following Health Promotion: Role of Health Beliefs, Social Support, and Self-Efficacy." *Social Science and Medicine*, 32 (3), 311–320.

Park, Denise C. 2000. "The Basic Mechanisms Accounting for Age-Related Decline in Cognitive Function." In *Cognitive Aging: A Primer*, ed. Denise C. Park and Norbert Schwarz, 3–22. Philadelphia: Psychology Press.

Reber, Rolf, and Norbert Schwarz. 1999. "Effects of Perceptual Fluency on Judgments of Truth." *Consciousness and Cognition*, 8 (3), 338–342.

Rothman, Alexander J., and Norbert Schwarz. 1998. "Constructing Perceptions of Vulnerability: Personal Relevance and the Use of Experiential Information in Health Judgments." *Personality and Social Psychology Bulletin*, 24 (10), 1053–1064.

Schwarz, Norbert. 2004. "Metacognitive Experiences in Consumer Judgment and Decision Making." *Journal of Consumer Psychology*, 14 (4), 332–348.

Schwarz, Norbert, Herbert Bless, Fritz Strack, Gisela Klumpp, Helga Rittenauer-Schatka, and Annette Simons. 1991. "Ease of Retrieval as Information: Another Look at the Availability Heuristic." *Journal of Personality and Social Psychology*, 61 (2), 195–202.

Schwarz, Norbert, Lawrence J. Sanna, Ian Skurnik, and Carolyn Yoon. 2007. "Metacognitive Experiences and the Intricacies of Setting People Straight: Implications for Debiasing and Public Information Campaigns." *Advances in Experimental Social Psychology*, 39, 127–161.

Schwarzer, Ralf. 1999. "Self-Regulatory Processes in the Adoption and Maintenance of Health Behaviors: The Role of Optimism, Goals, and Threats." *Journal of Health Psychology*, 4 (2), 115–127.

Skurnik, Ian, and Benoit Monin. 2010. "Fluency, Familiarity, and Truth in Rhyming Statements." Manuscript in preparation.

Skurnik, Ian, Norbert Schwarz, and Piotr Winkielman. 2000. "Drawing Inferences from Feelings: The Role of Naive Beliefs." In *The Message Within: The Role of Subjective Experience in Social Cognition and Behavior*, ed. Herbert Bless and Joseph P. Forgas, 162–175. Philadelphia: Psychology Press.

Skurnik, Ian, Carolyn Yoon, Denise C. Park, and Norbert Schwarz. 2005. "How Warnings about False Claims Become Recommendations." *Journal of Consumer Research*, 31 (4), 713–724.

Skurnik, Ian, Carolyn Yoon, and Norbert Schwarz. 2010. "Choice Behavior and the Illusion of Truth." Manuscript in preparation.

Song, Hyunjin, and Norbert Schwarz. 2008a. "Fluency and the Detection of Distortions: Low Processing Fluency Attenuates the Moses Illusion." *Social Cognition*, 26 (6), 791–799.

———. 2008b. "If It's Hard to Read, It's Hard to Do: Processing Fluency Affects Effort Prediction and Motivation." *Psychological Science*, 19 (10), 986–988.

———. 2009. "If It's Difficult to Pronounce, It Must Be Risky: Fluency, Familiarity, and Risk Perception." *Psychological Science*, 20 (2), 135–138.

Sparks, Paul, Carol A. Guthrie, and Richard Shepherd. 1997. "The Dimensional Structure of the Perceived Behavioral Control Construct." *Journal of Applied Social Psychology*, 27 (5), 418–438.

Strecher, Victor J., Brenda McEvoy DeVellis, Marshall H. Becker, and Irwin M. Rosenstock. 1986. "The Role of Self-Efficacy in Achieving Health Behavior Change." *Health Education and Behavior*, 13 (1), 73–92.

Strecher, Victor J., Gerard H. Seijts, Gerjo J. Kok, Gary P. Latham, Russell Glasgow, Brenda DeVellis, Ree M. Meertens, and David W. Bulger. 1995. "Goal Setting as a Strategy for Health Behavior Change." *Health Education and Behavior*, 22 (2), 190–200.

Tversky, Amos, and Daniel Kahneman. 1973. "Availability: A Heuristic for Judging Frequency and Probability." *Cognitive Psychology*, 5 (2), 207–232.

Unkelbach, Christian. 2007. "Reversing the Truth Effect: Learning the Interpretation of Processing Fluency in Judgments of Truth." *Journal of Experimental Psychology: Learning, Memory, and Cognition*, 33 (1), 219–230.

Weaver, Kimberlee, Stephen M. Garcia, Norbert Schwarz, and Dale T. Miller. 2007. "Inferring the Popularity of an Opinion From Its Familiarity: A Repetitive Voice Can Sound Like a Chorus." *Journal of Personality and Social Psychology*, 92 (5), 821–833.

CHAPTER 7

HOW THE BODY TYPE OF OTHERS IMPACTS OUR FOOD CONSUMPTION

BRENT MCFERRAN, DARREN W. DAHL, GAVAN J. FITZSIMONS, AND ANDREA C. MORALES

Obesity and unhealthy food consumption are major public health issues, especially in North American society. In the United States, an estimated 66 percent of adults and nearly one-third of preschoolers are overweight or obese (National Health and Nutrition Examination Survey [NHANES] 2004), and increasingly similar numbers exist in the United Kingdom (Pfanner 2008) and around the globe. This epidemic has serious consequences, as people who are overweight are at a greater risk of cardiovascular disease, sleep apnea, hypertension, gallbladder disease, type 2 diabetes, osteoarthritis, and various cancers (Bianchini, Kaaks, and Vainio 2002; U.S. Department of Health 2000). The economic cost of obesity to the U.S. health-care system is more than $92.6 billion dollars annually (Finkelstein, Fiebelkorn, and Wang 2003). According to the World Health Organization (WHO), by 2030 obesity will be the number one cause of death among the world's poor (see Kielburger and Kielburger 2008). Although a relatively recent problem, obesity is rapidly becoming a preeminent public concern. Data show that among adults, the percentage of those either overweight or obese doubled from 1980 to 2004, and rates for children exceeded those of adults (NHANES 1980, 2004), foreshadowing even more dire problems to come. Worldwide, the United Nations indicates that for the first time, there are now more overweight people in the world than people who are starving.

What has caused such a sharp rate of increase in the prevalence of obesity? While some authors point to an increasingly sedentary lifestyle (Blair and Brodney 1999) or genetics (Comuzzi and Allison 1998), most research tends to point to a marked increase in consumption of energy as the main driver of obesity (Dehghan, Akhtar-Danesh, and Merchant 2005; Young and Nestle 2002). While the human body has developed excellent responses to being underfed, it has comparatively weak systems to cope with overconsumption (Hill and Peters 1998). Human genes are not changing at such a rate that could possibly explain the increase in overweight and obesity rates in recent decades (Hill, Pagliassotti, and Peters 1994; Stunkard et al. 1990), and people's activity levels have remained stable over decades while obesity rates have increased (Young and Nestle 2002). What has changed is society's food choices.

Making healthy food choices is clearly an important part of maintaining a healthy body weight. Today, Americans eat at least 200 more calories a day than they did in 1980 (e.g., Chandon and Wansink 2007; NHANES 2004), often at increasingly available establishments offering relatively inexpensive, convenient, and calorically dense foods (Hill and Peters 1998). Consumers make over 200 food choices per day (Wansink 2006), and thus it is important to understand the antecedents to unhealthy food choices. However, little research in marketing has examined why consumers make the food choices they do. For instance, once inside a restaurant, what causes them to purchase the burger instead of the salad, or the large fries over the small ones? Such small decisions actually have large caloric consequences, as the difference between a sixteen-ounce McDonald's Swamp Sludge McFlurry and a McDonald's Low Fat Ice Cream Cone is 560 calories (McDonald's 2006). Portion size and unhealthy choices are linked to obesity (Young and Nestle 2002), and people who select larger portions tend to eat more than those given small portions. This is true even when the food is of poor taste or consumers are not even hungry (Wansink 2006).

In the domain of food consumption, the presence and behavior of other people (also known as social influence) have been argued to be a "major, if not the preeminent, influence on eating behavior" (Johnston 2002, 21; see also de Castro 1994; Goldman, Herman, and Polivy 1991). This research will review how the choices of other people may influence consumers' own choices in terms of the quantity they select and ultimately consume. We will also review recent research examining how the effect of social influence on consumption is moderated by the body type of the other consumer. In other words, observing an obese versus a thin consumer order food, or overhearing such a server make a recommendation, will have differential effects on the quantity of food a consumer chooses and consumes. In general, we focus on quantity of food eaten, rather than on specific (healthy versus unhealthy) food choices, although in a final study we do examine choice. Across a series of studies, we demonstrate

1. that people are sensitive to the quantity choices made by others, eating more food as those around them select larger portion sizes;
2. that these effects depend on the body type of the others around them, such that consumers are more influenced by food selections of thin companions than they are of obese ones;
3. that these effects are particularly pronounced for those dissatisfied with their physical appearance and when cognitive resources are not constrained; and
4. that noneating others' body types can also affect consumption, but that these effects are moderated by the eater's propensity toward restrained eating.

SOCIAL INFLUENCES AND SELECTION OF PORTION SIZE

Past research has shown that consumption decisions are influenced by those who are physically present. People are sensitive to the behavior of others in a retail context (Argo and Main 2008; Bearden and Etzel 1982; Dahl, Manchanda, and Argo 2001; Moschis 1976). Given that people eat many meals in the company of others and research shows that people's behavior is subject to social influences, understanding how others and their body types affect people's consumption choices is essential to understanding why consumers make the food choices they do.

Studies have found that social influence can have either a facilitating or attenuating effect on eating behavior, depending on the context (see Herman, Roth, and Polivy 2003 for an excellent review). On the one hand, the social facilitation literature has found that the presence of others leads to an increase in consumption (e.g., de Castro 1994; see also Conger et al. 1980; Johnston 2002; Rosenthal and Marx 1979) because the duration of the meal increases. De Castro (1990, 1994) finds that people eat about 35 percent more calories if they eat with just one other person and nearly twice as much in a group of seven or more, and more with friends and family than with other companions. The length of time people sit at the table strongly predicts how much they intake. If they spend a long time at the dinner table, they tend to eat more food. One need only imagine a Thanksgiving dinner or wedding reception that goes on for hours, while all the guests complain that they ate too much. More time spent with food results in increased consumption. Additionally, attenuation effects are also realized if people justify that they can eat more and still not be excessive when the other person eats a very small amount (Nisbett and Storms 1974) or is in some way not like them (Rosekrans 1967).

On the other hand, Herman, Roth, and Polivy (2003) argue that food choice is influenced by a desire to convey a certain impression or adhere to social norms (Leary and Kowalski 1990; Roth et al. 2001). Making a good impression usually means eating less, rather than more, when in the company of others. Indeed, people who suffer from eating disorders often binge while alone, but eat minimally in the company of others (Herman and Polivy 1980). In a social setting, few want to be the person who orders a steak for lunch when everyone else goes with the salad. This line of reasoning has led to a series of important experiments, known as the modeling or mimicry studies, in which the social other's choices are directly manipulated. In these studies (see Herman, Roth, and Polivy 2003), the participants' behavior is observed after they overhear or see another person (a confederate) choose her portion. The results of these studies consistently show that social influence can have either a facilitating or attenuating effect on consumption, depending on how much the confederate eats. Participants in these studies follow the norms the confederate sets, eating more (or less) in parallel with the confederate. These norm effects are particularly poignant: the confederate does not even have to be physically present (Roth et al. 2001); those who are naturally inclined to eat large portions sometimes eat less in the presence of others, while those who normally eat very little eat more.

In other words, as the group size increases, no one wants to stand out, and people increasingly conform to the group average (Bell and Pliner 2003). Following this logic, Wansink (2006) recommends that if you are a light eater, you should eat by yourself, and if you eat heavily, you should seek out a group to eat with if your goal is to lose weight, so as to avoid consuming too many calories.

According to the research discussed, there is an effect on eating behavior as a function of social influence; however, the literature is relatively agnostic with respect to who the "other" person or people are that one might be ordering (thereby choosing a portion) or eating alongside. According to theory from this literature, it should make no difference if the people one might be sharing a meal with are very thin or very obese, so long as they eat the same amount. However, research suggests that a consumer does not perceive obese individuals and normal-weight individuals in the same way and thus may not react in the same manner to their food choices.

OBESITY AND CONSUMPTION

While many of the social influence studies (see De Luca and Spigelman 1979; Johnston 2002 for exceptions) focus on the quantity, rather than the body type of the social other, the obesity studies take the opposite approach: ignoring what choices the other people have made and focusing only on their body type, concluding that eating with those who are overweight will lead to an increase in one's food consumption or that people emulate others they are close to.

For example, priming people with images of overweight consumers has been shown to lead to an increase in quantity consumed (Campbell and Mohr 2008). Using assimilation/contrast as a theoretical framework, these authors reported that people eat more when primed with overweight, but not obese consumers.

In a very interesting study, Christakis and Fowler (2007; see Cohen-Cole and Fletcher 2008 for a rebuttal) found that a person's chance of becoming obese significantly increased when a close other (e.g., friend, sibling, spouse) became obese. Moreover, the effect persisted even if the two people were not living in the same city, suggesting that social distance was a better predictor of influence than physical distance. Effects were not seen in neighbors in the same area. The authors' calculations show that a person who became obese gained seventeen pounds and this newly obese person's friends gained five on average.

However, it is important to note that obesity is something most people wish to avoid, so it seems counterintuitive that in the presence of conscious thought consumers would choose to mimic portion choices of someone who is overweight when they themselves (presumably) do not consciously desire to be overweight. Most cultures currently place a high value on thinness, and those who are overweight or obese are often victims of stereotyping or stigmatization (Shapiro, King, and Quinones 2007). Research shows that the obese are stereotyped as less hardworking, lacking self-control and restraint, slower, sloppier, and lazier than individuals who are not obese (Bacon, Scheltema, and Robinson 2001; Ryckman et al. 1989; Shapiro, King, and Quinones 2007). However, unlike some stigmas, blame for being obese is attributed directly to individuals, the assumption being that they are in full control of their weight (e.g., Crandall 1994; DeJong 1993; Rothblum 1992; Weiner, Perry, and Magnusson 1988). This bias exists even among physicians, resulting in a reluctance to solicit treatment, a higher likelihood of being denied treatment, and vulnerability to depression, anxiety, low self-esteem, social rejection, and suicidal thoughts (Kirkey 2008; Puhl and Bronwell 2001).

In the social influence literature more generally, the effects of the social "other" have been shown to be moderated by whether that individual is a member of an aspirational or dissociative group (Berger and Heath 2007, 2008; Berger and Rand 2008; Escalas and Bettman 2003, 2005; White and Dahl 2006, 2007). Given the stigmatization that the obese endure, it seems unlikely that people would intentionally model the eating patterns of obese people, but that is precisely what some research suggests. But are you really equally likely to order the cheeseburger after first hearing it ordered by someone who is obese (vs. thin)? Does seeing an obese person order a large amount of food really influence you to order more food yourself, or might it put you off? What if you see a thin girl order a very small salad for lunch? Or what if an obese server recommends something unhealthy? Past research suggests that the extent to which one is a chronic dieter might make a difference in answering these questions.

THE ROLE OF RESTRAINED EATING

As concerns over their weight and physical appearance increase, many people seek to manage their eating through dieting. The dieting industry is now worth over $40 billion annually in the United States alone (Reisner 2008; Sherrid 2003), and one out of three women and one out of every four men are on a diet at any given time (Crossen 2003; Fetto 2002).

In academic research, investigations of chronic dieting commonly use a measure of restrained eating developed by Herman and Polivy (1980). Restrained eating is defined as "the deliberate effort to combat the physiologically based urge to eat in order to lose weight or maintain a reduced weight" (Fedoroff, Polivy, and Herman 1997, 34). Their scale captures consumers' concern for dieting ("How often are you dieting?"), weight fluctuation ("In a typical week, how much does your weight fluctuate?"), and social eating behavior (e.g., "Do you eat sensibly in front of others and splurge alone?"). Restrained eaters, compared to unrestrained eaters, are continuously aware of their eating behavior (Herman and Mack 1975). Past research has shown that dieters (restrained eaters) and nondieters differ substantially in their food choices, with dieters sometimes exhibiting backfire effects, eating more (rather than less) following a "preload" of calories, more in anticipation of an impending diet (or anticipating a preload), or more after exposure to a food aroma (see Herman and Polivy 2004). Restrained eaters are also more likely to increase their consumption in high-stress situations (Heatherton and Baumeister 1991) or those that raise anxiety levels (Herman et al. 1987).

In one recent study, Scott et al. (2008) found that food size and package size also influenced how restrained eaters consumed. While both restrained and unrestrained eaters tend to label bite-sized food in small packages as "diet" as well as "high-calorie," these foods (e.g., 100-calorie minipacks) can cause high levels of stress among restrained eaters. The researchers found that restrained eaters consumed more calories from small food in small packages, while unrestrained eaters consumed more (or at least as many) calories from large food in a large package. Importantly, the restrained eaters could reduce their consumption by engaging their cool system (i.e., by thinking about food in terms of surrounding objects and spatial dimensions), rather than focusing on the emotions and feelings that food normally triggers for this group.

In a series of studies, we examine the roles of each of these factors in turn. We first report results of a pilot study we conducted that was designed to examine if consumers ever recall altering their food portions as a result of the choices of other consumers and/or their body type. We then extend this research to examine how the extent to which people are dissatisfied with their physical appearance or are dieting might moderate the effects.

PILOT STUDY

Method, Stimuli, and Procedures

To examine this question, critical incident analysis was used. Critical incident analysis, which has been used in emotion research (e.g., Keltner and Buswell 1996) as well as in marketing (e.g., Dahl, Honea, and Manchanda 2003), generally asks participants to write about a single incident that deals with a particular research question. For our study, 318 respondents from a large western university participated in the study, which was administered as a short survey instrument for partial course credit.

The instrument first asked participants the following question: "When at a restaurant or food establishment (an ice cream shop, pretzel stand, etc.) of any kind, have your choices of food items ever been influenced by what the person in front of you ordered, the size or weight of the person in front of you, or a combination of the two?" Participants indicated yes or no if they had experienced such a scenario, followed by some basic demographic information (age, gender, major, country of birth, height, weight). One hundred and fifty-seven participants (49 percent) indicated that they had experienced such a situation, and only data from their responses were analyzed. Sixty-six of these (42 percent) were female, and the average age of respondents was 21.53. Two trained research assistants, blind to the purposes of the study, coded the open-ended responses. Initial inter-rater agreement was 93.2 percent and disagreements were resolved by one of the authors.

Results and Discussion

While people claimed their choices were influenced by both heavy ($n = 37$) and thin ($n = 23$) others, the common response to seeing this other person order was to change their order to something smaller ($n = 21$) or healthier ($n = 37$). It seems from the critical incidents participants recalled, generally the presence of others led to a more modest portion choice, albeit for different reasons. In the case of a thin other, people reported ordering less ($n = 6$) or a healthier menu option ($n = 13$) as a result. Common reasons cited were that they envied the other person's figure and this reminded them that in order to lose weight, they needed to make smaller or healthier choices, not because she ordered something unhealthy or large (e.g., "I saw a skinny person ordering [a] lunch size salad that really [motivated] me to order the salad instead of pasta"; "I was going to order a regular soda drink even though I am [used] to ordering diet but a little skinny person in front of me ordered diet so I did too"; "If someone very thin orders something really healthy, I feel guilty for ordering something less healthy"; "I really wanted a Blizzard [ice-cream treat from Dairy Queen], but a very tiny person in front of me ordered just a small ice cream cone, and when it came my time to order, I ordered the same").

The most frequent situation participants recalled was seeing an obese other person order either a large quantity ($n = 11$) or an unhealthy menu option ($n = 20$). This resulted in participants reporting a worry about becoming obese (e.g., "at McDonald's a heavier person ordered an enormous amount of food and I have ordered less because I didn't want to end up that size"; "When I see an overweight person order something unhealthy it reminds me to stay healthy"). Consistent with research on dissociative groups, the choices of the obese were deliberately avoided (e.g., "if the person in front of me is overweight I will not get what they get"; "I might think I would then look like them if I ate that too"; "I think, 'don't order that or you'll end up like them'"). As a result, participants commonly chose a smaller ($n = 14$) or less indulgent ($n = 26$) menu item (e.g., "One time, at the movie theatre, the most gigantically obese woman I had ever seen ordered the XXL popcorn with extra butter, two large Coca Cola classics (not diet), a box of cookie dough bite sized candies, and a cinnamon sugar pretzel. When she finished paying and it was my turn to order, I asked for a water cup instead of getting concessions"; "I was at a restaurant last night and the table next to me had an overweight lady and man who ordered a whole bunch of food and I decided not to get dessert because of them"; "I went to McDonald's once and I noticed a man close to 300 lbs ordering a lot of food. He supersized his meal and I was unsure if all the food was for him or for others as well. Nevertheless, I did not order nearly as much as I would have. I was afraid that if I supersized my meal, I might end up eating too much and increase my weight size"; "if an overweight person orders something really fattening that may steer me to order something healthy"; "there was a rather large person in front of me who basically ordered the whole menu. I did not want to end up looking like them so I ordered less").

Interestingly, consumers' perceptions of how healthy a specific food choice is were influenced by the person choosing the item (e.g., "if it was a large person, I would order something different because I would perceive what they ordered as having the possibility of making me fat"; "If a skinny person ordered something, I kind of wanted to order it too because I associate that menu choice with being skinny"; "If I see an overweight person eating a sundae at McDonald's it is a turn off to those establishments. I don't want to be fat").

While the most common scenario participants recalled was paring back potentially indulgent choices, a few participants ($n = 6$) mentioned ordering more or something less healthy as a result of the thin other person, demonstrating a licensing effect: ("If the person is skinny and they order something fattening there is a good chance I will also. However if they are heavy then I probably will not"; "I wouldn't normally eat a lot of fatty foods [ice cream, muffins, etc.] but if a slender person orders it I usually follow suit. I never buy snacks at a gas station but during my spring break I broke my rule because my friend who was itzy bitzy bought a ton of candy"; "Also I can be influenced the opposite way [if a thin person orders something less healthy] to a less healthy choice because I feel like it is more justified").

Only one participant reported intentionally eating something more indulgent as a result of the obese person's order ("I saw a small but heavy-set guy in front of me order 4 foot-long subs. I was [deciding] between ordering one sandwich or two. After looking at this man I concluded that since he ordered 4, it wouldn't hurt for me to order half of what he did. So I did!"), and only one person claimed that thin people cause her to order more rather than less regardless of what they order ("I become jealous of good metabolism. If the person is skinny yet ordered a lot . . . I generally order a heavier meal because I want to show how I don't care about my weight . . . I can do it too").

The pilot study provides initial evidence that people were able to recall a situation in which they changed their food order as a function of the body type of others. The events participants recalled provide evidence for social comparison processes. The most frequent response centered on participants choosing to order a smaller or healthier food after overhearing a heavy person order an indulgent portion of food or a thin person ordering something modest. People recalled consciously deciding to pare back, stating that they wanted to avoid having a figure like the other person. The heavy person's choice was associated with the outcome of becoming overweight, and the thin person's choice reminded participants that they need to make healthy choices if they are to achieve their desired figure.

However, there remains a natural confound in our data: participants more often reported behaviors that were stereotype consistent (versus inconsistent), namely heavy people ordering a large or unhealthy portion or thin people ordering less. What would happen if the heavy other ordered a small salad for lunch? Perhaps this does happen less in practice (and thus participants were less likely to recall it), or when it happens it is just less conspicuous. The results of this study extend the research outlined above, which has tended to focus either on consumers' reactions to how much others eat or on how the body type of others impacts consumption, but not on the influence of the two jointly. Our recent work (McFerran et al. 2010a) has sought to examine how people react to another consumer's body type and food order by explicitly manipulating these factors in a controlled laboratory setting, with the aim of showing that people's choices are shaped by the selections of others (consistent with the social influence literature), but also that such effects are moderated by the body type of these other people (consistent with the obesity and reference group literature).

I'LL HAVE WHAT SHE'S HAVING

While some scholars (De Luca and Spigelman 1979; Johnston 2002) have looked at how obese others might impact participants' consumption, what has been lacking are tighter empirical controls and a strong theoretical explanation for such effects (as suggested by Herman, Roth, and Polivy 2003). We (McFerran et al. 2010a) sought to advance this quest by experimentally manipulating the weight of a single confederate, achieved with a professionally constructed obesity prosthesis, custom-designed for the confederate's body by an Academy Award–winning costume studio. Identical clothes were tailored in large (16) and small (00) sizes along with the prosthesis. This novel methodology allowed a single confederate to portray both a thin and obese consumer, thus controlling for any possible third variables that may have been operating in other research that used thin and heavy confederates.

In this series of studies, we had the confederate (portraying either a thin or heavy patron) first take a food selection, and then we measured what the participant subsequently took (and ate). Sometimes the confederate was instructed to choose a large portion, other times a small one, and sometimes there was no confederate at all (to establish a baseline). We then compared whether people's consumption differed as a function of (1) the choice, and (2) the body type of the confederate.

Theoretically, we presented and tested a parsimonious model based on anchoring and adjustment (Wansink, Kent, and Hoch 1998). What we found was that consumers anchor on the quantities others around them select, but that these portions are adjusted according to the body type of the other consumer. Study 1 first documented the effect, showing that people choose a larger portion following another consumer who first selects a large quantity, but that this portion is significantly smaller if the other is obese than if she is thin. However, we also tested whether this pattern would differ between foods perceived to be healthy versus those that are perceived as unhealthy. To test this, we used a manipulation borrowed from Wansink and Chandon (2006), where the experiment was run with half of the participants given granola as a snack, and half given M&Ms. These foods are similar in caloric density but differ strongly in health perception. Results showed that although obesity is linked more strongly to unhealthy foods (Weiner, Perry, and Magnusson 1988), the effect replicated with both types of food: participants took significantly less when the other consumer was obese than when she was thin.

In Study 2, we manipulated both how much the confederate took and her body type. We found strong evidence of participants' use of the confederate's choice as an anchor—choosing less (or more) as the confederate did first. This is conceptually consistent with what has been found in the modeling studies we reviewed above. However, we extend that research by identifying body type as a moderator of this effect. We replicated the finding that after seeing a large portion chosen by the other, consumers adjusted their consumption downward from the high-quantity anchor to a greater degree when the confederate was obese than when she was thin. However, we also found that rather than further decrease consumption when seeing an obese person choose a small portion, participants *increased* their portion choice. This ironic backfire effect is consistent with a greater upward adjustment from a low anchor when the confederate was obese than when she was thin. In other words, participants consistently followed the anchor that the confederate set more closely when she was thin than when she was heavy.

Study 3 showed further evidence of the process, using a scenario methodology. Results showed that the adjustment from the anchor was more pronounced for consumers low versus high in appearance self-esteem (Heatherton and Polivy 1991) and is attenuated when cognitive processing resources are constrained. In all of the studies, participants' own body mass index (BMI) did not impact results, showing that the effect is driven psychologically by dissatisfaction with one's appearance rather than physiologically by one's actual body type. We also measured and controlled for participants' orientation toward restrained eating (dieting), as numerous studies (outlined above) have shown how the food choices among dieters and nondieters differ.

Our second series of studies examines the role of restrained eating directly. While our earlier paper (McFerran et al. 2010a) examined the situation where one sees another consumer make an order, this paper examines the case where the obese (vs. thin) other is a server, rather than a fellow consumer. We show that dieting orientation moderates consumers' reaction to this situation.

EFFECTS OF NON-EATING OTHERS

While people eat many of their meals with companions (e.g., friends, coworkers), might the body type of a restaurant server alone alter their consumption choices? Research in marketing suggests that such social influences may have an effect, even if such a person is physically present and engages the consumer only in a limited way (Argo, Dahl, and Manchanda 2005; Zhou and Soman 2003). Might an obese (vs. a thinner) server influence diners to consume more (or less) food? What if she recommended an indulgent choice, or something very healthy? Might this influence the diner's choice? In this series of studies, we investigated how people's food choices can be shaped by the body type alone of others around them, and how dieters and nondieters differ. We (McFerran et al. 2010b) also examined how recommendations made by this other (whose consumption is not seen as she is a server) result in consumers making differing choices.

We again used the same prosthesis as we did in our earlier set of studies (McFerran et al. 2010a), but in this instance the confederate played the role of a server in a taste test study, rather than a fellow patron. In Study 1, we manipulated whether the server was obese or thin, and we measured participants' dieting orientation. Since overeating is associated with obesity, it would be reasonable to predict that people would eat less after seeing a heavy server. However, we found that dieters and nondieters exhibited opposite effects. While nondieters ate more when she was thin, dieters ate more snacks when the experimenter was heavy, a finding we claim supports the backfire effect.

In Study 2, we isolated our focus to dieters, manipulating both the servers' body type and the food she recommended (unhealthy cookies or healthy raw carrots). While persuasion research suggests that the thin server would be more persuasive, the backfire effect would predict that dieters would be less likely to choose an item recommended by a thin server than one who is obese. Indeed, this is what we found: when cookies were recommended, dieters chose cookies more often when the server was heavy than when she was thin (73 percent vs. 53 percent), but when carrots were recommended, they selected cookies with a greater frequency when she was thin than when she was heavy (53 percent vs. 79 percent). Instead of shunning the recommendation of the obese server, dieters were *more* persuaded by her recommendation, choosing both the healthy and the unhealthy snack more often when it was recommended to them. Collectively, these studies build on research showing that people's food choices may be shaped not only by what others eat, but also simply by others being physically present.

IMPLICATIONS AND CONCLUSIONS

Drawing on social psychological theories, our research, as well as numerous other excellent papers, explains how social influences, stemming from the choices and body types of others, may impact what people eat themselves. Our results replicate research that shows that people are more likely to eat greater portions when in the presence of others who do likewise; we also extend these results to show that this effect is even greater when the other person is thin rather than heavy.

Our findings strongly suggest, counter to other research, that in many cases the most dangerous people to eat with are not those who are overweight, but rather those who are thin but are heavy eaters. A heavy-set colleague who eats a lot is a better lunch partner than a thin colleague who orders the same dish. On the other hand, thin colleagues who eat lightly are more likely to cause others around them to order less. Thus, from the perspective of self-regulation, it is important for consumers to recognize situations in which they are likely to be vulnerable to overconsumption. As a matter of maintaining a healthy body weight, such small food-intake decisions have a larger impact than people realize. For instance, people could lower their caloric intake by 250 calories by eliminating sugared drinks or caloricity-dense liquids alone (e.g., one 591-ml bottle of cola), but would need to cycle for over an hour just to burn off that one bottle (Nutristrategy 2007, based on a 130-pound person pedaling less than 10 mph). Removing 250 calories a day could allow an obese person to shed thirty pounds in only one year (Wansink 2006).

Our results are also consistent with the recommendations of Wansink (2006), who suggests that small-portion eaters should eat by themselves, but large-portion eaters should seek out a group. Our research finds that, compared to eating alone, large portions chosen by others lead to greater consumption, and smaller portion choices by others are associated with eating less. However, we show this is qualified by the weight of the other person. Indeed, in our studies, the quantity that the confederate selected still overshadowed her body type, predicting what others took to a greater degree.

We also find that, for dieters, recommendations from overweight servers are more persuasive than those of thin servers. Our research suggests that discrimination against the obese may be counterproductive to certain businesses. However, we also find that servers' body types may influence those around them in significant ways, which may result in more or less consumption.

The general question of how the body type of others impacts people's food consumption is clearly a complicated one. We do have some preliminary evidence (from the pilot study) that seeing those who are obese or thin can trigger both self-focused thoughts (heightened concern about becoming obese after seeing an obese person) and other-focused thoughts (about the portion choices a thin person must select in order to stay thin). The latter are attributions made by others that would be an interesting avenue to explore further. For instance, in our studies, perhaps the thin person taking a large portion created an expectancy disconfirmation that led to cognitions focused on licensing (a belief that because she took a lot and is thin, I can too). On the other hand, seeing an obese person take a small portion might suggest that he is on a diet and needs to eat less, and this might similarly allow consumers to cognitively justify a larger selection. It is important to realize that these attributions may be focused on the other consumer's individual characteristics (e.g., "she must have good genes" or "must have just come from the gym" or "must not be hungry"), as well as on the food itself ("it must not be that bad for me, if the thin girl is taking so much"). Of course, in this case the authors constructed the "quotes," and one challenge of this type of research is getting respondents to admit that another person affected their choice, which, we have found, they are generally reluctant to do.

Another limitation of our research paradigm is that the confederate (other consumer or server) could not be known by participants in the research; otherwise the validity of the use of the prosthesis would be compromised. This raises an interesting question: how might social connectedness moderate our effects? Clearly eating with one's boss or a date triggers different impression management concerns than eating with family members. We could imagine a scenario where a person eats more (or less) to make another person feel good (or bad), perhaps depending on whether that other person is thin or heavy-set. It remains very possible (perhaps probable) that people may eat differently around others depending on who the other is, but scant research (see Herman, Roth, and Polivy 2003) has examined this question in the context of the body types of others.

From a communications perspective, this research also has significant implications for health organizations. While research has shown that people are less likely to overeat if overeating is associated with a dissociative outgroup (see also Chapter 11 in this volume), the fact that an outgroup does the behavior is not a given. For instance, if overeating large quantities of junk food became what the cool peers did (or simply normalized), that behavior could be expected to increase. On the other hand, if cool kids are seen as undereating, that behavior might increase as well. In developing communications, our research would suggest that "normalizing" heavier body types might have the unintended consequence of increasing consumption of those around them. However, the thin spokesperson for an unhealthy fast-food chain may prompt people to believe "because she can eat it and stay thin, so can I," even though their metabolism or exercise patterns are not the same as the spokesperson's. Every body is unique, and looking for cues about what to eat from other people can have mixed outcomes. It is important to note that our research is grounded on the assumption that the obese are a stigmatized group. As body type norms change over time (toward larger BMIs), this stigma may be attenuated. As a result, our research would suggest that eating with such individuals could be detrimental, assuming that they are indeed eating quantities of food that would induce obesity.

While research on body types has begun to emerge, it is still at the point of demonstrating effects rather than developing cogent theoretical explanations for them. Still, being aware of the situational factors that determine consumption, even if the reasons are not fully understood, is important if people wish to lower their caloric intake, given that many findings suggest that having knowledge or a mental awareness of how others might influence their choices may enable correction.

REFERENCES

Argo, Jennifer J., Darren W. Dahl, and Rajesh V. Manchanda. 2005. "The Influence of a Mere Social Presence in a Retail Context." *Journal of Consumer Research*, 32 (September), 207–212.
Argo, Jennifer J., and Kelley Main. 2008. "Stigma-by-Association in Coupon Redemption: Looking Cheap Because of Others." *Journal of Consumer Research*, 35 (December), 559–572.
Bacon, Jane G., Karen E. Scheltema, and Beatrice E. Robinson. 2001. "Fat Phobia Scale Revisited: The Short Form." *International Journal of Obesity*, 25 (2), 252–257.
Bearden, William O., and Michael J. Etzel. 1982. "Reference Group Influence on Product and Brand." *Journal of Consumer Research*, 9 (September), 183–194.
Bell, Rick, and Patricia L. Pliner. 2003. "Time To Eat: The Relationship Between the Number of People Eating and Meal Duration in Three Lunch Settings." *Appetite*, 41, 215–218.
Berger, Jonah, and Chip Heath. 2007. "Where Consumers Diverge From Others: Identity Signaling and Product Domains." *Journal of Consumer Research*, 34 (August), 121–134.

————. 2008. "Who Drives Divergence? Identity Signaling, Outgroup Dissimilarity, and the Abandonment of Cultural Tastes." *Journal of Personality and Social Psychology*, 95 (3), 593–607.

Berger, Jonah, and Lindsay Rand. 2008. "Shifting Signals to Help Health: Using Identity Signaling to Reduce Risky Health Behaviors." *Journal of Consumer Research*, 35 (August), 509–518.

Bianchini, France, Rudolf Kaaks, and Harri Vainio. 2002. "Overweight, Obesity, and Cancer Risk." *Lancet Oncology*, 3 (9), 565–574.

Blair, Steven N., and Suzanne Brodney. 1999. "Effects of Physical Inactivity and Obesity on Morbidity and Mortality: Current Evidence and Research Issues." *Medicine and Science in Sports and Exercise*, 31 (11) (Supplement), S646–S662.

Campbell, Margaret C., and Gina S. Mohr. 2008. "Seeing Is Eating: How an Overweight Prime Influences Consumer Behavior." Working paper, University of Colorado.

Chandon, Pierre, and Brian Wansink. 2007. "The Biasing Health Halos of Fast Food Restaurant Health Claims: Lower Calorie Estimates and Higher Side-Dish Consumption Intentions." *Journal of Consumer Research*, 34 (October), 301–314.

Christakis, Nicholas A., and James H. Fowler. 2007. "The Spread of Obesity in a Large Social Network Over 32 Years." *New England Journal of Medicine*, 357 (4), 370–379.

Cohen-Cole, Ethan, and Jason M. Fletcher. 2008. "Is Obesity Contagious? Social Networks vs. Environmental Factors in the Obesity Epidemic." *Journal of Health Economics*, 27 (5), 1382–1387.

Comuzzi, Anthony G., and David B. Allison. 1998. "The Search for Human Obesity Genes." *Science*, May 29, 1374–1377.

Conger, Judith C., Anthony J. Conger, Philip R. Costanzo, K. Lynn Wright, and Jean Anne Matter. 1980. "The Effect of Social Cues on the Eating Behavior of Obese and Normal Subjects." *Journal of Personality*, 48 (2), 258–271.

Crandall, Chris S. 1994. "Prejudice Against Fat People: Ideology and Self-Interest." *Journal of Personality and Social Psychology*, 66 (5), 882–894.

Crossen, Cynthia. 2003. "Americans Are Gaining, But 'Ideal' Weight Keeps Shrinking." *Wall Street Journal*, July 16.

Dahl, Darren W., Heather Honea, and Rajesh V. Manchanda. 2003. "The Nature of Self-Reported Guilt in Consumption Contexts." *Marketing Letters*, 14 (3), 159–171.

Dahl, Darren W., Rajesh V. Manchanda, and Jennifer J. Argo. 2001. "Embarrassment in Consumer Purchase: The Roles of Social Presence and Purchase Familiarity." *Journal of Consumer Research*, 28 (December), 473–481.

de Castro, John M. 1990. "Social Facilitation of Duration and Size But Not Rate of the Spontaneous Meal Intake of Humans." *Physiology and Behavior*, 47 (6), 1129–1135.

————. 1994. "Family and Friends Produce Greater Social Facilitation of Food Intake Than Other Companions." *Physiology and Behavior*, 56 (3), 445–455.

Dehghan, Mahshid, Noori Akhtar-Danesh, and Anwar T. Merchant. 2005. "Childhood Obesity, Prevalence and Prevention." *Nutrition Journal*, 4, 4–24.

DeJong, William. 1993. "Obesity as a Characterological Stigma: The Issue of Responsibility and Judgments of Task Performance." *Psychological Reports*, 73 (3, Pt. 1), 963–970.

De Luca, Rayleen V., and Manly N. Spigelman. 1979. "Effects of Models on Food Intake of Obese and Non-Obese Female College Students." *Canadian Journal of Behavioral Science*, 11 (2), 124–129.

Escalas, Jennifer Edson, and James R. Bettman. 2003. "You Are What They Eat: The Influence of Reference Groups on Consumer Connections to Brands." *Journal of Consumer Psychology*, 13 (3), 339–348.

————. 2005. "Self-Construal, Reference Groups, and Brand Meaning." *Journal of Consumer Research*, 32 (December), 378–389.

Fedoroff, Ingrid C., Janet Polivy, and C. Peter Herman. 1997. "The Effect of Pre-Exposure to Food Cues on the Eating Behavior of Restrained and Unrestrained Eaters." *Appetite*, 28 (1), 33–47.

Fetto, John. 2002. "A Moment on the Lips." *American Demographics*, 24 (3), 18.

Finkelstein, Eric A, Ian C. Fiebelkorn, and Guijing Wang. 2003. "National Medical Spending Attributable to Overweight and Obesity: How Much, and Who's Paying?" *Health Affairs*, W3, 219–226.

Goldman, Samuel J., C. Peter Herman, and Janet Polivy. 1991. "Is the Effect of Social Influence on Eating Attenuated by Hunger?" *Appetite*, 17, 129–140.

Heatherton, Todd F., and Roy F. Baumeister. 1991. "Binge Eating as an Escape From Self Awareness." *Psychological Bulletin*, 110 (1), 86–108.

Heatherton, Todd F., and Janet Polivy. 1991. "Development and Validation of a Scale for Measuring State Self-Esteem." *Journal of Personality and Social Psychology*, 60 (6), 895–910.

Herman, C. Peter, and Deborah Mack. 1975. "Restrained and Unrestrained Eating." *Journal of Personality*, 43 (4), 647–660.

Herman, C. Peter, and Janet Polivy. 1980. "Restrained Eating." In *Obesity*, ed. Albert J. Stunkard, 208–225. Philadelphia: Saunders.

———. 2004. "Sociocultural Idealization of Thin Female Body Shapes: An Introduction to the Special Issue on Body Image and Eating Disorders." *Journal of Social and Clinical Psychology*, 23 (1), 1–6.

Herman, C. Peter, Janet Polivy, Cynthia N. Lank, and Todd F. Heatherton. 1987. "Anxiety, Hunger, and Eating Behavior." *Journal of Abnormal Psychology*, 96 (3), 264–269.

Herman, C. Peter, Deborah A. Roth, and Janet Polivy. 2003. "Effects of the Presence of Others on Food Intake: A Normative Interpretation." *Psychological Bulletin*, 129 (6), 873–886.

Hill, James O., Michael J. Pagliassotti, and John C. Peters. 1994. "Non-genetic determinants of obesity and body fat topography." In *Genetic Determinants of Obesity*, ed. C Bouchard, 35–48. Boca Raton, FL: CRC Press.

Hill, James O., and John C. Peters. 1998. "Environmental Contributions to the Obesity Epidemic." *Science*, 1371–1374.

Johnston, Lucy. 2002. "Behavioral Mimicry and Stigmatization." *Social Cognition*, 20 (1), 18–35.

Keltner, Dacher, and Barbara N. Buswell. 1996. "Embarrassment: Its Distinct Form of Appeasement Functions." *Physiology and Behavior*, 122 (3), 250–270.

Kielburger, Craig, and Mark Kielburger. 2008. "Obesity Becoming World Crisis." *Toronto Star*, February 4.

Kirkey, Sharon. 2008. "Doctors Show 'Serious' Weight Bias." *Ottawa Citizen*, February 3.

Leary, Mark R., and Robin M. Kowalski. 1990. "Impression Management: A Literature Review and Two-Component Model." *Physiology and Behavior*, 107 (1), 34–47

McDonald's. 2006. "McDonald's USA Nutrition Spotlight." www.mcdonalds.com/usa/eat/nutrition_info.html.

McFerran, Brent, Darren W. Dahl, Gavan J. Fitzsimons, and Andrea C. Morales. 2010a. "I'll Have What She's Having: Effects of Social Influence and Body Type on the Food Choices of Others." *Journal of Consumer Research*, 36 (April), 915–929.

———. 2010b. "Might an Overweight Waitress Make You Eat More? How the Body Type of Others Is Sufficient to Alter Our Food Consumption." *Journal of Consumer Psychology*, 20 (3) 146–151.

Moschis, George P. 1976. "Social Comparison and Informal Group Influence." *Journal of Marketing Research*, 13 (3), 237–244.

National Health and Nutrition Examination Survey (NHANES). 1980. U.S. Centers for Disease Control. www.cdc.gov/nchs/nhanes.htm.

————. 2004. U.S. Centers for Disease Control. www.cdc.gov/nchs/nhanes.htm.

Nisbett, Richard E., and Michael D Storms. 1974. "Cognitive and Social Determinants of Food Intake." In *Cognitive Alteration of Feeling States*, ed. Harvey S. London and Richard E. Nisbett, 190–208. Chicago: Aldine.

Nutristrategy. 2007. "Calories Burned During Exercise." www.nutristrategy.com/activitylist4. htm.

Pfanner, Eric. 2008. "In Britain, a Campaign Against Obesity Is Snarled in Controversy." *New York Times*, February 11.

Puhl, Rebecca, and Kelley D. Brownell. 2001. "Bias, Discrimination, and Obesity." *Obesity Research*, 9 (12), 788–805.

Reisner, Rebecca. 2008. "The Diet Industry: A Big Fat Lie." *Business Week Debate Room.* www.businessweek.com/debateroom/archives/2008/01/the_diet_indust.html.

Rosekrans, Mary A. 1967. "Imitation in Children as a Function of Perceived Similarity to the Social Model and Vicarious Reinforcement." *Journal of Personality and Social Psychology*, 7 (3), 307–315.

Rosenthal, Barbara, and Robert D. Marx. 1979. "Modeling Influences in the Eating Behavior of Successful and Unsuccessful Dieters and Treated Normal Weight Individuals." *Addictive Behaviors*, 4 (3), 215–221.

Roth, Deborah A., C. Peter Herman, Janet Polivy, and Patricia Pliner. 2001. "Self-Presentational Conflict in Social Eating Situations: A Normative Perspective." *Appetite*, 36, 165–171.

Rothblum, Esther D. 1992. "The Stigma of Women's Weight: Social and Economic Realities." *Feminism and Psychology*, 2 (1), 61–73.

Ryckman, Richard M., Michael A. Robbins, Linda M. Kaczor, and Joel A. Gold. 1989. "Male and Female Raters' Stereotyping of Male and Female Physiques." *Personality and Social Psychology Bulletin*, 15 (2), 244–251.

Scott, Maura L., Stephen M. Nowlis, Naomi Mandel, and Andrea C. Morales. 2008. "Do 100-Calorie Packs Lead to Increased Consumption? The Effect of Reduced Food Sizes and Packages on the Consumption Behavior of Restrained Eaters and Unrestrained Eaters." *Journal of Consumer Research*, 35 (October), 391–406.

Shapiro, Jenessa R., Eden B. King, and Miguel A. Quinones. 2007. "Expectations of Obese Trainees: How Stigmatized Trainee Characteristics Influence Training Effectiveness." *Journal of Applied Psychology*, 92 (1), 239–249.

Sherrid, Pamela. 2003. "Piling on the Profit: There's No Slimming Down for Companies Selling Diet Products." *U.S. News and World Report*, June 8.

Stunkard, Albert J., Jennifer R. Harris, Nancy L. Pedersen, and Gerald E. McClearn. 1990. "The Body-Mass Index of Twins Who Have Been Reared Apart." *New England Journal of Medicine*, 322, 1483–1487.

U.S. Department of Health and Human Services, National Institutes of Health. 2000. *Clinical Guidelines on the Identification, Evaluation, and Treatment of Overweight and Obesity in Adults: The Evidence Report*, NHLBI document 98–4083.

Wansink, Brian. 2006. *Mindless Eating: Why We Eat More Than We Think*. New York: Bantam-Dell.

Wansink, Brian, and Pierre Chandon. 2006. "Can 'Low-Fat' Nutrition Labels Lead to Obesity?" *Journal of Marketing Research*, 43 (November), 605–617.

Wansink, Brian, Robert J. Kent, and Stephen J. Hoch. 1998. "An Anchoring and Adjustment Model of Purchase Quantity Decisions." *Journal of Marketing Research*, 35 (February), 71–81.

Weiner, Bernard, Raymond P. Perry, and Jamie Magnusson. 1988. "An Attributional Analysis of Reactions to Stigmas." *Journal of Personality and Social Psychology*, 55 (5), 738–748.

White, Katherine, and Darren W. Dahl. 2006. "To Be or Not Be: The Influence of Dissociative Reference Groups on Consumer Preferences." *Journal of Consumer Psychology*, 16 (4), 404–413.

———. 2007. "Are All Outgroups Created Equal? The Influence of Consumer Identity and Dissociative Reference Groups on Consumer Preferences." *Journal of Consumer Research*, 34 (December), 525–536.

Young, Lisa R., and Marion Nestle. 2002. "The Contribution of Expanding Portion Sizes to the US Obesity Epidemic." *American Journal of Public Health*, 92 (2), 246–249.

Zhou, Rongrong, and Dilip Soman. 2003. "Looking Back: Exploring the Psychology of Queuing and the Effect of the Number of People Behind." *Journal of Consumer Research*, 29 (March), 517–530.

PART III

COMMUNICATION STRATEGY AND TACTICS

CHAPTER 8

THE RELATIVE EFFECTIVENESS OF GAIN-FRAMED AND LOSS-FRAMED PERSUASIVE APPEALS CONCERNING OBESITY-RELATED BEHAVIORS

Meta-Analytic Evidence and Implications

DANIEL J. O'KEEFE AND JAKOB D. JENSEN

Obesity is a significant national health problem. The prevalence of obesity has been increasing (Ogden et al. 2006), and obesity has significant undesirable health consequences, though estimates of the magnitude of effect vary (e.g., Flegal et al. 2005; Mokdad et al. 2004).

A variety of persuasive communications and interventions have been explored as possible means to prevent or reduce obesity. One persuasive message variation that has been of interest to researchers in this domain is the contrast between gain-framed and loss-framed appeals. A gain-framed appeal emphasizes the advantages of compliance with the advocated action (e.g., "if you exercise regularly, it will be easier to maintain a healthy body weight"); a loss-framed appeal emphasizes the disadvantages of noncompliance ("if you don't exercise regularly, it will be harder to maintain a healthy body weight"). For example, Bannon and Schwartz (2006) compared the effects of gain- and loss-framed messages on the snack choices of kindergarteners, and Jones, Sinclair, and Courneya (2003) examined the relative persuasiveness of gain- and loss-framed appeals for encouraging exercise by college students.

This chapter provides a meta-analytic review of the accumulated experimental research concerning the relative persuasiveness of gain-framed and loss-framed appeals for influencing various obesity-related behaviors. A meta-analytic review of this research offers natural advantages over the typical primary-research design, precisely because a meta-analysis synthesizes results from a number of different studies using different concrete instantiations of the general message contrast of interest (see Jackson 1992).

GENERAL BACKGROUND

Previous research has undermined a number of otherwise plausible hypotheses about the persuasive effects of message framing variations. For example, one hypothesis has been that in general, loss-framed appeals will be more persuasive than gain-framed appeals (e.g., Johnson, Maio, and Smith-McLallen 2005, 640). This hypothesis was made plausible by findings that negative information is often more powerful than parallel positive information (e.g., Rozin and Royzman 2001) and that people are more willing to take a risk to avoid (or minimize) losses than to obtain gains (e.g., Kuhberger, Schulte-Mecklenbeck, and Perner 1999). This hypothesis is not supported by the research evidence. O'Keefe and Jensen's (2006) review of 165 gain-loss message framing studies found no significant general difference in persuasiveness between the two forms of appeal.

A second approach invokes a distinction between disease detection behaviors and disease prevention behaviors. The hypothesis is that loss-framed appeals will be more persuasive than gain-framed appeals for encouraging disease detection behaviors, whereas gain-framed appeals will be more persuasive than loss-framed appeals for encouraging disease prevention behaviors (see, e.g., Rothman and Salovey 1997; Salovey and Wegener 2003).

This hypothesis is also unsupported. Concerning the suggestion that loss-framed appeals will be more persuasive than gain-framed appeals for disease detection: O'Keefe and Jensen's (2009) meta-analysis found that across fifty-three framing studies (with over 9,000 participants) focused on disease detection behaviors, there was a trivially small effect (corresponding to $r = -.04$) favoring loss-framed messages—but that effect was attributable to the large number of studies ($k = 17$) concerning breast cancer detection behaviors (which exhibited a small effect, $r = -.06$). The remaining thirty-six disease detection studies yielded no statistically significant difference in persuasiveness between gain-framed and loss-framed appeals, despite excellent statistical power. So the supposition that loss-framed appeals will generally have a persuasive advantage concerning disease detection behaviors is not tenable.

Concerning the suggestion that gain-framed appeals will be more persuasive than loss-framed appeals for disease prevention: O'Keefe and Jensen's (2007) meta-analysis found that across ninety-three framing studies (with over 21,000 participants) focused on disease prevention messages, there was a trivial effect (corresponding to $r = .03$) favoring gain-framed appeals—but that effect was due to a large effect ($r = .15$) for studies of dental hygiene behaviors ($k = 9$). The remaining eighty-four disease prevention studies yielded no statistically significant difference in persuasiveness between gain-framed and loss-framed appeals, again despite excellent statistical power. So the supposition that gain-framed appeals will generally have a persuasive advantage concerning disease prevention behaviors is not tenable.

SPECIFIC FOCUS

Even if there are not broad-scale differences in persuasiveness between gain- and loss-framed appeals (e.g., such that loss-framed appeals are more persuasive for disease detection behaviors), it is still possible that such a difference might emerge for some more specific behavioral domain (e.g., dental hygiene). This report is concerned specifically with obesity-relevant behaviors. Researchers have compared the persuasiveness of gain- and loss-framed appeals for two such behaviors, namely, exercise and healthy eating practices. In our earlier review (O'Keefe and Jensen 2007), there was no statistically significant difference in the persuasiveness of gain- and loss-framed appeals for either domain. However, there were too few studies of exercise behaviors ($k = 8$) to provide more than modest (.59) statistical power—and since that earlier review a number of additional studies have been completed.

Hence, this report offers an updated review of research concerning differences in the relative persuasiveness of gain- and loss-framed appeals for obesity-relevant behaviors. We were interested in estimating the size of any overall difference between gain- and loss-framed appeals in this domain, and in estimating such differences separately for messages advocating greater physical activity and those advocating healthy eating practices. We also wanted to explore the possible moderating role of an aspect of the phrasing of the appeals, namely, the linguistic representation of the "kernel state" of the consequence under discussion (O'Keefe and Jensen 2006). The kernel state is the basic, root state mentioned in the message's description of the consequence. A given framing form might mention either desirable or undesirable kernel states. For example, a gain-framed appeal might take the form "if you exercise, you'll increase your chances of having a healthy heart" (where the kernel state, "healthy heart," is a desirable one) or the form "if you exercise, you'll reduce your risk of heart disease" (where the kernel state, "heart disease," is an undesirable one). Several commentators have suggested that this variation might influence the relative persuasiveness of gain- and loss-framed appeals (e.g., Dillard and Marshall 2003).

METHOD

Identification of Relevant Investigations

Relevant research reports were located through personal knowledge of the literature, examination of previous reviews, and inspection of reference lists in previously located reports. Reports were also identified through computerized database searches through at least February 2009 of ABI-INFORM, CINAHL (Cumulative Index of Nursing and Allied Health Literature), Current Contents, Dissertation Abstracts, EBSCO, ERIC (Educational Resources Information Center), Linguistics and Language Behavior Abstracts, MEDLINE, and PsycINFO, using various appropriate combinations of terms such as *framing, framed, frame, appeal, message, persuasion, persuasive, gain, positive, positively, benefit, loss, negative, negatively, threat,* and *valence.*

We included a study if it met three criteria. First, the study had to compare gain-framed and loss-framed persuasive messages. A gain-framed message emphasizes the desirable consequences of compliance with the advocated view; a loss-framed message emphasizes the undesirable consequences of noncompliance. This criterion was applied so as to exclude imperfect realizations of this message contrast; for examples of such excluded studies, see Lockwood et al. (2005), Parrott et al. (2008), van den Heuvel (1982), and van Kleef, van Trijp, and Luning (2005).

Second, the messages had to advocate behaviors potentially relevant to obesity, such as undertaking regular exercise or engaging in healthy eating practices.

Third, appropriate quantitative data relevant to persuasive effects (e.g., attitude change, intention, or behavior) had to be available, either in the report or from authors. Excluded by this criterion were reports of effects on other outcome variables and studies for which appropriate quantitative information could not be obtained (e.g., Horgen and Brownell 2002; Siu 2004; van't Riet et al. 2009, Experiment 1; Yi and Baumgartner 2007).

Outcome Variable and Effect Size Measure

The outcome variable was persuasion, as assessed through attitude change, post-communication agreement, behavioral intention, behavior, and the like. When multiple indices of persuasion were available, we averaged the effects to yield a single summary. Most studies reported only immediate (short-term) effects; where both immediate and delayed effect size information was available (e.g., Jones, Sinclair, and Courneya 2003), only immediate effects were included to maximize comparability across studies.

Every comparison between a gain-framed message and its loss-framed counterpart was summarized using *r* as the effect size measure. When not reported as correlations, results were converted to *r* using formulas provided by Johnson (1993) and Rosenthal (1991). Differences indicating greater persuasion with gain-framed messages were given a positive sign. When correlations were averaged (e.g., across several indices of persuasive effect), we computed the average using the *r*-to-*z*-to-*r* transformation procedure, weighted by *n*.

Moderating Factors

Advocated Behavior

Cases were classified by the kind of behavior advocated, with three broad categories distinguished: healthy eating behaviors, physical activity (e.g., exercise), and other (or multiple different) obesity-relevant behaviors (e.g., attending a weight control class).

Kernel State Phrasing

The kernel states in each appeal were identified. As described earlier, a kernel state is the basic, root state mentioned in the message's description of the consequence under discussion. We coded each appeal as containing exclusively desirable kernel states, exclusively undesirable kernel states, a combination of desirable and undesirable kernel states, or as indeterminate with respect to kernel-state phrasing (as when insufficient detail was available about the messages).

Unit of Analysis and Meta-Analytic Procedures

The unit of analysis was the message pair, that is, the pair composed of a gain-framed message and its loss-framed counterpart. We recorded an effect size for each distinguishable message pair. When a message pair was used in more than one study (Bibby 2008, Study 1 and Study 2), an effect size estimate was initially computed for each study and then these multiple estimates were averaged to yield a single summary estimate. When a study reported data separately for multiple message pairs, each pair provided a separate effect size estimate (e.g., van Assema et al. 2001). When a given investigation was reported in more than one outlet, it was treated as a single study and analyzed accordingly. The collected effect sizes were analyzed using random-effects procedures (specifically, those of Borenstein and Rothstein 2005).

RESULTS

Overall Effects

Effect sizes were available for forty-three cases, with a total of 5,154 participants. Details for each included case are contained in Table 8.1. Across all forty-three cases, the mean correlation was .083, a statistically significant persuasive advantage for gain-framed appeals ($p = .002$); see Table 8.2. This overall effect, of course, averages results across rather different behaviors (even if all are in some way obesity-relevant). Hence, the more illuminating analyses are those that examine effects for different varieties of advocated actions.

Specific Obesity-Relevant Behaviors

For messages that encouraged physical activity, gain-framed appeals were significantly more persuasive than loss-framed appeals. Across eighteen cases, the random-effects weighted mean correlation was .171 ($p = .001$); see Table 8.2.

For messages that encouraged healthy eating practices, there was no significant difference in persuasiveness between gain-framed and loss-framed appeals. Across twenty-one cases, the random-effects weighted mean correlation was .017

Table 8.1

Cases Analyzed

Study	r	N	Codings[a]
Arora and Arora (2004)	.088	267	1/2/4
Bannon and Schwartz (2006)	.016	32	1/1/2
Bibby (2008)	−.147	121	1/2/1
Brug, Ruiter, and van Assema (2003), Study 2	.039	149	1/4/4
Brug, Ruiter, and van Assema (2003), Study 3	−.061	92	1/4/4
Cesario, Grant, and Higgins (2004), prevention	−.169	53	1/3/3
Cesario, Grant, and Higgins (2004), promotion	.115	53	1/1/2
Gray (2008), narrative	.160	132	2/3/3
Gray (2008), statistical	.222	143	2/1/3
Hashimoto (2002)	−.013	166	1/2/1
Hsiao (2002), exercise-prevention	.546	49	2/3/3
Hsiao (2002), exercise-detection	−.378	51	2/3/3
Jayanti (2001)	.007	69	1/4/4
Jones, Sinclair, and Courneya (2003)	.048	192	2/3/3
Jones, Sinclair, Rhodes, and Courneya (2004)	.020	413	2/3/3
Kroll (2004)	.063	192	2/3/3
Latimer, Rench et al. (2008)	.336	97	2/4/4
Latimer, Rivers et al. (2008)	.148	155	2/4/4
Lawatsch (1990)	.071	72	1/1/3
Lee and Aaker (2004), Experiment 3, high risk	−.312	45	1/3/3
Lee and Aaker (2004), Experiment 3, low risk	.382	36	1/3/3
Levin, Gaeth, Evangelista, Albaum, and Schreiber (2001)	−.127	224	1/2/1
Levin, Gaeth, Schreiber, and Lauriola (2002)	.021	102	1/2/1
Looker and Shannon (1984)	.006	227	1/1/1
McCall and Ginis (2004)	.311	29	2/3/3
Meyers-Levy and Maheswaran (2004)	.270	147	1/3/3
Nan (2007), Experiment 1, desirable-gain, desirable-loss	−.121	75	2/1/2
Nan (2007), Experiment 1, desirable-gain, undesirable-loss	.055	74	2/1/1
Nan (2007), Experiment 1, undesirable-gain, desirable-loss	.029	81	2/2/1
Nan (2007), Experiment 1, undesirable-gain, undesirable-loss	.197	80	2/2/2
Robberson and Rogers (1988), health	−.190	24	2/3/3
Robberson and Rogers (1988), self-esteem	.537	24	2/1/3
Shannon and Rowan (1987)	.031	138	3/4/4
Shen (2005), Study 1, obesity	.157	286	3/3/3
Simmering (1993), non-social	−.030	78	3/3/1
Simmering (1993), social	.027	77	3/1/3
Tsai (2007)	−.002	458	1/1/1
Tykocinski, Higgins, and Chaiken (1994)	.029	39	1/4/4
van Assema, Martens, Ruiter, and Brug (2001), low-fat	.035	75	1/3/1
van Assema, Martens, Ruiter, and Brug (2001), fruit and vegetable	.068	66	1/3/1
van't Riet, Ruiter, Werrij, Candel, and de Vries (2009), Experiment 2	.087	129	1/3/1
Whitbourne and Lachman (2003), appearance	.477	93	2/1/3
Whitbourne and Lachman (2003), health	.506	92	2/1/3

Notes: [a]The coding judgments, in order, are: specific obesity-relevant behavior (1 = healthy eating, 2 = physical activity, 3 = other obesity-relevant behavior); gain kernel-state language (1 = desirable states, 2 = undesirable states, 3 = both desirable and undesirable states, 4 = indeterminate); loss kernel-state language (1 = undesirable states, 2 = desirable states, 3 = both desirable and undesirable states, 4 = indeterminate).

Table 8.2

Summary of Results

	k	N	Mean r	95% CI	Power	Q (df)
All cases	43	5,154	.083	.030, .134	—	133.8(42)**
Advocated behavior						
Healthy eating	21	2,622	.017	−.036, .070	.95	32.9(20)*
Physical activity	18	1,953	.171	.068, .270	—	80.7(17)**
Other	4	579	.083	−.002, .167	.39	3.2(3)
Gain message kernel						
Desirable only	12	1,420	.158	.032, .278	—	52.9(11)**
Undesirable only	7	1,041	−.002	−.089, .086	.62	11.4(6)
Both	17	1,997	.073	−.014, .159	.88	51.4(16)**
Indeterminate	7	696	.082	−.019, .180	.45	10.1(6)
Loss message kernel						
Desirable only	4	241	−.001	−.130, .128	.19	1.8(3)
Undesirable only	12	1,800	−.006	−.053, .041	.84	10.9(11)
Both	19	2,150	.154	.051, .253	—	90.1(18)**
Indeterminate	8	963	.083	.003, .162	—	10.1(7)

$*p < .05; **p < .001$

($p = .527$), a nonsignificant effect despite excellent statistical power (.95); see Table 8.2. (Power values reported in this chapter are for detecting a population effect size of $r = .10$, assuming large heterogeneity, with a random-effects analysis, .05 alpha, and a two-tailed test [Hedges and Pigott 2001].) The various "healthy eating" behaviors were quite diverse, which limited the utility of further analyses. In four cases, the messages advocated eating more fruits and vegetables (Bibby 2008; Cesario, Grant, and Higgins 2004, prevention condition and promotion condition; van Assema et al. 2001, fruit and vegetable condition); across these cases, mean $r = -.049$ ($n = 293$), 95 percent CI limits of −.186 and .091 ($p = .495$), power = .22; $Q(3) = 4.1$, $p = .251$. In five cases, the messages advocated consumption of some form of dietary supplements (Brug, Ruiter, and van Assema 2003, Study 2 and Study 3; Hashimoto 2002; Lee and Aaker 2004, Experiment 3, high risk, and Experiment 3, low risk); across these cases, mean $r = -.003$ ($n = 488$), 95 percent CI limits of −.156 and .151 ($p = .972$), power = .34; $Q(4) = 10.3$, $p = .036$. In the remaining twelve cases, various other healthy-eating practices were encouraged, such as making wise snack food choices and reducing salt consumption; across these cases, mean $r = .038$ ($n = 1,841$), 95 percent CI limits of −.022 and .098 ($p = .215$), power = .85; $Q(11) = 16.3$, $p = .129$.

In four studies, the advocated action was some other obesity-relevant behavior (such as attending a weight control class) or multiple such behaviors (e.g., "regular exercise and a healthy diet"; Shen 2005). Across these four cases, the persuasive advantage for gain-framed appeals (mean $r = .083$) was not quite statistically significant ($p = .056$); see Table 8.2.

Kernel-State Phrasing

Kernel-State Phrasing in Gain-Framed Appeals

Gain-framed appeals were significantly more persuasive than loss-framed appeals when the gain-framed appeal had exclusively desirable kernel states (mean $r =$ .158, $p = .014$); see Table 8.2. Gain-framed appeals that had exclusively undesirable kernel states were not significantly more persuasive than loss-framed appeals (mean $r = -.002$, $p = .967$). The persuasive advantage (compared to loss-framed appeals) of gain-framed appeals using exclusively desirable kernel states (mean $r = .158$) was significantly different from the effect obtained when gain-framed appeals used exclusively undesirable kernel states (mean $r = -.002$); $Q(1) = 4.19$, $p = .041$.

Gain-framed appeals that combined desirable and undesirable kernel states were not significantly more persuasive than loss-framed appeals (mean $r = .073$, $p = .102$); see Table 8.2. The persuasive advantage (compared to loss-framed appeals) of gain-framed appeals using exclusively desirable kernel states (mean $r =$ .158) was not significantly different from the effect obtained when gain-framed appeals used a combination of desirable and undesirable kernel states (mean $r =$ .073); $Q(1) = 1.21$, $p = .272$.

Kernel-State Phrasing in Loss-Framed Appeals

Gain- and loss-framed appeals did not differ significantly in persuasiveness either when the loss-framed appeal had exclusively desirable kernel states (mean $r =$ −.001, $p = .987$) or when it had exclusively undesirable kernel states (mean $r =$ −.006, $p = .803$); see Table 8.2. These two mean effects were not significantly different [$Q(1) = .01$, p = .945].

When the loss-framed appeal had a combination of desirable and undesirable kernel states, gain-framed appeals had a significant persuasive advantage (mean r = .154, $p = .003$); see Table 8.2. This effect was not significantly different from the effect obtained using loss-framed appeals with exclusively desirable kernel states (mean $r = -.001$); $Q(1) = 3.40$, $p = .065$. It was, however, significantly larger than the effect obtained using loss-framed appeals with exclusively undesirable kernel states (mean $r = -.006$); $Q(1) = 7.70$, $p = .006$.

DISCUSSION

Broadly speaking, these results would appear to recommend the use of gain-framed appeals for encouraging obesity-relevant behaviors; across the whole set of studies, gain-framed appeals were significantly more persuasive than loss-framed appeals. And these results would seem to point specifically to the desirability of using gain-framed appeals that are expressed in terms of desirable kernel states; across the studies reviewed here, gain-framed appeals enjoyed their persuasive advantage when the appeals invoked exclusively desirable kernel states but not when the appeals invoked exclusively undesirable kernel states.

However, this characterization of these results is misleading. The advantage of gain-framed appeals over their loss-framed counterparts was obtained specifically for messages encouraging physical activity. No such advantage was obtained for messages encouraging healthy eating practices. In fact, the mean effect for physical-activity messages (mean $r = .171$) and that for healthy-eating messages (mean $r = .017$) are significantly different; $Q(1) = 6.70$, $p = .010$. So it will be useful to consider separately these two broad behavioral categories.

Healthy Eating Practices

The studies in which messages advocated various healthy eating practices are not narrowly relevant to obesity prevention or reduction. The advocated eating practices—such as consuming more fruits and vegetables, reducing salt intake or red meat consumption, taking dietary supplements, and so forth—are not aimed specifically at preventing or reducing obesity. We examined these studies because of their potential for shedding light on effective advocacy of other eating practices that *would* be directly relevant to obesity.

However—consistent with our earlier review (O'Keefe and Jensen 2007)—there is no evidence here that either gain- or loss-framed appeals enjoy any persuasive advantage in influencing healthy eating behaviors. Thus we think it unlikely to be profitable for researchers to investigate gain-loss framing variations for healthy eating behaviors that are more specifically targeted to obesity, and we think it unwise for designers of messages aimed at specifically obesity-relevant eating practices to worry very much about whether those messages are gain- or loss-framed.

Physical Activity

In our earlier review (O'Keefe and Jensen 2007), there was no significant difference between gain- and loss-framed appeals for encouraging physical activity, but there were relatively few studies (eight, as against the eighteen reviewed here) and correspondingly relatively poor statistical power (.59). But the current review makes it clear that advocates for increased physical activity should employ gain-framed rather than loss-framed appeals. Indeed, the advantage that loss-framed appeals have over gain-framed appeals in this domain (mean $r = .17$) is relatively large compared to the mean effect sizes observed for other persuasive message variations (see O'Keefe 1999). But this result naturally gives rise to two questions. First, if physical activity messages are to be gain-framed, are some forms of gain-framed appeals likely to be more persuasive than others? Second, what explains the persuasive advantage of gain-framed appeals for physical activity messages?

Enhancing the Persuasiveness of Gain-Framed Physical
Activity Appeals

There is no reason to suppose that all gain-framed physical activity appeals will
be equally persuasive. However, the data most relevant to this question will come
from designs that compare alternative forms of a gain-framed appeal.

Still, one might try to mine the current studies for some clues on this matter
by seeing whether the relative advantage of gain-framed appeals (concerning
physical activity) varies as a function of the kernel-state language in the appeal.
Unfortunately, the extant gain-loss message framing research literature is less
than ideal for this purpose—for two reasons. First, the existing studies are not
well distributed across different kernel-state phrasings of gain-framed appeals.
For example, of the eighteen studies of physical activity messages, only two had
gain-framed appeals with exclusively undesirable states. Second, the results of a
comparison of a given gain-framed version against a loss-framed message might
vary depending on the kernel-state phrasing of the *loss*-framed message—and
the extant studies are not well-distributed across different kernel-state phrasings
of loss-framed appeals.

These studies do permit one relatively clean contrast, between the effects
observed for gain-framed appeals that contained a combination of desirable and
undesirable kernel states and the effects observed for gain-framed appeals that
contained exclusively desirable kernel states, where the comparison loss-framed
appeal contained both desirable and undesirable kernel states. When the gain-framed
appeal contained both desirable and undesirable kernel states, the mean effect size
was $r = .079$ [$k = 8$, $n = 1,082$, 95 percent CI limits of $-.062$ and $.217$, $p = .274$;
$Q(7) = 29.2$, $p < .001$]. When the gain-framed appeal contained exclusively desirable kernel states, the mean effect size was $r = .421$ [$k = 4$, $n = 352$, 95 percent CI
limits of $.251$ and $.565$, $p < .001$; $Q(3) = 8.5$, $p = .037$]. These two mean effect sizes
are significantly different [$Q(1) = 9.26$, $p = .002$]. This evidence, although limited,
suggests that messages advocating physical activity should avoid appeals phrased
in terms of both desirable and undesirable kernel states and should instead phrase
appeals exclusively in terms of desirable kernel states.

It should not pass unnoticed that the contrast between desirable and undesirable kernel states in gain-framed appeals can be redescribed in term of a contrast
between "promotion-focused" and "prevention-focused" appeals (see, e.g., Higgins
1999). A promotion-focused appeal emphasizes (the obtaining of, or the failure to
obtain) positive states; a prevention-focused appeal emphasizes (the obtaining of,
or the avoidance of) negative states. Expressed that way, these data hint that for
physical activity messages, promotion-focused gain-framed appeals may be more
persuasive than gain-framed appeals that combine promotion- and prevention-
based appeals (for some discussions of the interplay of gain-loss framing and
promotion-prevention focus, see Lin 2007; Yi and Baumgartner 2008; Zhao and
Pechmann 2007).

Explaining the Persuasive Advantage of Gain-Framed Physical Activity Appeals

It is not immediately apparent what might explain the persuasive advantage that gain-framed appeals enjoy over loss-framed appeals for encouraging physical activity. One well-publicized explanatory framework, however, can be shown to be insufficient.

That explanatory framework is based on Kahneman and Tversky's (1979) prospect theory, which has often been interpreted as suggesting that the relative persuasiveness of gain- and loss-framed appeals will vary depending on the riskiness of the advocated behavior. The idea has been that for riskier behaviors, such as disease detection behaviors (e.g., cancer screenings), loss-framed appeals will be more persuasive than gain-framed appeals, whereas for low-risk behaviors, such as disease prevention behaviors (e.g., exercising or wearing sunscreen), gain-framed appeals will have the advantage (see, e.g., Rothman and Salovey 1997; Salovey, Schneider, and Apanovitch 2002). This account, though common, is arguably not entirely well thought out. In particular, it seems to depend on confusing dangerousness and uncertainty, which are two distinct possible senses of "risk" (see O'Keefe and Jensen 2006, 22–23).

As discussed above, these expectations have not been borne out by the research evidence. For disease detection behaviors, any advantage of loss-framed appeals may be limited to breast cancer detection behaviors (O'Keefe and Jensen 2009). For disease prevention behaviors (exercise apart), gain-framed appeals enjoy an advantage only when the messages advocate dental hygiene behaviors (O'Keefe and Jensen 2007). In short, the observed advantage of gain-framed appeals for physical activity messages cannot be explained simply by invoking some putatively general advantage of such appeals for encouraging disease prevention behaviors, because there is no such advantage.

The lack of a good explanation, of course, is no barrier to seeing the practical advice that issues from this result: those advocating greater physical activity should use gain-framed appeals rather than loss-framed appeals. At the same time, a good explanatory account would presumably provide a better grasp of the mechanisms underlying the observed effects—and that, in turn, could inform the development of even more effective messages.

REFERENCES

Note: References marked with an asterisk indicate studies included in the meta-analysis.

*Arora, Raj, and Alisha Arora. 2004. "The Impact of Message Framing and Credibility Finding for Nutritional Guidelines." *Services Marketing Quarterly*, 26 (1), 35–53.
*Bannon, Katie, and Marline B. Schwartz. 2006. "Impact of Nutrition Messages on Children's Food Choice: Pilot Study." *Appetite*, 46, 124–129.
*Bibby, Peter. 2008. "Effects of Gender on Gain and Loss Framed Messages for Eating Fruit and Vegetables." Paper presented at the second joint European and UK Health Psychology

Conference of the Division of Health Psychology of the British Psychological Society and the European Health Psychology Society, Bath, England.

Borenstein, Michael, and Hannah Rothstein. 2005. Comprehensive Meta-Analysis, Version 2.2.023 (computer software). Englewood, NJ: Biostat.

*Brug, Johannes, Robert A. C. Ruiter, and Patricia van Assema. 2003. "The (Ir)Relevance of Framing Nutrition Education Messages." *Nutrition and Health*, 17, 9–20.

*Cesario, Joseph, Heidi Grant, and Tory E. Higgins. 2004. "Regulatory Fit and Persuasion: Transfer from 'Feeling Right.'" *Journal of Personality and Social Psychology*, 86, 388–404.

Dillard, James P., and Linda J. Marshall. 2003. "Persuasion as a Social Skill." In *Handbook of Communication and Social Interaction Skills*, ed. John O. Green and Brant R. Burleson, 479–513. Mahwah, NJ: Lawrence Erlbaum.

Flegal, Katherine M., Barry I. Graubard, David F. Williamson, and Mitchell H. Gail. 2005. "Excess Deaths Associated With Underweight, Overweight, and Obesity." *Journal of the American Medical Association*, 293, 1861–1867.

*Gray, Jennifer B. 2008. "Framing the Evidence: A Test of an Integrated Message Strategy in the Exercise Context." PhD diss., University of Kentucky. *Dissertation Abstracts International*, 69 (2008), A. (UMI No. AAT-3315012).

*Hashimoto, Sayaka. 2002. "The Effect of Message Framing on College Women's Folic Acid Intake Attitudes, Intentions, and Behavior." Master's thesis, University of Cincinnati.

Hedges, Larry V., and Therese D. Pigott. 2001. "The Power of Statistical Tests in Meta-Analysis." *Psychological Methods*, 6, 203–217.

Higgins, E. Tory. 1999. "Promotion and Prevention as a Motivational Duality: Implications for Evaluative Processes." In *Dual-Process Models in Social Psychology*, ed. Shelly Chaiken and Yaakov Trope, 503–525. New York: Guilford Press.

Horgen, Katherine B., and Kelly D. Brownell. 2002. "Comparison of Price Change and Health Message Interventions in Promoting Healthy Food Choices." *Health Psychology*, 21, 505–512.

*Hsiao, Evana T.Y. 2002. "Using Message Framing to Promote Regular Physical Activity in College-Age Women and Men." PhD diss., Ohio State University. *Dissertation Abstracts International*, 63 (2003), 3461B. (UMI No. AAT-3059265).

Jackson, Sally. 1992. *Message Effects Research: Principles of Design and Analysis*. New York: Guilford Press.

*Jayanti, Rama. 2001. "Are Negative Frames More Persuasive Than Positive Frames for Senior Citizens? An Exploratory Investigation of Age Differences in Framing Effects." Paper presented at the meeting of the European Association for Consumer Research, Berlin, Germany.

Johnson, Blair T. 1993. DSTAT, Version 1.10 (computer software). Hillsdale, NJ: Lawrence Erlbaum.

Johnson, Blair T., Gregory R. Maio, and Aaron Smith-McLallen. 2005. "Communication and Attitude Change: Causes, Processes, and Effects." In *The Handbook of Attitudes*, ed. Dolores Albarracin, Blair T. Johnson, and Mark P. Zanna, 617–669. Mahwah, NJ: Lawrence Erlbaum.

*Jones, Lee W., Robert C. Sinclair, and Kerry S. Courneya. 2003. "The Effects of Source Credibility and Message Framing on Exercise Intentions, Behaviors, and Attitudes: An Integration of the Elaboration Likelihood Model and Prospect Theory." *Journal of Applied Social Psychology*, 33, 179–196.

*Jones, Lee W., Robert C. Sinclair, Ryan E. Rhodes, and Kerry S. Courneya. 2004. "Promoting Exercise Behaviour: An Integration of Persuasion Theories and the Theory of Planned Behaviour." *British Journal of Health Psychology*, 9, 505–521.

Kahneman, Daniel, and Amos Tversky. 1979. "Prospect Theory: An Analysis of Decision Under Risk." *Econometrica*, 47, 263–291.

*Kroll, Evan. 2004. "The Effects of Message Framing and Gender on Physical Exercise Communications to High School Students." PhD diss., Hofstra University. *Dissertation Abstracts International*, 66 (2005), 587B. (UMI No. AAT-3161768).

Kuhberger, Anton, Michael Schulte-Mecklenbeck, and Josef Perner. 1999. "The Effects of Framing, Reflection, Probability, and Payoff on Risk Preference in Choice Tasks." *Organizational Behavior and Human Decision Processes*, 78, 204–231.

*Latimer, Amy E., Tara A. Rench, Susan E. Rivers, Nicole A. Katulak, Stephanie A. Materese, Lisa Cadmus, Althea Hicks, Julie Keany Hodorowski, and Peter Salovey. 2008. "Promoting Participation in Physical Activity Using Framed Messages: An Application of Prospect Theory." *British Journal of Health Psychology*, 13, 659–681.

*Latimer, Amy E., Susan E. Rivers, Tara A. Rench, Nicole A. Katulak, Althea Hicks, Julie Keany Hodorowski, E. Tory Higgins, and Peter Salovey. 2008. "A Field Experiment Testing the Utility of Regulatory Fit Messages for Promoting Physical Activity." *Journal of Experimental Social Psychology*, 44, 826–832.

*Lawatsch, Deanna E. 1990. "A Comparison of Two Teaching Strategies on Nutrition Knowledge, Attitudes and Food Behavior of Preschool Children." *Journal of Nutrition Education*, 22, 117–123.

*Lee, Angela Y., and Jennifer L. Aaker. 2004. "Bringing the Frame into Focus: The Influence of Regulatory Fit on Processing Fluency and Persuasion." *Journal of Personality and Social Psychology*, 86, 205–218.

*Levin, Irwin P., Gary J. Gaeth, Felicitas Evangelista, Gerald Albaum, and Judy Schreiber. 2001. "How Positive and Negative Frames Influence the Decisions of Persons in the United States and Australia." *Asia Pacific Journal of Marketing and Logistics*, 13 (2), 64–71.

*Levin, Irwin P., Gary J. Gaeth, Judy Schreiber, and Marco Lauriola. 2002. "A New Look at Framing Effects: Distribution of Effect Sizes, Individual Differences, and Independence of Types of Effects." *Organizational Behavior and Human Decision Processes*, 88, 411–429.

Lin, Hui-Fei. 2007. "Framing Hedonic and Utilitarian Product Attributes in Advertisements: The Impact of Regulatory Fit on Persuasion." PhD diss., Pennsylvania State University. *Dissertation Abstracts International*, 68 (2007), 1718A. (UMI No. AAT 3266154).

Lockwood, Penelope, Carol Wong, Kelly McShane, and Dan Dolderman. 2005. "The Impact of Positive and Negative Fitness Exemplars on Motivation." *Basic and Applied Social Psychology*, 27, 1–13.

*Looker, Anne, and Barbara Shannon. 1984. "Threat vs. Benefit Appeals: Effectiveness in Adult Nutrition Education." *Journal of Nutrition Education*, 16, 173–176.

*McCall, Lori A., and Kathleen A. Martin Ginis. 2004. "The Effects of Message Framing on Exercise Adherence and Health Beliefs Among Patients in a Cardiac Rehabilitation Program." *Journal of Applied Biobehavioral Research*, 9, 122–135.

*Meyers-Levy, Joan, and Durairaj Maheswaran. 2004. "Exploring Message Framing Outcomes When Systematic, Heuristic, or Both Types of Processing Occur." *Journal of Consumer Psychology*, 14, 159–167.

Mokdad, Ali H., James S. Marks, Donna F. Stroup, and Julie L. Gerberding. 2004. "Actual Causes of Death in the United States, 2000." *Journal of the American Medical Association*, 293, 293–294.

*Nan, Xiaoli. 2007. "The Relative Persuasive Effect of Gain- Versus Loss-Framed Messages: Exploring the Moderating Role of the Desirability of End-States." *Journalism and Mass Communication Quarterly*, 84, 509–524.

Ogden, Cynthia L., Margaret D. Carroll, Lester R. Curtin, Margaret A. McDowell, Carolyn J. Tabak, and Katherine M. Flegal. 2006. "Prevalence of Overweight and Obesity in the United States, 1999–2004." *Journal of the American Medical Association*, 295, 1549–1555.

O'Keefe, Daniel J. 1999. "Variability of Persuasive Message Effects: Meta-Analytic Evidence and Implications." *Document Design*, 1, 87–97.

O'Keefe, Daniel J., and Jakob D. Jensen. 2006. "The Advantages of Compliance or the Disadvantages of Noncompliance? A Meta-Analytic Review of the Relative Persuasive Effectiveness of Gain-Framed and Loss-Framed Messages." *Communication Yearbook*, 30, 1–43.

———. 2007. "The Relative Persuasiveness of Gain-Framed and Loss-Framed Messages for Encouraging Disease Prevention Behaviors: A Meta-Analytic Review." *Journal of Health Communication*, 12, 623–644.

———. 2009. "The Relative Persuasiveness of Gain-Framed and Loss-Framed Messages for Encouraging Disease Detection Behaviors: A Meta-Analytic Review." *Journal of Communication*, 59, 296–316.

Parrott, Matthew W., Leo Keith Tennant, Stephen Olejnik, and Melanie S. Poudevigne. 2008. "Theory of Planned Behavior: Implications for an Email-Based Physical Activity Intervention." *Psychology of Sport and Exercise*, 9, 511–526.

*Robberson, Margaret R., and Ronald W. Rogers. 1988. "Beyond Fear Appeals: Negative and Positive Persuasive Appeals to Health and Self-Esteem." *Journal of Applied Social Psychology*, 18, 277–287.

Rosenthal, Robert. 1991. *Meta-Analytic Procedures for Social Research*. 2nd ed. Beverly Hills, CA: Sage.

Rothman, Alexander J., and Peter Salovey. 1997. "Shaping Perceptions to Motivate Healthy Behavior: The Role of Message Framing." *Psychological Bulletin*, 121, 3–19.

Rozin, Paul, and Edward B. Royzman. 2001. "Negativity Bias, Negativity Dominance, and Contagion." *Personality and Social Psychology Review*, 5, 296–320.

Salovey, Peter, Tamara R. Schneider, and Anne Marie Apanovitch. 2002. "Message Framing in the Prevention and Early Detection of Illness." In *The Persuasion Handbook: Developments in Theory and Practice*, ed. James P. Dillard and Michael Pfau, 391–406. Thousand Oaks, CA: Sage.

Salovey, Peter, and Duane T. Wegener. 2003. "Communicating About Health: Message Framing, Persuasion, and Health Behavior." In *Social Psychology Foundations of Health and Illness*, ed. Jerry M. Suls and Kenneth A. Wallston, 54–81. Oxford, UK: Blackwell.

*Shannon, Barbara, and Mary L Rowan. 1987. "Threat vs. Benefit Appeals for Motivating Adults to Participate in a Weight-Control Class." *Journal of the American Dietetic Association*, 87, 1612–1614.

*Shen, Lijiang. 2005. "The Interplay of Message Framing, Cognition and Affect in Persuasive Health Communication." PhD diss, University of Wisconsin-Madison. *Dissertation Abstracts International*, 66 (2005), 1561A. (UMI No. 3175536).

*Simmering, Melisande J. 1993. "Effects of Social and Non-Social Messages Regarding Weight on Women's Weight Loss Intentions as a Function of Self-Presentational Style." PhD diss., Columbia University. *Dissertation Abstracts International*, 54 (1993), 4447B. (UMI No. AAI-9333865).

Siu, Wanda Luen-wun. 2004. "The Integration of Prospect Theory, Priming and Source Factors in the Evaluation of Public Service Announcements." PhD diss., University of Minnesota. *Dissertation Abstracts International*, 65 (2005), 2821A. (UMI No. AAT-3144288).

*Tsai, Shu-Pei. 2007. "Message Framing Strategy for Brand Communication." *Journal of Advertising Research*, 47, 364–377.

*Tykocinski, Orit, E. Tory Higgins, and Shelly Chaiken. 1994. "Message Framing, Self-Discrepancies, and Yielding to Persuasive Messages: The Motivational Significance of Psychological Situations." *Personality and Social Psychology Bulletin*, 20, 107–115.

*van Assema, Patricia, Marloes Martens, Robert A.C. Ruiter, and Johannes Brug. 2001. "Framing of Nutrition Education Messages in Persuading Consumers of the Advantages of a Healthy Diet." *Journal of Human Nutrition and Dietetics*, 14, 435–442.

van den Heuvel, Karen. 1982. "Teaching Strategies in Preschool Nutrition Education." Master's thesis, Pennsylvania State University, University Park.

van Kleef, Ellen, Hans C.M. van Trijp, and Pieternel Luning. 2005. "Functional Foods: Health Claim–Food Product Compatibility and the Impact of Health Claim Framing on Consumer Evaluation." *Appetite*, 44, 299–308.

*van't Riet, Jonathan, Robert A.C. Ruiter, Marieke Q. Werrij, Math J.J.M. Candel, and Hein de Vries. 2009. "Distinct Pathways to Persuasion: The Role of Affect in Message-Framing Effects." Unpublished manuscript, Department of Health Promotion, University of Maastricht.

*Whitbourne, Stacey B., and Margie E. Lachman. 2003. "Promoting Exercise in Adults: Effects of Positive and Negative Message Frames." Paper presented at the 111th Annual Convention of the American Psychological Association, Toronto.

Yi, Sunghwan, and Hans Baumgartner. 2007. "Regulatory Focus as a Moderator of Persuasion in Message Framing: A Test of Three Accounts." In *European Advances in Consumer Research* 8, ed. Stefania Borghini, Mart A. McGrath, and Cele Otnes, 262–263. Duluth, MN: Association for Consumer Research.

———. 2008. "Motivational Compatibility and the Role of Anticipated Feelings in Positively Valenced Persuasive Message Framing." *Psychology and Marketing*, 25, 1007–1026.

Zhao, Guangzhi, and Cornelia Pechmann. 2007. "The Impact of Regulatory Focus on Adolescents' Response to Antismoking Advertising Campaigns." *Journal of Marketing Research*, 44, 671–687.

CHAPTER 9

PRACTICING WHAT YOU PREACH

Using Hypocrisy and Cognitive Dissonance to Reduce the Risk for Obesity

JEFF STONE

Obesity is one of the most critical health problems facing the United States today. It contributes to the spiraling costs of health care, and for those whose body mass index (BMI) exceeds the normal range, obesity reduces the quality of their life and increases their risk for coronary heart disease, hypertension and stroke, type 2 diabetes, and some forms of cancer (National Heart, Lung, and Blood Institute 1998; U.S. Department of Health and Human Services 2001). As the medical and social costs of obesity continue to rise, so does the need for new approaches to reducing its occurrence.

Research indicates that the high BMI of some people stems from genetic and metabolic antecedents over which they have little control. But many people become obese because they consume more calories than they use during physical activity. People can reduce the "energy imbalance" that leads them to gain too much weight if they consume fewer calories and engage in more physical activity. Thus, it is important to educate people about the importance of the energy balance and motivate them to control their levels of consumption and activity, so they can reduce their risk for obesity.

Health marketing and communication campaigns represent an especially useful approach for helping people change the consumption and activity behaviors that cause obesity. Health marketing and communication approaches to behavior change utilize traditional marketing principles to create and disseminate health information and interventions. For example, a traditional health marketing approach to reducing obesity might start by targeting the consumers (e.g., first-year college students) who have a specific obesity-related goal (e.g., weight control). A marketing strategy would then be devised to promote a target product (e.g., purchasing more fruits and vegetables) or service (using the student recreational center) that is available at a specific time and place (e.g., during lunch or a snack on campus) for achieving the goal. By implementing an appropriate marketing mix, health marketing and communication campaigns can motivate people to initiate and maintain the behaviors that lead to a healthy BMI.

The focus of this chapter is the use of hypocrisy as a promotional weapon for changing health behaviors such as those necessary for fighting obesity. Over a decade of research shows that when individuals are made aware that they do not practice health behaviors that they preach to others, their act of hypocrisy induces cognitive dissonance and the motivation to change their own health behavior (Stone and Fernandez 2008). When applied in a health marketing and communication campaign, hypocrisy represents an active and involving persuasive communication that motivates the target audience to take action; an act of hypocrisy inspires people to bring their poor health behavior into line with their positive attitudes and beliefs about good health. The use of hypocrisy incorporates all four elements of the marketing mix. For example, to get people to acquire a product or use a service that benefits their health, hypocrisy requires precise targeting and segmentation of the market, systematic construction of a message about the benefits, costs, and availability of the target health product, and careful attention to the channels of communication for delivery of the message. When applied properly, hypocrisy motivates target individuals to perform the behaviors that they were willing to advocate to others—it causes consumers to practice what they preach.

The goal of this review is fourfold: (1) to describe the theoretical assumptions that guide the use of hypocrisy for behavior change, (2) to review the laboratory and field evidence showing that hypocrisy motivates a wide variety of behavior change, (3) to present important limits to delivering hypocrisy in a behavior change campaign, and (4) to discuss the action-oriented implications of hypocrisy for public health communications, in particular for changing the consumption and physical activity behaviors that contribute to obesity.

USING THE DISSONANCE IN HYPOCRISY TO MOTIVATE BEHAVIOR CHANGE

The use of hypocrisy for motivating health behavior change takes advantage of well-documented social influence and persuasion strategies that are based on the need to maintain consistency between attitudes, beliefs, and behaviors. According to Festinger (1957), the perception of an inconsistency between behavior and belief induces a negative state of tension that is similar to how people feel when they are hungry or thirsty. The tension or discomfort subsequently motivates people to reduce it by restoring consistency among the relevant cognitions. Festinger believed that the psychological processes by which people restore consistency could lead to enduring and meaningful changes in the way they act.

Our work focuses on the utility of dissonance processes for promoting behavior change through the induction of *hypocrisy* (Aronson 1999; Aronson, Fried, and Stone 1991). In the hypocrisy approach, a targeted audience is made aware of an inconsistency between their beliefs and behavior through two carefully constructed tasks. First, consumers are asked to make a public advocacy about the importance of the target behavior. For example, they can deliver a brief statement or write an essay designed to convince others of the importance of a behavior that they believe will benefit the health and welfare of specific individuals or society in general. Whereas this task may induce a public commitment to the issue when consistent with their current attitudes and beliefs about the issue, the advocacy, by itself, should not cause the discomfort that leads to change (see below for a more detailed discussion). Dissonance and the motivation to reduce it via behavior change emerge when after the advocacy people are subsequently made aware that they themselves have failed to perform the target behavior in the past.

Second, mindfulness for past failures is accomplished by having consumers examine or generate a list of their reasons for not performing the behavior when they had the opportunity. Once they are made mindful of the inconsistency between their positive attitudes about the behavior and their past failures to perform the behavior, consumers feel the discomfort associated with cognitive dissonance, which they become motivated to reduce.

A key element of hypocrisy is that the dissonance motivates the target audience to focus on changing their behavior to reduce their discomfort. The vast majority of dissonance studies, beginning with Festinger and Carlsmith (1959), show that when behavior is inconsistent with attitudes and beliefs, people can reduce dissonance by changing their attitudes to be consistent with the discrepant behavior (Cooper and Fazio 1984). In other words, they justify the discrepant act in order to reduce their discomfort and the perception that they did anything wrong (Tavris and Aronson 2007). In contrast, a hypocritical discrepancy motivates people to literally "practice what they preach"; an act of hypocrisy motivates consumers to take the steps that are necessary to make their behavior consistent with the behavioral standards that they advocate to others. Thus, an act of hypocrisy arouses a form of dissonance that pushes consumers to take action.

There are two reasons why consumers will focus on behavior change as the primary strategy for dissonance reduction following hypocrisy. First, when they advocate prescribed, well-accepted normative standards for performing the target behavior, these cognitions can be difficult to distort or change. According to Festinger (1957), the considerations for how to reduce dissonance are constrained by perceptions of "reality." People often rely on their perception of the normative standards to define reality and to maintain their relationships with important others. Altering their perceptions of the norms for behavior to reduce a hypocritical discrepancy may not only imperil important relationships, but by contradicting well-prescribed norms, such changes may also create new inconsistencies that arouse more discomfort. As a result, attitudes and beliefs that are associated with widely accepted norms for appropriate conduct are more resistant to change than future behavior. Indeed, changing future behavior following an act of hypocrisy brings people into line with the perception of reality that they tend to share in common with important others.

Second, when people are made mindful of failures to uphold the advocated norms for behavior, the discrepancy activates highly important cognitions linked to perceptions of self-integrity. An act of hypocrisy presents a threat to core self-beliefs about honesty and sincerity, and to the degree that the target audience cares about being honest and sincere about the health behavior they advocate to others, then the hypocritical act motivates them to restore their perceptions of self-integrity. Thus, the most direct way for hypocrites to restore their self-integrity is to bring their behavior into line with the course for action they proposed to others.

THE EFFECT OF HYPOCRISY ON HEALTH BEHAVIOR CHANGE

With respect to the obesity epidemic, research has only recently started to examine the use of hypocrisy to change the various behaviors that impact the energy balance. For now, the best illustration of the use of hypocrisy to motivate health behavior change is found in studies designed to motivate sexually active college students to adopt the use of condoms to reduce their risk for sexually transmitted diseases like AIDS (Aronson, Fried, and Stone 1991; Stone et al. 1994). In the first experiment (Aronson, Fried, and Stone 1991), sexually active male and female college students were targeted to help develop an AIDS prevention and education program. Through random assignment, participants in the "advocacy" condition were asked to make a brief speech about the importance of practicing safer sex through condom use (all agreed). To help them construct the speech, they were supplied with information about the risks of unsafe sex and the benefits of using condoms. They then delivered their speech to a video camera. In order to manipulate their level of "mindfulness" for past failures to practice safe sex, some of the students were then asked to reflect on and describe the circumstances that led them to have unprotected sex (e.g., they forgot to acquire condoms). They then wrote down examples of when they failed to use a condom during intercourse.

The effectiveness of the hypocrisy procedure was measured via self-report responses collected during an interview with the experimenter. The results showed that hypocrisy about practicing safer sex motivated the students to increase their intentions to use condoms over control conditions (Aronson, Fried, and Stone 1991). In a follow-up study designed to measure whether those in the hypocrisy condition were serious about their intentions to use condoms, participants were provided with an opportunity to purchase condoms after the study was over (Stone et al. 1994). The results showed that more students in the hypocrisy condition (83 percent) were motivated to purchase condoms when the opportunity was present compared to students who only advocated the importance of condom use (33 percent), who were only made mindful of past failures (50 percent), or who were only exposed to information about the importance of condom use (44 percent). Thus, hypocrisy motivated the target audience to purchase the products they needed to perform the target health behavior.

Nevertheless, it is not clear from these studies whether purchasing condoms reflects a motivation to restore the perceptions of honesty and sincerity that underlie self-integrity. For example, if hypocrisy activates a more general goal to enhance self-worth, then performing an unrelated positive behavior, like helping another person in need, might resolve the discomfort, even if it does not directly restore perceptions of honesty and sincerity about condom use (Steele 1988). However, if an act of hypocrisy arouses dissonance because the behavior threatens self-views about honesty and sincerity, then in order to restore their self-integrity, participants should be motivated to change the discrepant behavior, even if other options for dissonance reduction are available. Thus, when provided a choice between performing the behavior that would reduce the hypocrisy and restore their self-integrity, or performing a behavior that will leave the discrepancy intact but enhance self-worth, most people should choose to perform the behavior that most directly reduces the hypocritical discrepancy.

Stone and colleagues (1997) tested these predictions by having sexually active college students commit an act of hypocrisy about their practice of safer sex. At the end of the study, some students were provided with the opportunity to donate to support a homeless shelter—a behavior that would reduce their dissonance via self-enhancement, but would not directly restore their sense of honesty and sincerity about the importance of safer sex. In another condition, some students were offered the opportunity to donate to the homeless, but were then also offered the opportunity to directly resolve the hypocritical discrepancy about safer sex by purchasing condoms. The results supported the self-integrity prediction: when offered only the enhancement option (donation), 83 percent of those in the hypocrisy condition used it. However, when students were offered a choice between the self-enhancing donation and the opportunity to restore their honesty and sincerity by purchasing condoms, 78 percent chose to purchase condoms and directly restore their self-integrity, whereas only 13 percent chose the self-enhancing donation option. A second experiment replicated the choice for directly resolving the hypocritical discrepancy even when an alternative option held more importance for self-worth than the integrity option. Together, the results indicate that when the only dissonance reduction opportunity available to hypocrites is a behavior that enhances global self-worth, they will take advantage of it. After all, people often do want to think and feel good about themselves, even if doing so does not solve the problem that caused their discomfort in the first place. However, when a behavior is available that directly resolves the hypocrisy and restores the attributes of honesty and sincerity, most consumers are motivated to perform the target behavior (see Fointiat 2004 for similar findings).

These studies indicate that unlike a general state of psychological ambivalence (Newby-Clark, McGregor, and Zanna 2002) or other cognitive discrepancies that cause discomfort (Cooper 2008), hypocrisy motivates a specific form of dissonance arousal and reduction that directs consumers toward changing their behavior. Once they advocate their beliefs about the benefits of a target health behavior and are then made mindful of past failures to uphold their beliefs, the threat to self-integrity motivates a desire to resolve the discrepancy by bringing their behavior into line with what they preach to others. Addressing the discrepancy directly appears to be the preferred mode of dissonance reduction, even when other options for reducing their discomfort are present.

OPTIMIZING THE DELIVERY OF HYPOCRISY

Across a variety of topics and settings, hypocrisy is an effective approach for motivating consumers to prepare for and perform behaviors that contribute to good health, sustainability, and improved interpersonal relationships (Stone and Fernandez 2008). The research examining when and how hypocrisy motivates behavior change reveals important parameters to using the procedure to motivate the target response. The next section describes factors in the delivery that moderate the influence of hypocrisy on behavior change.

Advocating Normative Standards and Commitment

Hypocrisy begins when consumers who hold positive attitudes and beliefs toward the target course of action advocate the importance of the behavior to others. The research indicates that the effect of hypocrisy on behavior change is greatest when consumers construct and deliver, either in writing or in a recording, a persuasive message about the importance of performing the target behavior. Just reading about the importance of performing the behavior (Aronson, Fried, Stone 1991; Stone et al. 1994) or constructing a speech but not delivering it (Stone et al. 1997) does not engender the same level of dissonance and behavior change as does the act of delivering the statement to an "audience," in conjunction with being made mindful of past failures. Advocating the importance of a behavior to others appears to be a necessary condition in the hypocrisy effect.

However, as noted earlier, the available data suggest that the effect of a prosocial public advocacy on the arousal of dissonance following hypocrisy may depend on whether or not consumers make a public commitment to perform the behavior when they advocate it to others. In studies showing a greater effect for hypocrisy over simply making the advocacy by itself (e.g., Fried 1998; Fried and Aronson 1995; Stone et al. 1994; Stone et al. 1997), the instructions for creating the videotaped or written statement did *not* ask advocates to predict or state that they would perform the behavior in the future. The speakers focused on talking about why it is important to perform the behavior without holding themselves up as an example now or in the future. This suggests that advocating the prosocial behavior without making a personal commitment to it does not, by itself, motivate consumers to perform the behavior. As reported above, several studies show that when people only publicly advocate the importance of a prosocial behavior, they are significantly less likely than those in the hypocrisy condition to perform the behavior when offered the opportunity later, and in some cases, the level of compliance has been less than in control conditions in which consumers are simply informed about the issue.

Advocating a course of action to others in the absence of a commitment may inhibit subsequent performance of the behavior through a number of mechanisms, such as inducing the perception of having established one's moral credentials on the topic (Monin and Miller 2001), or by inducing a positive illusion about how well one currently upholds the advocated behavioral standards. Breaking these inhibitory mechanisms appears to require that the advocate also be made aware of past failures to perform the target act. Thus, when consumers advocate a prosocial course of action without making a public commitment to perform the behavior themselves, they may not experience much dissonance unless they are also made mindful of their failures to perform the behavior in the past.

Nevertheless, other hypocrisy studies (e.g., Dickerson et al. 1992) indicate that when participants were asked to make a public commitment to the prosocial course of action, either by making a prediction or by signing a pledge, the advocacy alone may increase the motivation to perform the behavior. One explanation for this effect is that committing to perform the future behavior, while advocating it to others, automatically makes consumers mindful of past inconsistent behavior. For example, research on the self-prophecy effect (e.g., Spangenberg et al. 2003) shows that when consumers make a prediction regarding their intention to perform or not perform a prosocial behavior in the future, they are more likely to adopt the behavior compared to when they predict a different behavior or simply learn about the behavior. This suggests that a public commitment to a prosocial course of action, in and of itself, may be sufficient to cause the dissonance associated with hypocrisy.

An important limitation to this observation is the assumption that the act of making a public commitment to a future course of action will automatically activate knowledge of past failures. The bulk of the research does not directly show this to be the case. Given the potential limitations to how priming activates related constructs (see Bargh 2006), and the evidence that people sometimes uncouple their current and past self when they reflect back on negative experiences (Ross and Wilson 2002), it may be risky to assume that predicting the future will spontaneously bring to mind the past failures that induce hypocrisy. A more effective approach is to directly activate the discrepancy by making consumers mindful of past failures after they predict or commit to the target behavior.

Mindfulness: Private, Personal, and Easy

Several studies have identified factors that determine the impact of being made mindful of past failures on the motivation to perform the target behavior. For example, Stone and colleagues (1997) showed that recalling personal reasons for failing to practice safer sex caused significantly more consumers to perform the target behavior compared to consumers who recalled the reasons that other people give for failing to perform the behavior in the past. Thus, hypocrisy causes the greatest motivation to adopt the target behavior when the procedure is tailored to consumers' own personal failures to practice the behavior in the past.

Fried (1998) documented another important parameter to the use of hypocrisy for behavior change. In her research, after consumers videotaped (Study 1) or wrote a persuasive speech (Study 2) about the importance of recycling, they were then asked to list past failures to recycle bottles, cans, or newspapers. The level of publicity for past failures was varied by having some consumers complete the list anonymously; they were told not to sign it and to place it in an envelope ostensibly full of lists completed by other respondents. Those in an *identified* condition completed the list and included their name and phone number on it. They then signed it in front of the experimenter. The results showed that hypocrites who felt anonymous about their recycling failures donated more time to the recycling efforts (Study 1) and donated more money to the recycling program (Study 2) compared to hypocrites who were publicly identified with their past failures to recycle. Moreover, in Study 2, hypocrites who were publicly identified with their past failures reported significantly more *negative* attitudes toward recycling than hypocrites in the anonymous failure condition. The publicity of the past transgressions apparently pushed some to justify their past failures by changing their attitudes to be more negative toward the target behavior.

The research by Fried (1998; see also McKimmie et al. 2003) points to an important factor in the use of hypocrisy for motivating health behavior change. When publicly associated with past failures to uphold the standards or when presented with evidence that past failures are deviant, dissonance is aroused but it may be reduced differently than when consumers are allowed to consider their past failures in private. Publicly confronting consumers about past transgressions may activate cognitions in the dissonance ratio that direct them toward other avenues for dissonance reduction. For example, when identified publicly with failing to perform the target act, consumers may perceive that they are being humiliated or shamed for their past transgressions, which could cause anger and self-blame (Tangney and Dearing 2002; see Stone and Cooper 2001). Such self-directed thoughts and emotions may focus hypocrites on the fear of rejection by others, which could then make future behavior more resistant to change (Festinger 1957). As a result, consumers are forced to take the path of least resistance and change their attitudes about the importance of performing the behavior. Alternatively, allowing consumers to "discover" their past mistakes in private does not force them to save face; instead, it motivates them to resolve the discrepancy by bringing their behavior into line with their advocated beliefs.

There is also evidence to suggest that if consumers considering their past transgressions have difficulty coming up with past failures to perform the target behavior, they may conclude that they are not hypocritical about the issue. For example, in a study designed to reduce prejudice, Son Hing, Li, and Zanna (2002) targeted college students with aversive attitudes toward Asian Canadians and made them feel hypocritical about their past treatment of Asians. When asked to make recommendations for the campus budget, including the percentage of cuts recommended for the Asian Students Association (ASA), the aversive racists in the hypocrisy condition recommended significantly smaller budget cuts for the ASA compared to low-prejudiced individuals. Importantly, aversive racists also tended to recall more recent examples of biased behavior compared to low-prejudice individuals. The temporal difference suggests that if hypocrites have trouble recalling examples of past failure, they may conclude that past slips do not represent an important discrepancy from what they advocated to others. If recalling past failures is easy, in part because they represent recent examples, then consumers may be more likely to perceive that their past behavior is discrepant from their advocacy and be motivated to bring their actions into line with their beliefs.

Finally, a recent study examined the number of past failures that advocates need to recall in order to feel dissonance and the motivation to change their behavior (Fernandez and Stone, 2009). The original theory of cognitive dissonance predicts that after advocating the target behavior, recalling many past failures will cause more dissonance and more behavior change (Festinger 1957). However, when advocates are asked to recall past failures, recent research on self-validation processes (Tormala, Petty, and Brinol 2002) suggests that advocates may also recruit examples of when they successfully performed the behavior, especially when they are motivated and have the ability to think carefully about the past (i.e., high elaboration). If advocates carefully recall both failures and successes, it could balance the ratio of inconsistent to consistent cognitions, which would reduce the level of dissonance and need to change behavior following hypocrisy. Thus, under high elaboration conditions, when advocates are asked to recall many past failures to perform a health behavior, the self-validation process would reduce the level of dissonance and the motivation to change behavior. In contrast, carefully recalling few past failures would reduce the self-validation process and cause more behavioral change following hypocrisy.

When they are not highly motivated to think about past failures (i.e., low elaboration), if advocates focus primarily on the number of failures recalled without recruiting other relevant information (e.g., successes), then recalling many past failures will induce more dissonance and behavior change following hypocrisy than recalling few past failures. To test these predictions, female college students with positive attitudes toward the use of sunscreen were targeted and asked to advocate the importance of using sunscreen to reduce the risk of skin cancer. All were then asked to report past failures to use sunscreen. In the high elaboration condition, the women were told their responses were important because only a few people were being asked to report information about failures to use sunscreen. Women in the low elaboration condition were told that thousands of people were reporting information about past failures to use sunscreen. Then some were asked to recall only two past failures to use sunscreen whereas the other half were asked to recall eight past failures to use sunscreen. All were then offered an opportunity to order a sample of sunscreen from an independent organization.

The results revealed the predicted interaction between elaboration and the number of past failures participants recalled. Under high elaboration, significantly more students (82 percent) acquired a sample of sunscreen when they were asked to recall two past failures compared to those asked to recall eight past failures (52 percent). In contrast, under low elaboration, significantly more students (68 percent) acquired a sample of sunscreen when asked to recall eight past failures compared to those asked to recall two past failures (39 percent). Thus, it appears that in hypocrisy, the effect of recalling many past failures on behavior change is a function of how carefully advocates think about their past behavior. More is better when consumers do *not* think too carefully about their past failures.

In summary, the research reviewed in this section points to several important parameters to the use of hypocrisy for changing behavior. Specifically, the induction of hypocrisy appears to exert its greatest effect on behavior change when consumers *publicly advocate* the importance of the target course of action and then can *easily* but *privately* recall *personal* past failures to perform the target behavior. The data indicate that the hypocrisy procedure induces a lower level of discomfort or motivates the use of rationalization strategies for dissonance reduction when consumers simply learn or think about the behavior, focus on the failures of others, or are publicly identified with past personal failures to perform the target behavior.

FIELD AND MASS MEDIA PROMOTIONS

An important question regarding the use of hypocrisy to motivate behavior change is whether the strategy can produce the same level of behavior change in the field as typically seen in the carefully controlled laboratory studies. The answer appears to be yes. For example, in a field experiment designed to use hypocrisy to motivate water conservation, female swimmers were approached entering the women's locker room from a campus recreation pool (Dickerson et al. 1992). After establishing that the swimmers were in favor of water conservation, those in the hypocrisy condition completed a survey intended to make them aware of past failures to conserve water (e.g., "When you take showers, do you ALWAYS make them as short as possible, or do you sometimes linger longer than necessary?") and were then asked to publicly support campus conservation efforts by printing their name on a posted flyer that read: "Please conserve water. Take shorter showers. Turn showers off while soaping up. IF I CAN DO IT, SO CAN YOU!"

To measure their water conservation behavior, a female confederate unobtrusively recorded how long the swimmers allowed the water to run while they showered and the percentage that turned the shower off while they applied shampoo. As predicted, the results revealed that swimmers in the hypocrisy condition allowed the water to run for significantly less time, and were significantly more likely to turn off the shower while washing their hair, compared to swimmers in a no-treatment control condition.

Fointiat (2004) tested the effects of hypocrisy for motivating people who were out shopping to become safer drivers. In one study (Fointiat 2004), experimenters approached shoppers outside a supermarket parking lot and asked if they would participate in a road safety study. All shoppers first signed a flyer advocating driving at the posted speed limit, and then shoppers in the hypocrisy condition were made mindful when they wrote down times in the last two months in which they failed to obey the posted speed limit. The primary dependent measure was the percentage that then volunteered to have a tachometer installed in their car that would record their driving behavior. The results showed that significantly more shoppers in the hypocrisy condition volunteered to have their driving monitored (35 percent) compared to those in the advocacy-only condition (12 percent).

These studies suggest that hypocrisy can motivate consumers to adopt the target behavior when implemented in the hustle and bustle of their everyday lives. Nevertheless, the studies reviewed up to this point also rely heavily on the personal selling channel to achieve their behavior change goals. Whereas the face-to-face delivery of hypocrisy is effective, it also requires a somewhat costly level of time and effort for target individuals as they complete the activities that produce dissonance. Such costs may not be feasible or desirable, especially when the goal of a campaign is to influence a large audience quickly and for less cost.

There is evidence that hypocrisy can be induced through other communication channels, like mass media advertising, by modifying how people are made aware of the discrepancy. In one direct mail example, Kantola, Syme, and Campbell (1984) used a procedure similar to hypocrisy to influence energy conservation behavior. They first targeted homeowners in Australia who held a positive attitude toward the conservation of electricity and agreed to have their consumption of electricity monitored by the State Energy Commission. After a two-week base-line measure of their electricity use, homeowners were randomly assigned to receive one of four mailings from the energy commission: (1) a letter stating that they were high consumers of electricity and that they had previously said that they believed in conservation (i.e., the dissonance group); they also received an informational pamphlet on energy conservation, (2) a letter stating that they were high consumers of electricity plus a conservation pamphlet, (3) just the conservation pamphlet, and (4) a thank-you letter. All participants also received a postage-paid post card that they could return to receive more information about energy conservation. The primary measure of the intervention was the home's consumption of electricity over two sequential two-week periods. As predicted, homes assigned to the dissonance condition used significantly less electricity compared to the control conditions during both follow-up periods. This study suggests that it is possible to induce dissonance that motivates the target behavior change by providing consumers with feedback that, similar to hypocrisy, draws their attention to a discrepancy between their proconservation attitudes and their failures to conserve in the past.

Another potential mass media approach works by exposing consumers to the hypocritical behavior of another person. Stone and colleagues (2010) proposed that people could be motivated to adopt a new course of action by witnessing the hypocrisy of someone with whom they share a strong social identity. Specifically, when observers perceive that a hypocrite shares an important group identity with them, it will cause dissonance because the in-group member's hypocrisy challenges the observers' positive view of the group as having integrity—as being honest, principled, and sincere about important issues (Stone et al. 1997). Consequently, the threat to the group's integrity will motivate highly identified in-group perceivers to reduce their "vicarious" dissonance by seeking a way to maintain their positive image of the group's integrity. The most direct way to accomplish this goal is for in-group members to bolster attitudes and behavior to support the hypocrite's proposed course of action.

To test the effect of vicarious hypocrisy, the researchers targeted female college students who held positive attitudes about the use of sunscreen and were highly identified with their university campus. They then evaluated a recorded message by another female student about the importance of using sunscreen to reduce skin cancer. The speaker was portrayed as either an in-group (same university) or an out-group member (rival university). Perceived hypocrisy was created when the speaker admitted to previous failures to use sunscreen. The results showed that, as predicted, female students, who shared a strong social identity with the female hypocritical speaker, became significantly more favorable toward the regular use of sunscreen, and were more likely to acquire a sample of sunscreen, than female students exposed to an out-group speaker, and compared to male students who did not share the same level of similarity to the female speaker. These findings indicate that exposure to the hypocritical behavior of another person can motivate those who share an important social identity with the speaker to bolster their support for the cause. They also suggest that hypocrisy can be implemented to change attitudes and behavior through channels, like broadcast mass media, that are less costly and more efficient to implement.

USING HYPOCRISY AND COGNITIVE DISSONANCE TO REDUCE THE RISK FOR OBESITY

How can the use of hypocrisy and dissonance contribute to the battle to reduce obesity? There is some evidence that promotions based on dissonance, and hypocrisy in particular, can be applied successfully to motivate consumers to change their levels of consumption and physical activity. However, as will be detailed below, more research is needed to document the most effective marketing plan for using hypocrisy to motivate the initiation and maintenance of new dietary and exercise behavior.

In an early translation of dissonance principles to encourage weight loss, Axsom and Cooper (1985) designed a procedure to motivate overweight people to exercise and diet. The key element of the intervention was to have community members who were motivated to lose weight engage in a series of effortful cognitive tasks designed to cause dissonance and the need to justify participation in the weight loss program. Program participants also received information about exercise and healthy eating. The results showed that compared to a low-dissonance control group, the high-dissonance group was able to lose an average of six to seven pounds immediately following the intervention, and they sustained the weight loss for one full year after the program ended. Thus, by participating in the program, participants were faced with an inconsistency between the effort they put into the series of meaningless cognitive tasks and the wisdom of participating in what appeared to be a nonsensical weight loss program. To reduce dissonance and justify their effort, they apparently became more positive toward losing weight, which led them to initiate and maintain new exercise and healthy eating behaviors over time.

Stice and colleagues (2008) use an intervention based on dissonance to reduce the incidence of eating disorders like anorexia and bulimia. In their approach, women who are at risk for eating disorders engage in public advocacy and role-playing exercises that are inconsistent with their attitudes toward the "thin-ideal" body type. A recent meta-analytic review of sixteen clinical trials by Stice and Shaw (2004) reported that compared to other interventions and assessment-only control conditions, the use of the dissonance-based intervention showed stronger reduction of eating disorder risk factors and symptoms, and lower future risk for onset of the disorder, obesity, and the use of mental health resources, immediately after the intervention.

Both these approaches to using dissonance to motivate changes in diet and physical activity rely on getting the target audience to justify a series of inconsistent acts. In contrast, the use of hypocrisy does not rely on creating an inconsistency that necessitates self-justification; hypocrisy simply calls attention to an inconsistency that is already present in the minds of the target audience. That is, to the degree that the target audience subscribes to healthy eating and getting more exercise, but does not perform these behaviors as regularly as they can or should, then hypocrisy can be used to bring these two inconsistent sets of cognitions into their awareness. Consumers should then be motivated by dissonance to eat more healthy meals and exercise more regularly when the opportunity is present.

There are two studies that support the use of hypocrisy to motivate exercise behavior. For example, Barquissau and Stone (2000) targeted male and female college students who reported positive attitudes toward regular exercise. Half then made a videotaped advocacy about the positive benefits gained through regular exercise, whereas the other half warned others about the negative consequences avoided through exercise. All were then reminded of past failures to exercise that were due either to their own choice (high responsibility) or to circumstances beyond their control (low responsibility). The primary dependent measure was how far the students rode an exercise bicycle during a ten-minute exercise period. The results showed that after controlling for specific self-report emotions, those in the negative-outcome/high-responsibility condition rode significantly further than the negative-outcome/low-responsibility condition, with the positive consequence conditions falling in between. Thus, the greatest level of dissonance and motivation to exercise occurred when the proexercise message in the advocacy was framed in prevention or avoidance terms and when the students focused on their own responsibility for not exercising regularly in the past. However, this effect was only significant in the first three minutes of the bike ride; it dissipated by the end of the exercise period, suggesting that the benefit of focusing consumers on being hypocritical about disease prevention was short-lived.

Bator and Bryan (2009) recently reported a field study that supports the use of hypocrisy for promoting exercise behavior. The researchers approached 127 members of a college fitness center and, based on the delivery of hypocrisy created by Dickerson and colleagues (1992), asked them to provide reasons why they do not exercise regularly before asking them to sign a large poster advocating the regular use of the fitness facility. The results showed that members in the hypocrisy condition reported significantly higher intentions to exercise regularly and were more likely to use the facility during the next week than members in the control conditions.

On the other side of the energy balance, there are currently no published studies that use hypocrisy to motivate consumers to change their dietary behavior. In considering how to apply hypocrisy to motivate consumers to adopt a more healthy diet, it is useful to discuss market segmentation, especially as it relates to other contemporary models of behavior change like the theory of planned behavior (Ajzen 1991), the transtheoretical model (Prochaska, DiClemente, and Norcross 1992), the health belief model (Rosenstock, Strecher, and Becker 1988), and protection motivation theory (Maddux and Rogers 1983). These models generally recognized that consumers must move through a series of stages or steps in order to initiate a new behavior before they proceed through the stages or steps necessary to maintain the new behavior (Rothman 2000). Segmenting the target market by different stages of change and then applying hypocrisy to motivate the market's advance to the next stage of change are likely to improve the effectiveness of the promotion for encouraging dietary change. The assumptions that guide the use of hypocrisy are sufficiently flexible to permit targeting for specific stages of initiation and also the cultural tailoring of the materials to ensure that the hypocritical discrepancy includes cognitions that are important and relevant to the target market.

The current literature shows that the hypocrisy procedure is effective for motivating the target behavior when the consumers are knowledgeable about its benefits and hold positive attitudes toward performing it, but currently do not perform the behavior as often or as well as they could or should. In many contemporary models of health behavior change, this may represent the stages or steps where consumers have contemplated initiating change, prepared to take action, and may even have attempted to perform the behavior in a limited fashion. The research suggests that the induction of a hypocritical discrepancy may help consumers move from forming a goal for change toward taking the first steps necessary to achieving that goal.

Hypocrisy can also be crafted to influence the decision processes for consumers at other stages of initiation. For example, when consumers are in an earlier stage of initiation where they are unaware of how to change their diet, do not know about the benefits to be gained from eating smaller portions or more fruits and vegetables, or do not know how to prepare new foods, the hypocrisy procedure could be used as a "teachable moment" to motivate them to learn about the benefits of these behaviors and how to perform them (see McBride, Emmons, and Lipkus 2003). Making consumers hypocritical about knowing how to change their dietary behavior could be used to improve their memory for what foods to purchase and where to find them in a store. Thus, by adjusting what they advocate and are then made mindful about, hypocrisy can motivate consumers to move from the early stages of contemplation to the initial stages of performing the behavior.

Less is known about the effects of hypocrisy on the maintenance of a new health behavior once consumers have initiated it. Whereas some studies report that the effect did not last beyond the first performance of the target behavior (Fried and Aronson 1995), other studies report that an induction of hypocrisy led consumers to maintain the target behavior over an extended period of time (e.g., Bator and Bryan 2009; Kantola, Syme, and Campbell 1984). One reason for the mixed findings is that previous applications of hypocrisy have not focused specifically on motivating consumers to maintain the new behavior over time. With a few twists, tailoring the hypocrisy to focus consumers on performing the new target behavior regularly in the future has the potential to cause lasting change.

For example, once hypocrisy has been implemented to motivate consumers to initiate a new dietary behavior, like consuming more fruits and vegetables, follow-up promotions could then provide reminders of the previous hypocritical discrepancy about eating a healthy diet (see Dal Cin et al. 2006). The delivery of subtle cues about the previous failure to practice what was preached through direct mail or electronic media like email or text messaging may reinstate dissonance and the motivation to continue performing the new behavior (Higgins, Rhodewalt, and Zanna 1979).

It may also be effective to induce hypocrisy specifically about behavior maintenance. For example, the advocacy could be tailored toward emphasizing the benefits of eating smaller portions and more fruits and vegetables on a continuous basis, and the importance of carefully planning future meals and snacks to avoid relapses. In addition, the advocacy could stress the importance of practicing cognitive and behavioral skills that are designed to prevent behavioral lapses (Schwarzer 1992). After they advocate the benefits and mechanics of behavior maintenance, consumers could then be made mindful of how they recently failed to follow through on their own personal plans or failed to practice the relapse-avoidance skills as regularly as they could. The discrepancy between their beliefs about the importance of maintaining the new diet over time and their past failures to follow through should pose a challenge to self-integrity that is not easily resolved by performing the behavior only once or irregularly in the future. The most direct way to restore their honesty and sincerity about maintaining a healthy diet would be to take their own good advice and eat a more healthy diet on a regular basis over time. With a little ingenuity, the hypocrisy procedure may prove useful for just this purpose.

CONCLUSIONS

Behavior change will play a major role in reducing the rising tide of obesity in the United States. When used as a promotional tool in health marketing and communication programs, hypocrisy can be effective for motivating consumers to initiate and maintain the consumption and physical activity behaviors that reduce risk for obesity. The research suggests that the most effective personal selling delivery of hypocrisy is to have consumers (1) *publicly advocate* the importance of the target behavior and then (2) *easily* but (3) *privately* recall (4) *personal* past failures to follow their own good advice. With appropriate alterations, hypocrisy also shows promise for motivating behavior change when delivered through direct mail and broadcast media. Motivating consumers to be honest and sincere about important health issues can be a powerful way to help them bring their behavior into line with their positive attitudes and beliefs about good health.

REFERENCES

Ajzen, Icek. 1991. "The Theory of Planned Behavior." *Organizational Behavior and Human Decision Processes*, 50, 179–211.
Aronson, Elliot. 1999. "Dissonance, Hypocrisy, and the Self-Concept." In *Cognitive Dissonance: Progress on a Pivotal Theory in Social Psychology*, ed. Eddie Harmon-Jones and Judson Mills, 103–126. Washington, DC: American Psychological Association.
Aronson, Elliot, Carrie B. Fried, and Jeff Stone. 1991. "Overcoming Denial and Increasing the Use of Condoms Through the Induction of Hypocrisy." *American Journal of Public Health*, 81, 1636–1638.
Axsom, Danny, and Joel Cooper. 1985. "Cognitive Dissonance and Psychotherapy: The Role of Effort Justification in Inducing Weight Loss." *Journal of Experimental Social Psychology*, 21, 149–160.
Bargh, John A. 2006. "What Have We Been Priming All These Years? On the Development, Mechanisms, and Ecology of Nonconscious Social Behavior." *European Journal of Social Psychology*, 36, 147–168.
Barquissau, Marchelle, and Jeff Stone. 2000. "When Hypocrisy Induced Dissonance Encourages Exercise Behavior." Unpublished manuscript, University of Arizona.
Bator, Renee J., and Angela Bryan. 2009. "Revised Hypocrisy Manipulation to Induce Commitment to Exercise." Poster presentation at the 21st Annual Convention of the Association for Psychological Science, San Francisco, May 22–25.
Cooper, Joel. 2008. *Cognitive Dissonance: Fifty Years of a Classic Theory*. Thousand Oaks, CA: Sage.
Cooper, Joel, and Russell H. Fazio. 1984. "A New Look at Dissonance Theory." In *Advances in Experimental Social Psychology*, 17, ed. Leonard Berkowitz, 229–262. Hillsdale, NJ: Erlbaum.
Dal Cin, Sonya, Tara K. MacDonald, Geoffrey T. Fong, Mark P. Zanna, and Tara E. Elton-Marshall. 2006. "Remembering the Message: Using a Reminder Cue to Increase Condom Use Following a Safer Sex Intervention." *Health Psychology*, 25, 438–443.
Dickerson, Chris A., Ruth Thibodeau, Elliot Aronson, and Dayna Miller. 1992. "Using Cognitive Dissonance to Encourage Water Conservation." *Journal of Applied Social Psychology*, 22, 841–854.
Fernandez, Nicholas, and Jeff Stone. 2009. "When Less Failure Causes More Dissonance:

The Role of Self-Validation and Heuristics in Behavior Change Following Hypocrisy." Paper submitted for publication.

Festinger, Leon. 1957. *A Theory of Cognitive Dissonance*. Evanston, IL: Row, Peterson.

Festinger, Leon, and James M. Carlsmith. 1959. "Cognitive Consequences of Forced Compliance." *Journal of Abnormal and Social Psychology*, 58, 203–210.

Fointiat, Valerie. 2004. "'I Know What I Have to Do, But . . .': When Hypocrisy Leads to Behavioral Change." *Social Behavior and Personality*, 32, 741–746.

Fried, Carrie B. 1998. "Hypocrisy and Identification with Transgressions: A Case of Undetected Dissonance." *Basic and Applied Social Psychology*, 20, 145–154.

Fried, Carrie B., and Elliot Aronson. 1995. "Hypocrisy, Misattribution, and Dissonance Reduction." *Personality and Social Psychology Bulletin*, 21, 925–933.

Higgins, E. Tory, Frederick Rhodewalt, and Mark P. Zanna. 1979. "Dissonance Motivation: Its Nature, Persistence, and Reinstatement." *Journal of Experimental Social Psychology*, 15, 16–34.

Kantola, Steven J., Geoff J. Syme, and Norm A. Campbell. 1984. "Cognitive Dissonance and Energy Conservation." *Journal of Applied Psychology*, 69, 416–421.

Maddux, James E., and Ronald W. Rogers. 1983. "Protection Motivation Theory and Self-Efficacy: A Revised Theory of Fear Appeals and Attitude Change." *Journal of Experimental Social Psychology*, 19, 469–479.

McBride, Colleen M., Karen M. Emmons, and Isaac M. Lipkus. 2003. "Understanding the Potential of Teachable Moments: The Case of Smoking Cessation." *Health Education Research*, 18 (2), 156–170.

McKimmie, Blake M., Deborah J. Terry, Michael A. Hogg, Anthony S.R. Manstead, Russell Spears, and Bertjan Doosje. 2003. "I'm a Hypocrite but So Is Everyone Else: The Role of Social Support in the Reduction of Cognitive Dissonance." *Group Dynamics: Theory, Research, and Practice*, 7 (3), 214–224.

Monin, Benoit, and Dale T. Miller. 2001. "Moral Credentials and the Expression of Prejudice." *Journal of Personality and Social Psychology*, 81, 33–43.

National Heart, Lung, and Blood Institute. 1998. "Clinical Guideline on the Identification, Evaluation, and Treatment of Overweight and Obesity in Adults: The Evidence Report." Bethesda, MD: U.S. Department of Health and Human Services, National Institutes of Health, National Heart, Lung, and Blood Institute. www.nhlbi.nih.gov/guidelines/obesity/ob_gdlns.htm.

Newby-Clark, Ian R., Ian McGregor, and Mark P. Zanna. 2002. "Thinking and Caring About Cognitive Inconsistency: When and for Whom Does Attitudinal Ambivalence Feel Uncomfortable?" *Journal of Personality and Social Psychology*, 82, 157–166.

Prochaska, James O., Carlo C. DiClemente, and John Norcross. 1992. "In Search of How People Change: Applications to Addictive Behaviors." *American Psychologist*, 47, 1102–1114.

Rosenstock, Irwin M., Victor J. Strecher, and Marshall H. Becker. 1988. "Social Learning Theory and the Health Belief Model." *Health Education Behavior*, 15, 175–183.

Ross, Michael, and Anne E. Wilson. 2002. "It Feels Like Yesterday: Self-Esteem, Valence of Personal Past Experiences, and Judgments of Subjective Distance." *Journal of Personality and Social Psychology*, 82, 792–803.

Rothman, Alexander J. 2000. "Toward a Theory-Based Analysis of Behavioral Maintenance." *Health Psychology*, 19, 64–69.

Schwarzer, Ralf. 1992. "Self-Efficacy in the Adoption and Maintenance of Health Behaviors: Theoretical Approaches and a New Model." In *Self-Efficacy: Thought Control of Action*, ed. Ralf Schwarzer, 217–243. Washington, DC: Hemisphere.

Son Hing, Leanne S., Winnie Li, and Mark P. Zanna. 2002. "Inducing Hypocrisy to Reduce Prejudicial Responses Among Aversive Racists." *Journal of Experimental Social Psychology*, 38, 71–78.

Spangenberg, Eric R., David E. Sprott, Bianca Grohmann, and Ronn J. Smith. 2003. "Mass-Communicated Prediction Requests: Practical Application and a Cognitive Dissonance Explanation for Self-Prophecy." *Journal of Marketing*, 67, 47–62.

Steele, Claude M. 1988. "The Psychology of Self-Affirmation: Sustaining the Integrity of the Self." In *Advances in Experimental Social Psychology*, 21, ed. Leonard Berkowitz, 261–302. Hillsdale: Erlbaum.

Stice, Eric, and Heather Shaw. 2004. "Eating Disorder Prevention Programs: A Meta-Analytic Review." *Psychological Bulletin*, 130, 206–227.

Stice, Eric, Heather Shaw, Carolyn Black Becker, and Paul Rohde. 2008. "Dissonance-Based Interventions for the Prevention of Eating Disorders: Using Persuasion Principles to Promote Health." *Prevention Science*, 9, 114–128.

Stone, Jeff, Elliot Aronson, A. Lauren Crain, Matthew P. Winslow, and Carrie B. Fried. 1994. "Inducing Hypocrisy as a Means of Encouraging Young Adults to Use Condoms." *Personality and Social Psychology Bulletin*, 20, 116–128.

Stone, Jeff, and Joel Cooper. 2001. "A Self-Standards Model of Cognitive Dissonance." *Journal of Experimental Social Psychology*, 37, 228–243.

Stone, Jeff, and Nicholas C. Fernandez. 2008. "To Practice What We Preach: The Use of Hypocrisy and Cognitive Dissonance to Motivate Behavior Change." *Social and Personality Psychology Compass*, 2 (2), 1024–1051.

Stone, Jeff, Nicholas C. Fernandez, Joel Cooper, Michael Hogg, and Elizabeth Focella. 2010. "Vicarious Hypocrisy: Bolstering Attitudes and Taking Action After Exposure to a Hypocritical In-Group Member." Paper submitted for publication.

Stone, Jeff, Andrew W. Wiegand, Joel Cooper, and Elliot Aronson. 1997. "When Exemplification Fails: Hypocrisy and the Motive for Self-Integrity." *Journal of Personality and Social Psychology*, 72, 54–65.

Tangney, June Price, and Rhonda L. Dearing. 2002. *Shame and Guilt*. New York: Guilford Press.

Tavris, Carol, and Elliot Aronson. 2007. *Mistakes Were Made (But Not By Me): Why We Justify Foolish Beliefs, Bad Decisions, and Hurtful Acts*. New York: Harcourt.

Tormala, Zakary L., Richard E. Petty, and Pablo Brinol. 2002. Ease of Retrieval Effects in Persuasion: A Self-Validation Analysis." *Personality and Social Psychology Bulletin*, 28, 1700–1712.

U.S. Department of Health and Human Services. 2001. "The Surgeon General's Call to Action to Prevent and Decrease Obesity." Rockville, MD: U.S. Department of Health and Human Services, U.S. Public Health Service, Office of the Surgeon General. www.surgeon-general.gov/topics/obesity/calltoaction/CalltoAction.pdf.

CHAPTER 10

THE USE OF NEGATIVE EMOTIONS IN HEALTH COMMUNICATION

Implications for Fighting Obesity

IMÈNE BECHEUR AND PIERRE VALETTE-FLORENCE

Obesity is considered a serious health problem. In 2004, the U.S. Centers for Disease Control and Prevention (CDC) ranked obesity as the number one health risk facing America. According to the World Health Organization, obesity currently results in an estimated 400,000 deaths a year in the United States and costs the national economy nearly $122.9 billion annually. Obesity not only has an impact on lifestyle but also can lead to lower self-esteem, cause depression and discomfort in social situations, and significantly diminish quality of life. Obesity also increases a person's risk for developing serious obesity-related health conditions such as diabetes, heart disease, hypertension, metabolic syndrome, and polycystic ovary syndrome.

In most instances, emotions determine people's food choices, resulting in an experience full of emotions. We refer to this as "emotional eating." Research indicates that feelings of depression and anxiety lead to eating disorders (Killen et al. 1996; Stice 2001). Other studies show that women who reported eating disorder symptoms were more likely to use maladaptive methods to cope with these negative emotions (Bybee et al. 1996). Using negative emotions in messages to fight overeating disorders leading to obesity would reinforce the level of negative emotions already present among the targeted people. Hence, there is a need to give recommendations in the message on how to cope with these emotions in an adaptive way.

To shed light on how emotions relate to obesity and to messages combating obesity, we report here the findings of two studies investigating the use of negative emotions to fight alcohol abuse. The objective of our two studies on alcohol abuse was to demonstrate that even though the use of fear appeals is widespread in social welfare communications, other negative emotions, such as anger, sadness, shame, or guilt, might also lead to persuasion, given the adaptive role of these emotions.

We also investigate gender differences. As evidenced in psychological studies, women prove to be more sensitive to fear, shame, and guilt and have higher levels of emotional intensity than men.

The results of our research can be extrapolated to several other domains in public health. Our findings help us establish guidelines for managers on the concrete modalities of negative emotion appeals. Based on our research, we encourage the use of shame appeals to fight health risks for young people. Using our research, public agencies, advertising companies, or policy makers can utilize a framework for analyzing relevant elements before developing negative emotion appeals in order to fight excessive consumption of alcohol or any other health risk, especially obesity.

Because our studies, reported below, utilize different types of negative emotional appeals, we now review some of the relevant literature on the types and dimensions of emotions and the prior literature on the use of different negative emotions in persuasive messages.

EMOTIONS AND PERSUASION

Frijda (1987, 1989) defines emotions as "motivational states underlying behaviors and interactions with the environment." He argues that emotions are not simple reactions to the evaluation of events, but also include tendencies to act. This motivational characteristic of emotions has prompted advertisers to use emotional stimuli for persuasion.

Izard (1977) says emotions are "an intra-individual process characterized by a specific neurophysiological activity and a distinctive facial expression." He adds that every type of emotion is linked to a unique emotional state, expressed consciously. Izard therefore puts the emphasis on three aspects of emotion manifestations: neurophysiological, expressive, and phenomenological.

Classification of Emotions

Given the wide range of emotions and the lack of consensus on the nature and the structure of emotions, psychologists formulated valid methods to organize and structure emotions. One approach consists of finding a few dimensions that account for the main similarities and differences between emotions. The other approach classifies emotions based on typology.

Classification of Emotions Based on Dimensionality (Continuous Approach)

Lang (1994) and Russel (1980) posit that emotions are linked and do not form discrete categories. Thus, emotions can be placed on a multidimensional emotional map defined by two or more dimensions. The dimensions arise from consumers' evaluations of emotions. These evaluations are statistically analyzed to construct a few measures from a number of correlated emotions (factorial analysis) or to position emotions along a few dimensions, while preserving information about their similarities and differences (multidimensional scaling). These methods often show that only two dimensions, valence and activation level, are needed to account for the main differences between emotions (Parrott 2001).

Classification of Emotions Based on Typology (Discrete Approach)

Another approach for classifying emotions consists of analyzing the similarities between emotions using cluster analysis, which gives a hierarchical structure rather than a multidimensional one. Consequently, emotions are classified into groups according to the desired specificity level. Ekman (1993) expanded the list of basic emotions to sixteen: amusement, anger, contempt, contentment, disappointment, disgust, embarrassment, excitement, fear, guilt, pride, relief, sadness, sensory pleasure, shame, and surprise. Izard (1977) identified ten discrete or basic emotions—anger, contempt, disgust, distress, fear, guilt, interest, joy, shame, and surprise.

Bagozzi, Gopinath, and Nyer (1999) refer to Roseman's appraisal theory (1991) to specify the conditions leading to discrete emotional responses. This theory says that particular combinations of five appraisals determine which of sixteen unique emotions will be experienced in any given situation. The five appraisals are labeled motive consistent/motive inconsistent, appetitive/aversive, agency, probability, and power. Hence, fear and sadness are experienced differently, although they have the same valence (motive inconsistent). Fear is caused by an impersonal, uncertain circumstance under conditions of low coping potential, whereas sadness is experienced with high certainty under conditions of low coping power. It is perceived to be caused by impersonal circumstances.

Emotions and Gender

In their study, Allen and Haccoun (1976) asked young people "what they would feel" with regard to four emotions. The subjects did not express any differences in the frequency of emotions but rather in their intensity. Women expressed greater emotional intensity on three of four emotions—fear, sadness, and joy. Diener, Sandvik, and Larsen (1985) measured emotional intensity for subjects aged sixteen to sixty-eight and showed that women had higher levels of emotional intensity (positive and negative emotions) and extreme mood variations in comparison with men. Tangney (1998) showed that women express more shame and guilt than men. This result is a consequence of a weaker social status and less physical aggression. It results from the traditional and natural roles of women (taking care of children, maternal relationships), which require women to have more capacity for interpreting the emotional signals of others. On the other hand, anger, pride, and contempt are more present among men with regard to their need to be different, to compete with others, to minimize their vulnerability, and to maximize their chances of success (Brody and Hall 1993).

The Role of Negative Emotions in Public Health Communication

Fear Appeals Theory

Fear is considered a negatively valenced emotion, accompanied by a high level of arousal, and is elicited by a threat that is perceived to be significant and personally relevant (Easterling and Leventhal 1989; Witte 1992). Messages using fear appeals have been used in various domains such as road safety; prevention of drug, tobacco, and alcohol abuse; and prevention of AIDS. Since the pioneering study of Janis and Feshbach (1953) on dental hygiene, research on persuasion through fear appeals has led to contrasting results, revealing either strong positive effects (Arthur and Quester 2004; Bennett 1996) or little or no effects (Krisher, Darley, and Darley 1973; Schoenbachler and Whittler 1996) on persuasion.

Three theoretical models have been used to explain the role of fear in persuasion, and they correspond to three time periods (Dillard 1994): (1) fear drive models (Janis and Feshbach 1953; McGuire 1968), (2) parallel process models (Leventhal 1970), and (3) expectancy value theories (Rogers 1983; Sutton 1982; Tanner, Hunt, and Eppright 1991). Based on these theories, Witte (1992) proposes an extended parallel process model (EPPM), which is regarded as theoretically founded and empirically verified. This model shows that a fear appeal leads to two cognitive evaluation processes. The individual first evaluates the threat. If this leads to a perception of a moderate to important threat, then fear is activated (Easterling and Leventhal 1989). In this case, the individual is motivated to evaluate efficacy. A high level of efficacy (response efficacy and self-efficacy) leads to the success of the fear appeal. If, on the contrary, the threat is perceived as low, the individual has no motivation to process the message, the efficacy is not evaluated, and there is no reaction (or persuasion).

Recent Studies on Fear Appeals in Public Health Communication

Witte and Allen (2000) examined the previous studies conducted on fear appeals and identified a list of outcome variables, which they separated into two groups. The first group includes variables linked to the recommendation's acceptance (i.e., attitude, intention, and behavioral change), and the second relates to the recommendations' rejection variables (i.e., self-defense, message denial, reaction).

The majority of the recent studies show a positive relationship between fear and persuasion (Bécheur et al. 2007). Block and Keller (1997) evaluated the effects of a fear appeal containing vivid information on sexually transmitted diseases and skin cancer. Results show that the audience prefers vivid messages to neutral ones, and messages in which perceived self-efficacy is high. These results give more empirical validation to fear appeal models.

In the same context, Block and Keller (1995) showed that in the case of low perceived self-efficacy, people are forced to evaluate the results of compliance with the message's recommendation. In that case, negatively framed messages prove to be more efficient than positively framed messages. On the contrary, in the case of high perceived self-efficacy, positive and negative messages have identical effects. LaTour, Snipes, and Bliss (1996) found that the purchase intentions for a promoted gun brand were significantly higher for messages activating intense fear.

The variability of fear appeal effects according to culture was also studied. In this context, Laroche et al. (2001) showed that intentions to stop smoking were higher among Caucasians after being exposed to a fear appeal introducing physical threat versus social threat. Intentions to stop smoking among Chinese subjects did not vary according to the type of the threat presented in the message (social vs. physical).

Negative Emotions Other Than Fear

Most of the studies on the role of emotions in public health communication focus on the use of fear and neglect the impact of other negative emotions such as shame, guilt, anger, or sadness.

Although guilt appeals are used in many contexts (e.g., anti-alcohol campaigns, AIDS prevention, feminine hygiene product promotion), studies on the effectiveness of guilt in persuasion are limited (Bennett 1998). Some rare contributions appeared during the last three decades (Bécheur et al. 2007; Bennett 1998; Bozinoff and Ghingold 1983; Burnett and Lunsford 1994; Cotte, Coulter, and Moore 2005; Coulter and Pinto 1995).

Several types of guilt exist. Burnett and Lunsford (1994) identify four types often used in advertising persuasion: financial guilt, guilt related to health, moral guilt, and guilt related to social responsibility. Financial guilt occurs after unnecessary purchases. Guilt related to health occurs when a person feels she does not take care of herself properly (e.g., smoking during pregnancy, drinking and driving). Moral guilt implies a violation of personal moral standards. Finally, guilt related to social responsibility concerns other people (e.g., neglect of a close friend's birthday). Moreover, Coulter, Cotte, and Moore (1999) distinguish between anticipatory, reactive, and existential guilt. Huhmann and Brotherton (1997) say that anticipatory guilt is most used in commercial advertising.

Guilt appeals are often used in social marketing. The most common type of guilt in this case is existential guilt (Huhmann and Brotherton 1997), which results from a difference between one's own welfare and the welfare of others (Izard 1977). Some empirical studies that tested the impact of guilt had diverging results and affirm its positive effect on persuasion.

In this regard, Bozinoff and Ghingold (1983) point out that, although guilt is easily activated after exposure to guilt appeals, these messages prove to be inefficient in changing attitudes and behaviors. This failure could be due to a feeling of manipulation (Coulter, Cotte, and Moore 1999). In spite of these warnings against the use of guilt in persuasion, Bécheur et al. (2007) show that guilt is an emotion that enhances persuasion and motivates the adoption of the recommended actions in fighting alcohol abuse.

Finally, regarding shame appeals, research is again quite limited. Bennett (1998) compares the effects of shame and guilt in advertising persuasion. Results show that reactions to guilt appeals are more positive than reactions to shame appeals. Bennett argues that the distinction between shame and guilt often made in psychology is appropriate in advertising and that advertising based on guilt might be efficient, provided that shame is not activated. Moreover, Bécheur et al. (2007) recently showed that among the emotions of fear, shame, and guilt, shame is the most effective against alcohol abuse (Study 1).

TWO STUDIES USING NEGATIVE EMOTIONS TO FIGHT ALCOHOL ABUSE

We study the effects of negative emotions within the framework of health communication. Our two studies focus on the use of negative emotional appeals in advertising that targets an audience of young adults in order to prevent the physical and psychosocial risks linked to alcohol abuse. Based on Witte's (1992) framework, we built our model of persuasion by using the emotions of fear, guilt, and shame that we describe in Study 1. We chose to explore fear, shame, and guilt among all other negative emotions based on the results of a previous qualitative study. Indeed, when thinking about the risks associated with alcohol abuse, respondents reported experiencing not only fear, but also shame and guilt. In addition, the social threat leading to feelings of shame and guilt seems to be more relevant to young people.

Our first study (see Bécheur et al. 2007) tests the effects of fear, shame, and guilt on the persuasiveness of anti–alcohol abuse advertising directed at young people. Given the limitations of studying only three negative emotions, while research in psychology argues that a perceived threat activates a wide range of negative emotions, we decided to conduct a second study (see Bécheur, Dib, and Valette-Florence 2009). It examines the effects of nine basic emotions activated by a shocking message on drinking and driving, which are then measured by Izard's scale.

Study 1

First, we built a conceptual model explaining persuasion (Figure 10.1). Fear, shame, and guilt are correlated and result in negative affect (Lazarus 1991). A factor analysis on emotion data proves the existence of a superior factor [negative affect $\rightarrow$ fear (.485, $|t| = 12.814$); negative affect $\rightarrow$ guilt (.585, $|t| = 16.352$); negative affect $\rightarrow$ shame (.967, $|t| = 24.114$)].

Persuasion is directly affected by the stimulation of negative emotions (the more intense the negative emotions, the higher the persuasion) and by both the perceived

Figure 10.1 **Conceptual Model Tested in Study 1**

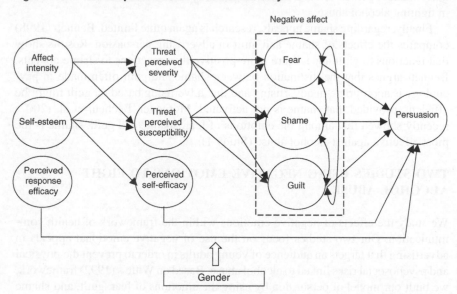

efficacy of the recommended solution (perceived response efficacy) and the perceived ability to adopt the recommended solution (perceived self-efficacy).[1] The level of activation of negative emotions is affected by the severity of the threat and the perceptions of the susceptibility to the threat. Affect intensity is hypothesized to have a positive impact on threat-perceived severity and threat-perceived susceptibility. Self-esteem is hypothesized to have a negative impact on the same constructs. In addition, self-esteem has a positive impact on perceived self-efficacy. We hypothesized that sensation seeking moderates the impact of negative emotions on persuasion.

In order to test our conceptual model, we created four anti-alcohol advertising messages, one for the fear and one for the guilt scenarios and two for the shame scenario (one for each gender). The ads aimed at generating perceptions of severe threat, high susceptibility to threat, efficacy of the solution, and high self-efficacy (Witte 1992).

We measured responses for all items on a seven-point Likert-type scale. Measurements of threat-perceived severity, threat-perceived susceptibility, perceived response efficacy, and perceived self-efficacy are adapted from Witte (1992). The emotion of fear is measured through five items adapted from Block and Keller (1995) and Laroche et al. (2001). Guilt is measured by three items adapted from Cotte, Coulter, and Moore (2005) and Izard (1977), and shame is measured by four items adapted from Rolland and De Fruyt (2003). Other measurements were drawn from existing scales: persuasion (Block and Keller 1997), self-esteem (Rosenberg [1965], from which we eliminated reverse items), affect intensity (second dimension of the Geuens and De Pelsmacker [2002] scale that corresponds to negative emotions), and sensation seeking

(Zuckerman et al. 1964). We collected 1,082 usable questionnaires (391, 401, and 290 for the fear, the guilt, and the shame scenarios, respectively).

To uncover differences between the three emotional situations (fear, guilt, and shame), we used a structural multigroup approach. We compared a model with free structural parameters to a model in which structural parameters were constrained to 1. We found a significant difference [$\Delta\chi^2(32) = 119.59$, $p < .001$].

Although the impact of perceived susceptibility on guilt is insignificant (for the guilt scenario), negative emotions appear to play a mediating role between threat perceptions and persuasion, which supports the importance of negative emotions and the conceptualization that a threat leads to negative emotions (fear, guilt, shame) that in turn determine behavior (Arthur and Quester 2004). In addition, negative emotions appear interdependent, such that the guilt scenario generates fear, and the shame scenario produces both of the other negative emotions. Persuasion therefore results from all these effects. In a shame scenario, persuasion occurs because all three emotions are activated in support of Lazarus's (1991) propositions about the role of shame. Shame motivates social behaviors and leads to conformance to social norms.

Gender Differences

Overall, in the samples of women compared to men, we notice stronger path coefficients in all conditions. Only the effect of perceived self-efficacy—that is, the ability to adopt the recommended solution—on persuasion was more important among men. Results show, for instance, that the impact of affect intensity on threat perceptions is greater for all scenarios among women. Similarly, in the sample of women, fear (guilt or shame) was more effective under the fear (guilt or shame) condition. In the case of the shame appeal, persuasion occurred because the three emotions studied were activated. All these emotions had stronger effects on persuasion in the sample of women. The effect of perceived response efficacy on persuasion was greater among women when exposed to the shame condition. Although the effect of perceived self-efficacy on persuasion was stronger among men in the case of the fear scenario, fear had a stronger impact on persuasion among women. This may suggest that the level of fear stimulated by the fear condition can be increased among men in order to provoke a better effect on persuasion.

In conclusion, compared to men, women showed higher levels of affect intensity and experienced more fear, shame, and guilt when exposed to our three conditions. This result confirms findings in psychological studies on emotion activation and gender differences (Tangney 1998). Negative emotions had a stronger impact on persuasion for women compared to men.

Study 2

In order to test our hypotheses, we created an advertising message featuring a disfigured woman whose face and hands are completely burned after an accident due to

Figure 10.2 **Conceptual Model Tested in Study 2**

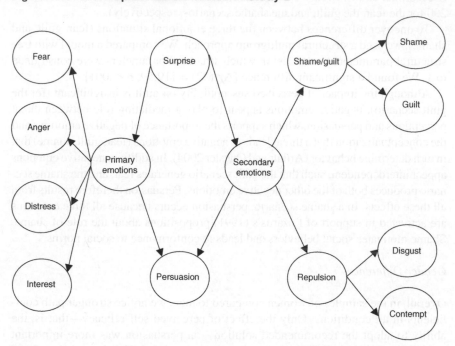

drinking and driving. The visual presents a photograph of the young woman before the accident and another after the accident; her father expresses painful emotions. A written message below the ad introduces a solution aimed at preventing such an accident (avoid threat): "Please don't let this happen to you!!! During a party, never drink more than three glasses of alcohol and stop drinking before driving."

We collected 167 usable questionnaires and measured responses for all items on a seven-point Likert-type scale. Emotions are measured through the Izard's (1977) differential emotions scale (DES). The DES I contains thirty adjective items, three to measure each of Izard's fundamental emotions. We eliminated the measurement of joy from the scale. Measurements of perceived self-efficacy are adapted from Witte (1992). Persuasion is drawn from Block and Keller (1997) (six items).

Before testing the effects of negative emotions on persuasion, an exploratory analysis was conducted to cluster these emotions into groups. A principal component analysis, with Promax rotation performed on the twenty-seven items of Izard's scale (without joy as a variable), resulted in three dimensions interpreted as primary emotions, secondary emotions, and surprise. Secondary emotions were composed of two subdimensions: repulsion and guilt or shame (Figure 10.2).[2] Considering the reduced size of our sample, the model was tested according to a PLS (partial least squares) approach.

Results show that primary emotions have direct positive effects on persuasion, while the effect of secondary emotions is insignificant. Because of this result, we decided to explore the effects of first-order dimensions of emotions. Fear was the most effective primary emotion on persuasion. The effects of distress and interest were also significant. However, and contrary to our assumption, all first-order secondary emotions did not have significant effects on persuasion. This result contradicts findings from our first study and emphasizes the need to conduct more experiments in this domain. Results also showed that after exposure to threat-related stimuli, the activation of surprise occurred before the activations of all the other negative emotions. We support Schutzwohl and Borgstedt's (2005) findings regarding the important role of surprise in the processing of negatively valenced stimuli.

This research supported the role of fear in the context of preventing drinking and driving and examined the role of other emotions—that is, interest, enjoyment, distress, anger, disgust, contempt, shame, and guilt. Our experimentation shows that after exposure to a threatening message, the audience became involved in a danger-control process and was motivated to control the danger rather than the negative emotions (Leventhal 1970). We prove that fear motivates the adoption of the solutions recommended in the ad, as other research has shown. Results support the theories of Leventhal (1970), Rogers (1983), and Witte (1992) that show that fear determines behavior, and extend findings on the role of fear to other emotions, particularly, interest.

However, recent articles (e.g., Gorn, Pham, and Sin 2001) argue that it is the arousal, not valence, of the emotions that influences ad evaluation. In other words, even emotions in the same valence (e.g., all negative) may influence people in different ways. This may explain why we found significant effects of some emotions but not others.

Gender Differences

To test the moderating impact of gender, we performed multigroup analysis with permutation tests. Results show that gender does not moderate the effects of primary and secondary emotions on persuasion.

IMPLICATIONS AND RECOMMENDATIONS

Conditions of Success of a Threatening Message on Obesity

An anti-obesity campaign based on negative emotions is doomed to failure if certain conditions are not met. First, the persons to whom the prospective, preventive message is addressed must consider the introduced threat due to obesity as serious and imminent (such as physical or social threats like cardiovascular diseases, hypertension, disdainful looks from others). Then, the message should announce a solution to the threat that is perceived as efficient and easy to implement. Following the recommendations of Witte et al. (1996), we suggest that if the perception of threat is superior to the perception of efficacy, people could become involved in a fear-control process, which leads to maladaptive behavior. It will then be necessary to reinforce their perception of efficacy by offering a simple, easy solution to prevent obesity. On the other hand, if the perception of the threat is lower than the perception of efficacy, individuals become involved in a danger-control process and therefore adopt the recommendations given by the ad. It will then be necessary to continue motivating them to become involved in the adaptive processes by emphasizing the perceptions of threat and efficacy. Finally, people who have a low perception of threat are not concerned by the problem. It is then necessary to break their "invulnerability barriers" by communicating high levels of perceived vulnerability. Pretesting the anti-obesity ad on a small sample of our targeted group allowed us to assess levels of threat and efficacy and adjust them so that they create positive effects on the audience.

The Role of Perceived Threat

Several methods are offered in the literature to increase threat perceptions. With regard to smoking, Rogers (1983) suggests increasing the amount of information and details in the ad about the serious consequences of the risky behavior (continuing the same consumption habits). Gallopel (2000) says that to be really threatening and produce the expected effect, antismoking ads should feature the physical deterioration of the smoker caused by various associated diseases. She explains that it is also necessary to speak about death along with the pain felt by people who lost a close relative due to smoking. We suggest doing the same with obesity, which means that the ad should show the physical and moral deterioration of the "victims," talk about death, and show the pain obesity causes not only to the potential victims, but also to their families, relatives, and friends.

Generalizing from this research on fighting alcohol abuse, we think that social threats (rejection of the group, feeling bad, loss of self-control, isolation) that provoke shame and guilt in particular would be efficient in preventing obesity. Moreover, to ensure that the person viewing the ad is concerned about the severity of obesity, the actors in the ad should have the same characteristics as the person (same age, gender, race, demographic characteristics, and so on).

The Role of Perceived Efficacy

Witte (1992) shows that these mechanisms of defense and reaction, which explain the failure of fear appeals, occur when perceptions of threat exceed perceptions of efficacy—that is, when people feel that neither they nor the recommendations in the message would be able to prevent the occurrence of the threat presented in the message. Self-efficacy is therefore particularly important for countering psychological reaction. In fact, people are motivated to assert their freedom when it appears that their freedom might be threatened or restricted (Eagle et al. 2004). It is possible, therefore, that attempted restrictions may encourage consumption rather than limiting it, if self-efficacy is low.

Thus, to increase response efficacy, solutions for reducing overconsumption (response efficacy) must also be presented to the prospects—for example, in the form of nutritional information. Garg, Wansink, and Inman (2007) manipulated specific emotional states to test the hypothesis that, in the absence of negative nutritional information, sad people consume more of a hedonic product than relatively happier people. They showed that among happy people, the presence of nutritional information does not drive consumption any lower, because they are already avoiding consumption. Conversely, in the absence of nutritional information, sad people overcome their negative state by consuming more. In addition, people in negative moods and states are more likely to overeat.

The integration of mixed emotions in the same ad is also possible, especially in television messages. Presenting the obesity threat in the first part of an ad creates negative emotions. Showing efficient solutions (exercising, eating small portions) would then stimulate the person's positive emotions and restore a state of equilibrium. In this context, Williams and Aaker (2002) show that persuasion appeals that highlight conflicting emotions (e.g., both happiness and sadness) lead to less favorable attitudes for individuals with a low propensity to accept duality (e.g., Anglo Americans, older adults). This effect appears to be due to increased levels of discomfort that arise for those with a lower, but not higher, propensity to accept duality when exposed to mixed emotional appeals.

The Role of Individual Variables

It seems necessary that advertisers must take into account individual and psychological characteristics of the obese people targeted. Results from Study 1 show, for example, that women exhibited higher levels of affect intensity and experienced more fear, shame, and guilt when exposed to our three conditions (fear, shame, and guilt). Practitioners should then consider this result when creating the threatening message. Hence, levels of induced negative emotions should be higher among men.

Further studies on gender effects should be conducted in the case of obesity. In fact, Garg, Wansink, and Inman (2007) did not find any gender effects in their studies. This implies that both men and women use consumption as a way to manage their affective state.

If certain individual variables are relevant in fighting alcohol abuse (e.g., seeking sensation), other individual and contextual variables, such as family environment, social class, introversion, source credibility, or ad repetition, might have an impact on the relationship between negative emotions and persuasion in the case of obesity and should be investigated. The levels of threat to be introduced in the different segments would be different.

Encouraging the Use of Shame in Anti-Obesity Campaigns

Results from Study 1 show that in the case of the shame scenario, persuasion occurs because the three emotions studied were activated. We confirm the proposition of Lazarus (1991) concerning the role of shame. Shame motivates a social behavior and leads to conformity to social norms. Contrary to Bennett (1998), who proposes that guilt messages may be persuasive if shame is not activated, our results show that a threatening message implying fear, guilt, and shame together might well be the most persuasive. Scherer (2006) says that it is not the shame that favors the control of the antisocial behaviors, but rather the fear of feeling ashamed.

Overweight, alcoholic populations, possibly having low levels of self-esteem and high levels of anxiety and depression, may be more predisposed to shame. The levels of threat to be addressed to these segments should then be lower. Pretests of the ads inducing shame or guilt should be preceded by an exam of the psychological profile of the audience (Bennett 1998).

Even though we tried in this work to present the elements that need to be present to maximize the efficacy of anti-obesity ads based on negative emotions, we remain convinced, as stipulated by Eagle et al. (2004), that the problem of obesity is complex and there is no simple solution. In addition to marketing communications, long-term initiatives from the government (such as public transportation to replace cars) should be envisioned, especially in the United States.

NOTES

1. Previous research indicates a positive correlation between perceived response efficacy and perceived self-efficacy (Tanner, Hunt, and Eppright 1991; Witte 1992). In addition, some recent studies on fear appeals show that perceived efficacy (response and self-efficacy) moderates the relationships between negative emotions and persuasion (see Block and Keller 1997). We chose not to study these relationships in order not to add more complexity to our model. We suggest doing it in future research.

2. First-order emotions are correlated, even though they are not shown in Figure 10.2.

REFERENCES

Allen, Jon G., and Dorothy M. Haccoun. 1976. "Sex Differences in Emotionality: A Multidimensional Approach." *Human Relations*, 29 (August), 711–722.

Arthur, Damien, and Pascale Quester. 2004. "Who's Afraid of That Ad? Applying Segmentation to the Protection Motivation Mode." *Psychology and Marketing*, 21 (September), 671–696.

Bagozzi, Richard P., Mahesh Gopinath, and Prashanth U. Nyer. 1999. "The Role of Emotions in Marketing." *Journal of the Academy of Marketing Science*, 27 (Spring), 184–206.

Bécheur, Imène, Hayan Dib, Dwight Merunka, and Pierre Valette-Florence. 2007. "The Effects of Fear, Guilt and Shame on Persuasiveness of Health Communication: A Study of Anti-Alcohol Messages." Paper presented at the Academy of Marketing Science Annual Conference, Miami, Florida (May).

Bécheur, Imène, Hayan Dib, and Pierre Valette-Florence. 2009. "Is Surprise Prior to the Activation of Negative Emotions? The Processing of a Shocking Ad on Drinking and

Driving." Paper presented at the 2009 AMA Winter Marketing Educators' Conference, Tampa, Florida (February).

Bennett, Roger. 1996. "Effects of Horrific Fear Appeals on Public Attitudes Towards AIDS." *International Journal of Advertising*, 15 (3), 183–202.

———. 1998. "Shame, Guilt and Responses to Non-Profit and Public Sector Ads." *International Journal of Advertising*, 17 (4), 483–499.

Block, Lauren G., and Punam A. Keller. 1995. "When to Accentuate the Negative: The Effects of Perceived Efficacy and Message Framing on Intentions to Perform a Health-Related Behavior." *Journal of Marketing Research*, 32 (May), 192–203.

———. 1997. "Effects of Self-efficacy and Vividness on the Persuasiveness of Health Communications." *Journal of Consumer Psychology*, 6 (1), 31–54.

Bozinoff, Lorne, and Morry Ghingold. 1983. "Evaluating Guilt Arousing Marketing Communications." *Journal of Business Research*, 11 (June), 243–255.

Brody, Leslie R., and Judy A. Hall. 1993. "Gender and Emotion." In *Handbook of Emotions*, ed. Michael Lewis and Jeannette M. Haviland-Jones, 447–460. New York: Guilford Press.

Burnett, Melissa S., and Dale A. Lunsford. 1994. "Conceptualizing Guilt in the Consumer Decision-Making Process." *Journal of Consumer Marketing*, 11 (3), 33–43.

Bybee, Jane, Edward Zigler, Dana Berliner, and Merisca Rolande. 1996. "Guilt, Guilt-Evoking Events, Depression, and Eating Disorders." *Current Psychology: Developmental, Learning, Personality, Social*, 15, 113–127.

Cotte, June, Robin H. Coulter, and Melissa Moore. 2005. "Enhancing or Disrupting Guilt: The Role of Ad Credibility and Perceived Manipulative Intent." *Journal of Business Research*, 58 (March), 361–368.

Coulter, Robin Higie, June Cotte, and Melissa Moore. 1999. "Believe It or Not: Persuasion, Manipulation and Credibility of Guilt Appeals." *Advances in Consumer Research*, 26, 288–294.

Coulter, Robin Higie, and Mary Beth Pinto. 1995. "Guilt Appeals in Advertising: What Are Their Effects?" *Journal of Applied Psychology*, 80 (December), 697–705.

Diener, Ed, Ed Sandvik, and Randy J. Larsen. 1985. "Age and Sex Effects for Emotional Intensity." *Developmental Psychology*, 21, 542–546.

Dillard, James P. 1994. "Rethinking the Study of Fear Appeals: An Emotional Perspective." *Communication Theory*, 4 (November), 295–323.

Eagle, Lynne, Sandy Bulmer, Philip Kitchen, and Jacinta Hawkins. 2004. "Complex and Controversial Causes for the 'Obesity Epidemic': The Role of Marketing Communications." *International Journal of Medical Marketing*, 4 (3), 271–287.

Easterling, Douglas V., and Howard Leventhal. 1989. "Contribution of Concrete Cognition to Emotion: Neutral Symptoms as Elicitors of Worry About Cancer." *Journal of Applied Psychology*, 74 (October), 787–796.

Ekman, Paul. 1993. "Facial Expression and Emotion." *American Psychologist*, 48 (4), 384–392.

Frijda, Nico H. 1986. *The Emotions: Studies in Emotion and Social Interaction*. New York: Cambridge University Press.

———. 1987. *The Emotions*. Cambridge: Cambridge University Press.

———. 1989. "Les Théories des Émotions: Un bilan." In *Textes de Base en Psychologie: Les Emotions*, ed. Bernard Rimé and Klaus Scherer, 21–72. Paris: Delachaux et Niestlé.

Gallopel, Karine. 2000. "Réflexions sur l'Utilisation de la Peur dans les Campagnes de Prévention des Comportements Tabagiques." Paper presented at the XVèmes journées des IAE, Bayonne-Biarritz, France (September).

Garg, Nikita, Brian Wansink, and Jeffrey J. Inman. 2007. "The Influence of Incidental Affect on Consumers' Food Intake." *Journal of Marketing*, 71 (January), 194–206.

Geuens, Maggie, and Patrick De Pelsmacker. 2002. "The Role of Humor in the Persuasion of Individuals Varying in Need for Cognition." *Advances in Consumer Research*, 29 (1), 50–56.

Gorn, Gerald, Michel Tuan Pham, and Leo Yatming Sin. 2001. "When Arousal Influences Ad Evaluation and Valence Does Not (and Vice Versa)." *Journal of Consumer Psychology*, 11 (1), 43–55.

Huhmann, Bruce A., and Timothy P. Brotherton. 1997. "A Content Analysis of Guilt Appeals in Popular Magazine Advertisements." *Journal of Advertising*, 26 (2), 35–45.

Izard, Carroll E. 1977. *Human Emotions*. New York: Plenum Press.

Janis, Irving L., and Seymour Feshbach. 1953. "Effects of Fear-Arousing Communications." *Journal of Abnormal and Social Psychology*, 48 (January), 78–92.

Killen, Joel D., C. Barr Taylor, Chris Hayward, K. Parish Haydel, Darrell M. Wilson, Lawrence D. Hammer, Helena Kraemer, Anne Blair-Greiner, and Diane Stachowski. 1996. "Weight Concerns Influence the Development of Eating Disorders: A Four-Year Prospective Study." *Journal of Consulting and Clinical Psychology*, 64, 936–940.

Krisher, Howard P., Susan A. Darley, and John M. Darley. 1973. "Fear Provoking Recommendations, Intentions to Take Preventive Actions and Actual Preventive Actions." *Journal of Personality and Social Psychology*, 26 (2), 301–308.

Lang, Peter J. 1994. "The Varieties of Emotional Experience: A Meditation of James-Lange Theory." *Psychological Review*, 101 (2), 211–221.

Laroche, Michel, Roy Toffoli, Quihong Zhang, and Frank Pons. 2001. "A Cross-Cultural Study of the Persuasive Effect of Fear Appeal Messages in Cigarette Advertising: China and Canada." *International Journal of Advertising*, 20 (3), 297–317.

LaTour, Michael S., Robin L. Snipes, and Sara J. Bliss. 1996. "Don't Be Afraid to Use Fear Appeals: An Experimental Study." *Journal of Advertising Research*, 36 (2), 56–67.

Lazarus, Richard S. 1991. *Emotion and Adaptation*. New York: Oxford University Press.

Leventhal, Howard. 1970. "Findings and Theory in the Study of Fear Communications." *Advances in Experimental Social Psychology*, 5, 119–186.

McGuire, William J. 1968. "Personality and Susceptibility to Social Influence." In *Handbook of Personality Theory and Research*, ed. Edward F. Borgotta and William W. Lambert, 1130–1187. Chicago: Rand McNally.

Parrott, W. Gerrod. 2001. "Emotions in Social Psychology: Volume Overview." In *Emotions in Social Psychology*, ed. W. Gerrod Parrott, 1–19. Philadelphia: Psychology Press.

Rogers, Ronald W. 1983. "Cognitive and Physiological Processes in Fear Appeal and Attitude Change: A Revisited Theory of Protection Motivation." In *Social Psychophysiology*, ed. John T. Cacioppo and Richard E. Petty, 153–176. New York: Guilford Press.

Rolland, Jean-Pierre, and Filip De Fruyt. 2003. "The Validity of FFM Personality Dimensions and Maladaptative Traits to Predict Negative Affects at Work: A Six Months Predictive Study in a Military Sample." *European Journal of Personality*, 17, 1–21.

Roseman, Ira J. 1991. "Appraisal Determinants of Discrete Emotions." *Cognition and Emotion*, 5, 161–200.

Rosenberg, Morris. 1965. *Society and the Adolescent Self-Image*. Princeton, NJ: Princeton University Press.

Russel, James A. 1980. "A Circumplex Model of Affect." *Journal of Personality and Social Psychology*, 39 (6), 1161–1178.

Scherer, Klaus. 2006. "Vers les Sciences Affectives." *Sciences Humaines*, 171, 42–43.

Schoenbachler, Denise D., and Tommy E. Whittler. 1996. "Adolescent Processing of Social and Physical Threat Communications." *Journal of Advertising*, 25 (Winter), 37–54.

Schutzwohl, Achim, and Kirsten Borgstedt. 2005. "The Processing of Affectively Valenced Stimuli: The Role of Surprise." *Cognition and Emotion*, 19 (4), 583–600.

Stice, Eric. 2001. "A Prospective Test of the Dual Pathway Model of Bulimic Pathology: Mediating Effects of Dieting and Negative Affect." *Journal of Abnormal Psychology*, 110, 124–135.

Sutton, Stephen R. 1982. "Fear-Arousing Communications: A Critical Examination of Theory and Research." In *Social Psychology Studies and Behavioral Medicine*, ed. Richard J. Eiser, 303–337. Chichester, UK: John Wiley.

Tangney, June P. 1998. "How Does Guilt Differ from Shame?" In *Guilt and Children*, ed. Jane Bybee, 1–17. San Diego: Academic Press.

Tanner, John F., Jr., James B. Hunt, and David R. Eppright. 1991. "The Protection Motivation Model: A Normative Model of Fear Appeals." *Journal of Marketing*, 55 (July), 36–45.

Williams, Patti, and Jennifer L. Aaker. 2002. "Can Mixed Emotions Peacefully Coexist?" *Journal of Consumer Research*, 28 (March), 636–650.

Witte, Kim. 1992. "Putting the Fear Back into Fear Appeals: The Extended Parallel Process Model." *Communication Monographs*, 59 (December), 329–349.

Witte, Kim, and Mike Allen. 2000. "A Meta-Analysis of Fear Appeals: Implications for Effective Public Health Campaigns." *Health Education and Behavior*, 27 (5), 591–615.

Witte, Kim, Cameron A. Kenzie, Janet K. McKeon, and Judy M. Berkowitz. 1996. "Predicting Risk Behaviors: Development and Validation of a Diagnostic Scale." *Journal of Health Communication*, 1, 317–341.

Zuckerman, Marvin, Elizabeth A. Kolin, Leah Price, and Leah Zoob. 1964. "Development of a Sensation Seeking Scale." *Journal of Consulting Psychology*, 28, 477–482.

CHAPTER 11

USING IDENTITY SIGNALING TO COMBAT OBESITY AND IMPROVE PUBLIC HEALTH

LINDSAY P. RAND AND JONAH BERGER

Over 50 percent of national health-care costs in the United States are due to three preventable conditions: heart disease, diabetes, and one issue that often underlies them both, obesity. Rates of obesity have increased by more than 60 percent among adults over the last twenty years (CDC 2006), and the American Academy of Pediatrics now warns that the number of overweight children in the United States has "reached epidemic proportions." There are many potential causes for this weighty trend, such as a more sedentary lifestyle (Blair and Brodney 1999) or certain genetic factors (Comuzzi and Allison 1998), but an increase in consumption—specifically of unhealthy foods and beverages—has more recently been cited as one of the most significant contributing factors (Chandon and Wansink 2007; Young and Nestle 2002). As the obesity epidemic becomes a widespread health crisis, it is critical that researchers, health professionals, and policy-makers develop new and creative methods for encouraging people to get healthy and reducing the consumption behaviors that are making Americans, and countries that imitate their Western diet, fat.

In this chapter, we will examine a novel strategy aimed at reducing rates of obesity-related health behaviors. Health and marketing research has shown that people will emulate the behaviors of aspiration groups (Englis and Solomon 1995). They will also diverge to avoid behaviors linked to dissociative reference groups (Berger and Heath 2007, 2008; White and Dahl 2006, 2007). By applying these concepts to consumption or obesity-related behavior choices, we believe that target populations can be encouraged to behave in ways that will positively impact their well-being. Put another way, our goal is to see whether campaigns that link obesity-related behaviors to dissociative reference groups can reduce rates of these behaviors and improve public health. First, we review some related research streams on which this perspective is based. Then we summarize the key findings from our own studies in the area, and finally we provide action-oriented implications of these findings for public health communications.

220

ROLE OF HEALTH EDUCATION

Public health campaigns designed to mitigate negative health behaviors (e.g., junk food consumption) often focus on raising risk awareness (Weinstein 1993). These campaigns are built on the notion that if people are educated about how behaviors may affect their future health, they will be inspired to make more intelligent health decisions today. Protection motivation theory (Rogers 1983), for example, suggests that people weigh the perceived severity of a disease or health outcome, and their vulnerability to that outcome, in considering whether to engage in unhealthy behavior.

However, increased risk awareness does not always lead to behavior change (Beck and Frankel 1981; Grier and Bryant 2005; Leventhal 1970). In reviewing dozens of protection motivation studies, for example, a recent meta-analysis found no significant relationship between risk perceptions and future behaviors (Milne, Paschal, and Orbell 2000). There are many reasons for this disconnect. Campaigns that rely on fear of future consequences tend to be threatening and yet ultimately ineffective. Informing consumers that unhealthy eating today may negatively impact their cardiovascular system or waistline in the future is useful, but it is hard for people to pass up the immediate gratification they get from consuming junk food in the present. Alternatively, to the degree that individuals want to continue to engage in unhealthy behaviors, they may use motivated reasoning and come to see the outcomes of negative health behaviors as less severe.

Rather than focusing on risk awareness, this chapter focuses on how shaping the meaning of consumption (Berger and Heath 2007, 2008) can make public health campaigns more effective. Health-related behaviors not only have consequences for well-being, but also they have symbolic meaning. Eating junk food may lead people to become obese, but it may also communicate particular social identities to others. The studies outlined in this chapter examine whether campaigns that work to shift the meaning of consumption, or, in this case, the social identity associated with junk food consumption, can improve consumer health by leading people to make healthier decisions.

THE ROLE OF MARKETING

Choices and behaviors often act as markers or signals of identity. People buy products not only for their functional value, but also for what they symbolize (Levy 1959). The clothes people wear, the cars they drive, and the behaviors in which they engage all signal useful information to others (Wernerfelt 1990). Importantly, however, the particular identity that people infer from the choices and behaviors of others depends on the behavior's meaning, which in turn depends on the set of people who engage in that behavior. Consequently, if people want to be associated with particular identities, or aspiration groups, they may adopt the tastes and behaviors linked to those identities (Englis and Solomon 1995).

Social marketing and public service messages are often designed to reinforce these associations and to "sell" a desirable behavior. For example, in 2009 the National Football League began to use several popular players in its "NFL Play 60" campaign, a marketing effort aimed at getting children and teenagers to be more physically active. For many kids, these players are an aspiration group. By associating professional football players with playground activities, campaign designers aimed to inspire their target audience to emulate the health and fitness habits of the players.

Linking popular or desirable groups with positive behaviors has frequently been shown to lead to an increase in these behaviors among members of a target audience. But what about dissociative identities (White and Dahl 2007), or groups that people want to avoid being associated with? Research on identity signaling and divergence (Berger and Heath 2007, 2008; also see White and Dahl 2006, 2007) has examined how people abandon tastes and behaviors when these preferences come to character- ize an identity that they no longer want to signal. Most behaviors are not inherently associated with any one particular identity. Rather they gain and lose meaning over time based on the set of people that hold them (Berger and Rand 2008). Across many identity-relevant decision domains, divergence research has demonstrated that when a taste or preference becomes associated with an undesired identity, individuals who used to hold that taste will abandon it to preserve meaningful signals of in-group identity and to avoid seeming like an undesirable "other."

One study, for example, demonstrated this type of divergence when a group of "geeky" undergraduates began wearing the popular yellow Livestrong wristbands (Berger and Heath 2008). For anyone unfamiliar with the Livestrong wristband, it is a yellow rubber bracelet used as a fundraising item for cancer research through the Lance Armstrong Foundation. In the study conducted by Berger and Heath, research assistants sold the bands to a target dorm of students and then returned a week later to sell the same bands to the academic theme dorm next door. Once students in the "geeky" dorm started wearing the wristbands, almost 33 percent of students in the original target dorm stopped wearing them. In this case, the desire to avoid looking like a geek led other students to abandon the item.

While work on divergence has tended to focus on behaviors in purchasing and product domains, there is some suggestion that the meaning of consumption also plays a role in health decision-making. The prototype model of risk behavior (Gib- bons and Gerrard 1995, 1997) contends that an individual's decision to adopt or avoid certain health behaviors is driven, in part, by the desire to acquire positive or avoid negative characteristics associated with that behavior. Because prototypes are interpersonal, a core assumption of the prototype/willingness model is that prototypes influence behavior via a social comparison process—comparing the self to the image of others (Gibbons and Gerrard 1997). Consequently, the deci- sion to engage in detrimental health behaviors may depend not only on the health consequences of those behaviors, but also on the identity that engaging in such behaviors signals to others (also see Berger and Heath 2008).

Research has shown that individuals are more likely to engage in unhealthy behaviors, for example, if they hold relatively favorable images of the kind of person who typically engages in the same behaviors. Social images have been shown to predict a change in specific health-related behaviors like smoking, drinking, and unprotected sexual intercourse (Ouellette et al. 2005). If teenagers think that cool kids drink and smoke, then they themselves may drink or smoke in an effort to appropriate that image into their own self-concept.

Though most prototype research has been correlational in nature, it suggests that if individuals are concerned with conforming to a specific identity, how favorably they perceive this identity and its associated behaviors can predict changes in their willingness to engage in those same behaviors over time (Oyserman 2009). Building on prior research, the following sections will examine whether campaigns that link risky health behaviors to dissociative social identities, or identities that consumers do not want to signal, can positively impact public health.

IDENTITY SIGNALING AND HEALTH BEHAVIORS

Food Choice

Recent research on identity signaling and health (Berger and Rand 2008) examined whether manipulating the social identity associated with a behavior could be a useful strategy for improving public health. In a preliminary investigation, participants were asked to make a number of real food choices from an array of healthy and unhealthy options. The social identity associated with junk food was manipulated to examine whether employing an identity-signaling strategy could encourage participants to make healthier choices.

Undergraduate participants were exposed to information that associated junk food consumption either with undergraduates (control condition) or with graduate students (out-group condition), a group with whom undergraduates did not want to be confused. Then, in the context of an ostensibly unrelated experiment, they made a number of real food choices (e.g., Coke vs. Pepsi) in a public pseudo-store environment among other study participants. In addition to some filler choices, some of the choice pairs were designed such that one option was obviously healthier than the other (e.g., an apple vs. a brownie).

Results indicated that linking junk food to a social identity that participants did not want to signal led them to make healthier choices. Compared to the participants in the control condition, those in the out-group condition chose almost 40 percent fewer junk food items.

Food Choice at the Vending Machine

One place people often make tough food choices is in front of vending machines. Vending machines provide quick and easy access to a snack, but are often not stocked with the healthiest food. Given the prevalence of food choices made from such convenience-driven outlets, another study examined whether an identity-signaling appeal could encourage healthier choices among vending machine patrons (Rand and Berger 2010). In particular, the study examined whether compared to a typical informational appeal, consumers would be more likely to avoid junk food when it was linked to a dissociative out-group.

Experimenters placed flyers on twenty different vending machines across a college campus. One of two flyer manipulations was placed on each machine. In the control condition, like so many informational public health campaigns, the flyer focused on the negative health consequences of consuming junk food. It showed a picture of an apple, listed some health-relevant facts like "consuming too much sodium is bad for your heart and kidneys," and reminded consumers to "pick health(y)." In contrast, in the identity-avoidance condition, the flyer focused on the identity communicated by choosing junk food. Specifically, it linked junk food consumption with computer gamers, an out-group with which most members of the target population did not want to be associated. The flyer showed a picture of a person playing games at a computer, the desk covered in junk food and wrappers, and below the picture a caption read, "This guy's a gamer. You know the type. Always at the computer. Desk covered in junk food. So, pick health(y) . . . Nobody wants to be mistaken for this guy."

The machines used in this study contained a standard assortment of snacks like chips and candy as well as some healthier options like granola and dried fruit. To measure food choice, an order sheet, purportedly from the vending machine company, was placed on each vending machine and patrons were asked to write down what they selected. At the conclusion of the study, two coders, blind to condition, rated all the food in the vending machines on a scale of -1 (unhealthy) to $+1$ (healthy). The healthiness of the selected options was then compared across condition.

As predicted, linking junk food consumption to a dissociative reference group led vending machine patrons to make seemingly healthier choices. It is important to note that this study was concerned with the perception of health value rather than the actual health value of each person's choice, as people cannot read nutrition facts for products trapped inside a vending machine. While a granola bar is actually very high in sugar and calories from fat, it is typically believed to be healthier than a chocolate bar or a bag of Cheetos. People often misestimate the health value of food items that seem healthy, or carry a "health halo" (Chandon and Wansink 2007). Because there was no way for participants to confirm their perceptions about the items in the vending machine by reconciling what they thought with what was on the label, the results of this study center around whether people would select items they believed to be healthier as a result of the manipulation.

As expected, compared to control participants (i.e., those who had been exposed to an informational appeal), participants exposed to an appeal linking junk food to an avoidance group tended to avoid junk food, selecting items generally rated as healthier ($M = -.21$ as opposed to $M = -.58$).

These results are particularly interesting because they contrast an identity-signaling approach with a traditional informational appeal. We do not mean to suggest that informational appeals should never be used, but the findings outlined above underscore the notion that information is not always enough. Whether consumers have become so used to informational appeals that they ignore them or because these appeals do not attack all roots of the problem, it is clear that identity-signaling approaches may sometimes be more effective.

This study illustrates that identity-signaling appeals can lead consumers to select options they perceive to be healthier, but given the interest in improving public health, our next study also examines the actual nutritional content of the items selected. Will consumers actually choose less fattening items, for example, when they are linked to dissociative reference groups?

Food Choice in an Eating Establishment

This study examined choice in a natural environment where diners were making real food choices in the presence of many peers (Berger and Rand 2008). Patrons were approached between the hours of 10 p.m. and 1 a.m. on their way into an all-hours on-campus eating establishment and, to provide a cover story for the manipulation, were asked to rate the writing style of a few newspaper articles. For participants in the experimental condition, one of the articles was a story that associated junk food consumption with a dissociative out-group (online gamers). For those in the control condition, all the articles were about innocuous control topics unrelated to health or food choice. Participants then went into the dining hall to order food, and a separate research assistant unobtrusively recorded what each participant ordered.

The results of this study further support the conclusions of the vending machine study. As predicted, even in a diner-type environment, an identity-signaling manipulation led people to choose healthier food. Compared to the control condition, participants in the avoidance group condition not only selected items they perceived to be healthier but items that were actually better for them, containing, on average, one-third fewer calories from fat. Similar effects were also found calculating total grams of fat per order.

In addition, the study investigated the role of individual differences in social-sensitization among participants. The self-monitoring scale (Snyder 1974) describes differences in how people monitor and control their behavior to achieve a desired public image. If the effects seen in this study were driven by the desire to avoid signaling certain identities to others, one would expect the modulation of behavior to occur most strongly among people who care most about how they appear. Consequently, linking junk food consumption to an avoidance group should have a greater effect on the food choices made by people identified as high self-monitors.

To test this possibility, participants were also asked to complete a self-monitoring scale before entering the dinning establishment.

As expected, results revealed that the effects were stronger among high self-monitors. Compared to the control condition, high self-monitors exposed to information linking junk food consumption to a generally dissociative out-group chose options that they perceived to be healthier and that were actually healthier for them.

This study further demonstrates the utility of identity-avoidance campaigns to mitigate risky consumer behaviors. Merely reading an article that linked an avoidance group to junk food consumption led many participants to make healthier decisions. The up-modulation by high self-monitors also corroborates the hypothesized role of identity signaling in this process. Consistent with the notion that the effects are driven by concerns of signaling to others, they occurred most strongly among people who are most sensitive to how others view them.

Taken together, these studies illustrate that identity-signaling appeals can encourage consumers to make healthier choices. In the context of related research, these results provide some important action-oriented conclusions that can be applied to help reduce rates of obesity in this country.

GENERAL DISCUSSION

Public health campaigns have made significant strides in addressing many of our nation's health concerns, but there is still much work to be done in combating the causes of child and adult obesity. While campaigns that present consumers with risk information may successfully increase awareness, such campaigns do not always lead to corresponding effects on behavior. Yet as millions of dollars are spent annually on caring for and treating people who are suffering from the side effects of being overweight, public health officials continue to spend money disseminating healthy eating tips and outlining dietary guidelines.

In contrast to campaigns that focus on raising risk awareness, this chapter has focused on the meaning of consumption, or what engaging in a particular behavior communicates about a person both to themselves and to those around them. Research has shown that choices and preferences are not only driven by functional utility, but also based on the image they will project. When dissociative out-group members adopt behaviors that someone once held, he or she may abandon that behavior to avoid being associated with the adopting group.

The work described in the preceding sections examines how to apply all these findings to health-relevant behaviors, specifically those that pertain to obesity. The three studies described in this chapter demonstrate not only that people are attending to the identity that their consumption choices are signaling, but also that they will alter their behavior depending on the identity their choices might convey. When consumption of an unhealthy snack was associated with an out-group, as in the vending machine study, participants made the decision to purchase healthier food. When junk food consumption was linked to an avoidance group in a diner-style setting, people who cared the most about how they appeared to others chose healthier options.

By shifting the social identity associated with junk food consumption, three simple, small-scale campaigns were able to impact the eating behavior of their target audiences. Addressing the meaning of consumption and what engaging in a behavior represents may be a new and powerful way to make public health campaigns more effective.

PUBLIC HEALTH CAMPAIGNS AND ADOLESCENT AUDIENCES

Using an out-group identity to motivate behavior change, especially as it pertains to food choice, may be particularly effective among teens and young adults, as their segment of the population is more likely to engage in social comparisons. Teens care a lot about fitting in, making friends, and appearing attractive to potential romantic partners. Consequently, they care a great deal about what their behavior communicates regarding their place in the social hierarchy. While this increased emphasis on identity and being "cool" means that adolescents may be more tempted to engage in detrimental health behaviors (like smoking and drinking), it may also mean that an identity-signaling strategy could facilitate a very successful intervention among members of this demographic. In the case of the obesity epidemic, as adult-onset, obesity-related illnesses like diabetes and hypertension become more prevalent among teens and children, their segment of the population deserves special attention.

Consider programs in another health domain waged against smoking and drug use among American teens. Campaigns like "wreckED" and "Above the Influence" tend to use the shock value of graphic images and staggering statistics to relay the message that smoking and using drugs can be risky and dangerous. The trouble with using scare tactics to reach young people is that often they are the least likely to respond by changing their behavior. In an age bracket where rebelliousness rules and mortality is hardly salient, it is especially difficult to influence teens to abandon behaviors they view as cool or that carry consequences to which they feel immune. The impact of a health message is often lost on their demographic because information they perceive to be unnecessary or patronizing tends to go in one ear and out the other (Burns, Ruland, and Finger 2004).

However, the usually unreachable adolescent audience may be the very demographic where identity-signaling appeals could be most useful. As we have seen, food choice is sometimes influenced by a desire to convey a certain impression or adhere to social norms (Leary and Kowalski 1990; Roth et al. 2001). As research has also shown, people attend to their public image more or less actively depending on factors relating to self-monitoring (Snyder 1974). Because teens and young adults are a segment of the population that typically scores high on the self-monitoring scale, this type of identity-signaling appeal may work especially well.

DESIGNING EFFECTIVE IDENTITY-SIGNALING CAMPAIGNS

One important consideration when designing an identity-relevant health campaign is what social identity should be used as the relevant out-group. As shown in the eating establishment study, people who are most concerned about how others view them are also the most likely to avoid engaging in behaviors that might signal that they are members of an undesired out-group. However, people who do not mind signaling the identity linked to the unhealthy behavior may be unaffected (and could conceivably show perverse effects). Thus, policy-makers should try to select out-groups for which most members of the target population hold dissociative attitudes. In order for an identity-signaling campaign to be effective, the desire to diverge from the out-group must inspire a change in behavior.

Policy-makers must also be careful about the out-group identities they select. The aim of this type of appeal is not to denigrate or marginalize the out-group chosen. An out-group should never be used to propagate negative stereotypes and it is not necessary to present out-groups in a negative light for dissociative influence to be effective. Additionally, the use of humor, when appropriate, may make any group associations central to the campaign even more memorable (Kotler and Lee 2007). By putting these ideas into practice, the studies outlined in this chapter demonstrate that the simple and lighthearted association of the consumption of junk food with groups that undergraduates had a predisposed motivation to avoid was enough to lead to a change in behavior.

The choice of out-group will also affect the credibility of the manipulation. In our studies, we found two groups that were not only avoidance groups, but also were plausible in the context of our manipulations. To find these groups, participants from the same population as the main studies were given a list containing a variety of social groups (e.g., sorority members, faculty members, graduate students, online video game players) and were asked: "For each of the groups below, how would you feel if people thought you were a member of that group?" Of the groups on the list, members of our population wanted to avoid being confused with graduate students and online gamers most strongly. In reality, some graduate students do not have very healthy eating habits and some computer gamers eat a lot of junk food, which made the associations in our manipulations reasonably credible. When selecting an out-group, if the link between the out-group and the target behavior seems tenuous, people may doubt the creditability of the message and, consequently, the campaign may be unsuccessful. Thus, policy makers must not only be socially conscious when designing a campaign of this nature, but also make sure it is believable. By employing a generally dissociative out-group like "deadbeat dads" or "tax evaders," policy-makers increase the likelihood that their campaign will have the desired effect. However, these groups may not be relevant to campaigns targeting health issues like obesity. Thus, it is also worth noting the value of "local fit" in designing identity-shifting campaigns.

By targeting audiences on a smaller, even individual level, policy-makers can tailor their campaign for maximum impact. Successfully applying an identity-signaling approach to a large-scale or national-level obesity prevention campaign would be extremely challenging because the associations with various out-groups change at the local level. The type of identity that teenagers in Missouri would want to avoid being associated with is likely quite different from one that high schoolers in south central Los Angeles would want to avoid. While we certainly cannot deny that obesity has become a national, even global concern, identity-signaling appeals can be more effective when they target a smaller audience. Finding a believable out-group for the population at large of the whole state of Mississippi, America's heaviest state, would be much more difficult than finding a relevant out-group for overweight Mississippi teens in rural schools, a far more specific and homogeneous population.

The fact that this type of campaign works best with a small target audience is not necessarily a limiting factor as eating is frequently a social behavior. In regular advertising, companies often try to reach as wide an audience as possible with their message because the belief is that consumers will not buy a product like Pepsi or Doritos unless they see an ad. In cases where behavior depends on the meaning of consumption, however, behavior is interdependent. People's decision about whether or not to engage in a behavior depends on who it is associated with, which depends in part on the other people engaging in the behavior. Thus a campaign that changes the behavior of some may have a cascading effect, ultimately influencing the behavior of many others. For example, if our obesity-relevant health campaign is intended to reach only 10 percent of a population, but it affects their behavior, some portion of the other 90 percent of this population may also change their behavior because they saw the first 10 percent doing so.

Consequently, the dynamic nature of the identity association process could actually serve to make identity-relevant health campaigns self-fulfilling. By changing the identity that a group of people associates with a negative health behavior and subsequently diminishing their likeliness to engage in that behavior, campaigns may come to affect an audience well beyond their original target group. A message does not need to reach everyone directly, as there can be indirect effects. For example, if mothers of elementary school students were successfully targeted by an identity-signaling campaign and subsequently made changes in their dietary behavior, they might also influence changes in the diet of their children by changing what they pack for lunch or prepare as an after-school snack. For campaigns that target an issue as widespread as obesity, this trickle-down process is certainly one major benefit of a campaign based on social influence. By shifting the behavior of some, we might be able to change the behavior of many. Additionally, recent research has shown that obesity is contagious to the degree that it spreads among populations and networks of people who know each other (Christakis and Fowler 2009). If obese people tend to associate with other obese people, the ability to affect a large overweight population by changing the behavior of a few overweight individuals becomes even more possible.

In addition to considering the inherent limits on the size and diversity of the target population for this type of manipulation, there is a question of temporal persistence. In our manipulations, the identity associated with junk food consumption was made salient at the point of purchase. While health manipulations have often been shown to have a measured effect on concurrent behaviors, they have proven less useful in predicting future behavior (Milne, Paschal, and Orbell 2000). However, in a field study that applied an identity-signaling strategy to the problem of underage drinking (Berger and Rand 2008), the observed change in behavior persisted more than three weeks after the manipulation materials were taken down. In this study, flyers were posted in restrooms of four all-freshmen dorms on a college campus. The avoidance group manipulation used in this study linked graduate students (out-group) to binge drinking behavior. Three weeks later, dorm members reported their recent alcohol consumption and their desire to avoid seeming like a variety of social groups, including graduate students. As predicted, undergraduates who did not want others to think they were akin to graduate students reported drinking significantly less. While it remains to be seen whether obesity-related campaigns will have the same lifespan, these results suggest that by changing the meaning of the behavior itself, shifting the identity associated with a risky health behavior can have a strong and persistent impact even when the behavior is temporally separated from the campaign material.

CONCLUSION

This chapter has focused on using identity-signaling appeals to improve public health. People of all ages attend to issues of identity when they determine how to behave, whether the question is how to act at a party or how much to eat from a buffet. While public health campaigns to date have made important strides in disseminating information to enable the American populace to make good decisions when it comes to their diet and fitness, information by itself may not solve the problem. Americans, especially young Americans, just keep getting larger and sicker.

As we have shown, it is among members of this very demographic where identity-signaling campaigns might have the greatest utility. Young people typically care a great deal about how they appear in the social world and they regularly monitor their behavior to fit a desired image. As our work demonstrates, individuals who care what their choices represent are more likely to change their behavior to diverge from an undesired out-group. While the applicability of an identity-signaling appeal is somewhat limited by the size and diversity of the target population, there is a chance that, by choosing an appropriate out-group, a campaign will indirectly affect many people beyond the original target audience.

Because of the implications for actual and widespread behavior change, policymakers who hope to mitigate identity-relevant risk behaviors like the decision to eat junk food should consider designing campaigns that link these obesity-relevant behaviors to identities that individuals at greatest risk for becoming obese do not want to signal. If this type of appeal can successfully reach at-risk populations, the question then becomes: *Should we eat junk food?* And the answer: *Not if they're doing it.*

REFERENCES

Beck, Kenneth, and Arthur Frankel. 1981. "A Conceptualization of Threat Communications and Protective Health Behavior." *Social Psychology Quarterly*, 44 (3), 204–217.

Berger, Jonah, and Chip Heath. 2007. "Where Consumers Diverge from Others: Identity Signaling and Product Domains." *Journal of Consumer Research*, 34, 121–134.

———. 2008. "Who Drives Divergence? Identity-Signaling, Outgroup Dissimilarity, and the Abandonment of Cultural Tastes." *Journal of Personality and Social Psychology*, 95 (3), 593–607.

Berger, Jonah, and Lindsay Rand. 2008. "Shifting Signals to Help Health: Using Identity-Signaling to Reduce Risky Health Behaviors." *Journal of Consumer Research*, 35, 509–518.

Blair, Steven N., and Suzanne Brodney. 1999. "Effects of Physical Inactivity and Obesity on Morbidity and Mortality: Current Evidence and Research Issues." *Medicine and Science in Sports and Exercise*, 31 (11, Supplement), S646–S662.

Burns, Arlene A., Claudia Ruland, and William Finger. 2004. "Reaching Out-of-School Youth with Reproductive Health and HIV/AIDS Information and Services." *Family Health International, Youth Issues Paper*, (4), 3–34.

Centers for Disease Control and Prevention (CDC). 2006. "State-Specific Prevalence of Obesity Among Adults—United States, 2005." *MMWR Weekly*, 55 (36), 985–988.

Chandon, Pierre, and Brian Wansink. 2007. "The Biasing Health Halos of Fast Food Restaurant Health Claims: Lower Calorie Estimates and Higher Side-Dish Consumption Intentions." *Journal of Consumer Research*, 34 (3), 301–314.

Christakis, Nicholas A., and James H. Fowler. 2009. *Connected: The Surprising Power of Our Social Networks and How They Shape Our Lives*. New York: Little, Brown.

Comuzzi, Anthony G., and David B. Allison. 1998. "The Search for Human Obesity Genes." *Science*, May 29, 1374–1377.

Englis, Basil G., and Michael R. Solomon. 1995. "To Be and Not to Be? Lifestyle Imagery, Reference Groups, and the Clustering of America." *Journal of Advertising*, 24 (Spring), 13–28.

Gibbons, Frederick X., and Meg Gerrard. 1995. "Predicting Young Adults' Health Risk Behavior." *Journal of Personality and Social Psychology*, 69, 505–517.

———. 1997. "Health Images and Their Effects on Health Behavior." In *Health, Coping and Well-Being: Perspectives from Social Comparison Theory*, ed. Bram P. Buunk and Frederick X. Gibbons, 63–94. Mahwah, NJ: Lawrence Erlbaum.

Grier, Sonya, and Carol A. Bryant. 2005. "Social Marketing in Public Health." *Annual Review of Public Health 2005*, 26, 319–339.

Kotler, Philip, and Nancy R. Lee. 2007. *Social Marketing: Influencing Behaviors for Good.* 3rd ed. Los Angeles: Sage.

Leary, Mark R., and Robin Kowalski. 1990. "Impression Management: A Literature Review and Two-Component Model." *Psychological Bulletin*, 107 (1), 34–47.

Leventhal, Howard. 1965. "Fear Communications in the Acceptance of Preventative Health Practices." *New York Academy of Medicine*, 41, 1144–1168.

———. 1970. "Findings and Theory in the Study of Fear Communications." *Advances in Experimental Social Psychology*, 5, 119–186.

Levy, Sidney J. 1959. "Symbols for Sale." *Harvard Business Review*, 33, 117–124.

Milne, Sarah, Sheeran Paschal, and Sheina Orbell. 2000. "Prediction and Intervention in Health-Related Behavior: A Meta-Analytic Review of Protection Motivation Theory." *Journal of Applied Social Psychology*, 30, 106–143.

Ogden, Cynthia L., Margaret D. Carroll, Lester R. Curtin, Margaret A. McDowell, Carolyn J. Tabak, and Katherine M. Flegal. 2006. "Prevalence of Overweight and Obesity in the United States, 1999–2004." *Journal of the American Medical Association*, 295 (13), 1549–1555.

Ouellette, Judith A., Robert Hessling, Frederick Gibbons, Monica Reis-Bergen, and Meg Gerrard. 2005. "Using Images to Increase Exercise Behavior: Prototypes Versus Possible Selves." *Personality and Social Psychology Bulletin*, 31 (5), 610–620.

Oyserman, Daphna. 2009. "Identity-based Motivation: Implications for Action-Readiness, Procedural-readiness, and Consumer Behavior." *Journal of Consumer Psychology*, 19, 250–260.

Rand, Lindsay, and Jonah Berger. 2010. "Who Do You Think I Am? Using Identity Signaling to Positively Influence Health Behaviors." Work in progress.

Rogers, Ronald W. 1983. "Cognitive and Psychological Processes in Fear Appeals and Attitude Change: A Revised Theory of Protection Motivation." In *Social Psychophysiology: A Sourcebook*, ed. John T. Cacioppo and Richard E. Petty, 153–176. New York: Guilford Press.

Roth, Deborah A., Peter C. Herman, Janet Polivy, and Patricia Pliner. 2001. "Self-Presentational Conflict in Social Eating Situations: A Normative Perspective." *Appetite*, 36, 165–171.

Snyder, Mark. 1974. "Self-Monitoring of Self-Expressive Behavior." *Journal of Personality and Social Psychology*, 30, 526–537.

Snyder, Mark, and Steve Gangestad. 1986. "On the Nature of Self-Monitoring: Matters of Assessment, Matters of Validity." *Journal of Personality and Social Psychology*, 51, 125–139.

Wechsler, Henry. 2001. *Binge Drinking on America's College Campuses: Findings from the Harvard School of Public Health College Alcohol Study*. Boston: Harvard School of Public Health.

Weinstein, Neil D. 1993. "Testing Four Competing Theories of Health-Protective Behavior." *Health Psychology*, 12 (4), 324–333.

Wernerfelt, Birger. 1990. "Advertising Content When Brand Choice Is a Signal." *Journal of Business*, 63, 91–98.

White, Kate, and Darren Dahl. 2006. "To Be or Not Be? The Influence of Dissociative Reference Groups on Consumer Preferences." *Journal of Consumer Psychology*, 16 (4), 404–414.

———. 2007. "Are All Outgroups Created Equal? Consumer Identity and Dissociative Influence." *Journal of Consumer Research*, 34 (4), 525–536.

Young, Lisa, and Marion Nestle. 2002. "The Contribution of Expanding Portion Sizes to the U.S. Obesity Epidemic." *American Journal of Public Health*, 92 (2), 246–249.

CHAPTER 12

DEVELOPING AND VALIDATING MOTIVATIONAL MESSAGE INTERVENTIONS FOR IMPROVING PRESCRIPTION DRUG ADHERENCE WITH CONSUMERS CONFRONTING CHRONIC DISEASES

Gary L. Kreps, Melinda M. Villagran, Xiaoquan Zhao,
Colleen McHorney, Christian Ledford,
Melinda Weathers, and Brian Keefe

A multimethodological multiphase applied research program was conducted to examine the unique factors that influence chronic disease patients' decisions not to follow medication prescription recommendations; the program also developed and tested evidence-based motivational messages designed to address consumer concerns about prescribed medications and encourage consumers to follow medication recommendations. Poor adherence to prescription medications is a serious and pervasive problem in the delivery of health care. The high rates of medication nonfulfillment (Gadkari and McHorney 2010) and nonpersistence (Haynes, McDonald, and Garg 2002; Osterberg and Blaschke 2005; WHO 2003) transcend time, geography, disease, sociodemographic characteristics, and health-care financing and organization. Lack of adherence with medication recommendations limits treatment effectiveness and thwarts the ability of patients to achieve their clinical goals (Bangsberg et al. 2001; Blouin et al. 2008; Breekveldt-Postma et al. 2008; DiMatteo 2004; Faught et al. 2008; Ho et al. 2008; Jackevicius, Li, and Tu 2008; Krapek et al. 2004). Concerted strategic efforts must be taken to increase patients' adherence to prescribed medication recommendations in order to improve individual and public health.

This is an especially difficult problem for obese health-care consumers, since they suffer at a disproportionately high rate from many serious chronic health problems (such as diabetes, hypertension, high cholesterol, sleep apnea, and depression) and depend upon a number of prescribed medications to manage these

233

chronic health problems. It is very important to help these obese consumers with chronic diseases to adhere to medication recommendations if they are to achieve their best health outcomes.

Suboptimal patient adherence with prescribed medications is a complex health-care problem that is influenced by a range of entrenched patient, provider, health-care system, and environmental factors (Hulka et al. 1976; Osterberg and Blaschke 2005). While no single adherence intervention strategy has been shown to work effectively with all patients, a large body of research suggests that improving patient adherence depends upon establishing a realistic assessment of patients' knowledge, understanding, and beliefs about the recommended regimen and engaging in targeted clear, sensitive, and motivating communication with patients to address their perceived impediments to adherence (Aladesanmi 2007; Haynes et al. 2002; Haynes, McKibbon, and Kanani 1996; Horne et al. 2007; McDonald, Garg, and Haynes 2002). The research program reported herein is designed to improve on past intervention strategies by developing evidence-based and theoretically grounded communication interventions to promote prescription medication adherence for patients with chronic disease.

THEORETICAL GROUNDING

Making good decisions about prescribed medications is a complex and highly equivocal health-care situation for many patients (Belcher et al. 2006; Benson and Britten 2002). Patients often need relevant information to help them address uncertainties they may have about prescription medications (Barber et al. 2004; Gardner et al. 1988; Haynes et al. 2002). Weick's model of organizing provides a useful framework for examining the questions and concerns patients have about their prescription medications (Kreps 2009; Weick 1979). Weick's model describes how cycles of communication can reduce the uncertainties of complex situations that individuals confront, empower informed decision-making about these complex situations, and establish rules for guiding future responses to similar complex situations. Strategic communication interventions can promote access to relevant information to help patients increase their understanding about the value and correct use of prescription medications, while helping to resolve concerns they may have that can serve as barriers to medication adherence (Kreps 2008).

This research program follows Weick's model by gathering data about patients' concerns about their prescription medications; using these data to guide development and implementation of evidence-based targeted communication strategies (communication cycles) to help patients address their key impediments to taking medications; and motivating these consumers to adhere to recommended prescription medication regimens. The model suggests three phases for helping patients cope with complex, equivocal problems, such as following medication recommendations. The first phase—enactment—suggests examining the unique information issues that make decisions complex for patients. The second phase—selection—suggests providing insightful information to help decision-makers address the complex issues they face. The final phase—retention—suggests developing strategies for preserving helpful information to guide future decisions. In this research program, we examined the unique information concerns that chronically ill patients encounter in making decisions about following medication recommendations (enactment). We developed and tested message strategies for helping chronically ill patients address the concerns they have about medication recommendations (selection). In future research, we plan to test interventions to provide and preserve helpful information to encourage chronically ill patients to follow medication recommendations now and in the future.

Although Weick's model is appropriate for examining differences in patient decision-making processes, this study also employed the framing postulate of prospect theory to examine how specific message content impacts adherence decisions (Tversky and Kahneman 1981). Prospect theory asserts that patients may respond differently to factually similar adherence messages based on the implied gain or loss inherent in the message. Positive and negative frames may work in conjunction with Wieck's model to create a decision framework for adherence.

This research program is also grounded in several behavior change theories, including the theory of reasoned action (Ajzen and Fishbein 1980), the health belief model (Becker 1974), and message framing theory (Keller, Lipkus, and Rimer 2003). The theory of reasoned action describes how behavioral intentions, attitudes, and social norms influence the adoption of health behaviors. The health belief model describes how the beliefs that consumers hold about a health behavior influence their adoption and maintenance of those behaviors. Message framing theory examines how messages that stress personal benefits from adopting a behavior (gain-framed messages) and messages that stress personal detriments from not adopting a behavior (loss-framed messages) influence the adoption of health behaviors. The formative research described in this chapter gathered data about the behavioral intentions, attitudes, social norms, and beliefs held by chronic disease patients who were not adhering to medication recommendations in order to assess the influences of these psychological variables on their medication behaviors. Motivational messages were developed to address the specific psychological orientations of consumers concerning their prescribed medications. In addition, the study examined whether gain framed or loss-framed messages were more effective in motivating medication adherence.

RESEARCH PHASE 1

Method

The first phase of this research program examined the uncertainties and concerns that led patients not to follow recommendations about prescription medications, identified message intervention topics for addressing these concerns, and developed, prioritized, and refined motivational messages for promoting medication adherence. In-depth personal interviews were conducted with chronically ill patients who self-reported not adhering to medication recommendations in order to understand their concerns and barriers about prescription medications. A convenience sample of thirty interview respondents was recruited from local health clinics referred to the research team by members of the Fairfax County (Virginia) Health Literacy Initiative collaborative. Respondents were screened to ensure that they had at least one major chronic health condition and all confirmed being nonadherent with medication recommendations. Interviews lasted between fifteen and forty minutes each, and the interviews were transcribed for analysis. Each interview sought to inductively explore patients' commitment to the need for medication, concerns about potential side effects and long-term safety, and ability to afford the costs of medication, hereafter referred to as "the 3Cs" of commitment, concerns, and cost (McHorney 2009).

The interviews were followed up with a series of focus groups with nonadherent patients with chronic disease to discover the key information and support they wanted to help them address their medication concerns. Four focus groups were conducted: one all-male group over fifty years of age, one all-male group under fifty years of age, one all-female group over fifty years of age, and one all-female group under fifty years of age. Each focus group included individuals who self-identified as having at least one chronic health condition. Participants were asked to discuss both barriers to adherence and potential solutions to increase adherence to medication. A male member of the research team facilitated the two men's focus groups, while a female member of the research team facilitated the two women's focus groups. All focus groups used the same interview guide.

Coding Procedures for the Interviews and Focus Groups

Using a grounded-theory approach, the modeling feature of NVivo was used for axial coding and tagging data into relevant themes (Glaser and Strauss 1967) that created an axis among the variables of interest. Axial coding results were reflexively compared via visual inspection to actual data to assess the potential operational definition of each theme. NVivo textual analysis software was used to create a graphic display of codes and subcodes within each 3C dimension. Finally, the transcripts from the interviews and focus groups were analyzed using NVivo qualitative data analysis software, and a library of draft motivational messages was crafted to address patient concerns about following prescribed medication recommendations.

Q-Sort Analysis and Panel Interview

A Q-sort analysis of the motivational messages was conducted with health and information professionals ($n = 8$) who work with chronically ill patients to assess the extent to which each message reflected the construct or theme from which it was created. The experts were leaders of the Fairfax County Health Literacy Initiative, representing major health-care delivery systems, rehabilitation centers, medical libraries, public health departments, and consumer advocacy organizations. Each expert respondent was provided with a stack of cards with a motivational message printed on each card to assess the content validity of the messages. Participants examined each message to consider the extent to which it reflected one of the 3C message types (commitment, concerns, and cost) and either a positive or negative message frame. Based upon the expert recommendations, the messages were refined to eliminate confusing or contradictory language within specific messages.

Results

Participant Characteristics

Seventeen males and thirteen females participated in the in-depth interviews; the average age of the participants was forty-six. Participants reported having a variety of chronic conditions, including high blood pressure, multiple sclerosis, hypertension, diabetes, depression, HIV, and asthma.

The focus groups were composed of twenty-eight participants (eleven women, seventeen men). Their average age was fifty-six. Chronic conditions included heart disease, high blood pressure, high cholesterol, sleep apnea, diabetes, asthma, post-traumatic stress disorder, depression, osteoarthritis, irritable bowel syndrome, Sjogren's syndrome, chronic obstructive pulmonary disease, and multiple sclerosis.

Analysis

Analysis of the interview and focus groups transcripts resulted in several interesting findings about medication adherence related to the 3Cs (see Table 12.1). First, lack of commitment about the need for and importance of the medication was the most commonly discussed reason for nonadherence, with 57 percent of participants reporting moderate or strong feelings about the need for the medication. Commitment seemed to be related to (1) the physician's communication regarding the importance of the medication; (2) lifestyle changes recommended by the physician and not met by the patient; and (3) trying different medications and/or combinations of medications that led to experienced side effects. It appears that shared decision-making and patient-centered approaches to trial and error led to lower commitment about the importance of the medication, especially when the trial and error stage was prolonged, unsuccessful in reducing symptoms, or caused greater side effects.

Concerns about side effects were dependent on (1) their impact on day-to-day

Table 12.1

Qualitative 3C Themes in Interviews

Theme 1: Commitment about the need for medicine (57 percent of participants)

Sources of strong commitment	Sources of weak commitment
Significant symptoms prior to diagnosis	Few symptoms prior to diagnosis
Reduction in symptoms after taking medication	Too much trial and error to find the appropriate medication
	Observed side effects from medication

Theme 2: Concern about side effects and long-term safety (30 percent of participants)

Sources of strong concern	Sources of weak concern
Changes in medications, such as the process of determining the right dosages and combinations of medications	Observation of side effects in other individuals, which motivated compliance
Side effects experienced as a result of missing medicine	Side effects never experienced, even during times of noncompliance
Potential interactions with existing prescriptions	Concern about dependency
Awareness of need to take vitamin supplements, but failure to follow through	

Theme 3: Cost of medicine (13 percent of interview participants)

Strong concern about cost	Weak concern about costs
Concern that dosage will increase and lead to more expense	No immediate concern; future concern related to changes in income or employment
Single prescription not a worry, but multiple prescriptions (for other conditions) create burden and worry	No immediate concern because expense is covered by health insurance
Concern about refills and purchasing flexibility that would help defray costs	

activities and (2) whether or not the participants had symptoms related to their diagnosis. Thus, there was low concern about side effects if they were tolerable and did not affect day-to-day activities. For example, concerns about the influences of medications on liver function were mentioned, but not stressed, by those patients with low concern. Low concern for side effects was triggered by symptomatic experiences. Thus, participants who had noticeable disease-related symptoms prior to diagnosis were less concerned about side effects of medication after diagnosis, as long as the medication helped resolve their existing health problems. These patients were more concerned about the reoccurrence of disease-related symptoms without long-term dependence on medication.

The cost of medication was surprisingly less important to participants than either commitment or concerns, since it is widely believed that the perceived cost of medication is a primary factor leading to poor medication adherence (Mojtabai and Olfson 2003). Specifically, cost was mentioned by only 13 percent of participants and was most often discussed in terms of future costs if medications increased in price or if the participant changed jobs and/or health insurance. Worry about the cost of medicine was not related to one particular prescription; rather, cost was an issue when participants considered changes in their income (retirement) or prescription (dosage). The cost of medication appeared to be an isolated issue unrelated to commitment and concern about side effects.

Motivational Message Drafts

Draft messages were created based upon the in-depth personal interviews and focus-group discussions. They were created through an iterative process of examining themes from the data reflecting barriers to adherence and concurrent themes reflecting potential solutions to increase adherence. Emergent categories and subcategories were further defined to ensure that each barrier or solution was addressed by at least one potential draft message. As a result, twenty-three "agnostic" messages (that covered multiple conditions and target audiences) were drafted. Because framing was mentioned by participants in the qualitative research as a potentially important issue in adherence messaging, the twenty-three messages were each further adapted to create a positive frame (illustrating potential gains that consumers would encounter from following prescribed medication recommendations) and a negative frame (illustrating potential losses that consumers would encounter from not following prescribed medication recommendations). The final message library thus included a total of forty-six messages.

The results of the Q-sort were used to confirm the content validity of the positive- and negative-frame variations of each message. The result was 100 percent agreement among the panel members about the framing of all messages. In other words, all the participants sorted all negatively framed messages into the negative-frame pile and all positively framed messages into the positive-frame pile. Based on panel feedback, slight wording changes were made to a few messages to improve the clarity and consistency of the language. For example, the word "commitment" related to taking medication was used interchangeably with the word "conviction" in the draft messages, so the wording was edited to create parallel language across the message set.

RESEARCH PHASE 2: EXPERIMENTAL TESTS OF CONSUMER RESPONSE TO MESSAGES

The second phase of the research program experimentally tested the refined motivational messages with a large sample of chronically ill patients. While the primary purpose of the Phase 2 study was to evaluate the motivational messages, a secondary purpose was to explore whether message framing (positive vs. negative) would influence message evaluation and impact.

Method

Participants

Participants in this study were recruited from the Harris Interactive Chronic Illness Panel. This online panel has over 6 million members worldwide who have opted-in and voluntarily agreed to participate in various online research studies. A short questionnaire was used to screen panel members into this study. To qualify for this study, individuals must be forty years of age or older and have one of six chronic diseases (asthma, diabetes, hyperlipidemia, hypertension, osteoporosis, or depression). Participants self-identified as medication adherers, nonfulfillers (received a new prescription in the past year and did not fill it), or nonpersisters (stopped taking a prescription medication in the past year without their doctor instructing them to do so) for one of the index diseases. In the end, 693 adherers, 914 nonpersisters, and 361 nonfulfillers participated in this study (N = 1,968). Because the tested messages were designed primarily for nonadherent patients, only nonpersisters and nonfulfillers were used for data analysis. This working sample included 1,275 individuals, who were 67.5 percent female and 90.1 percent white, with a mean age of 55.33 (SD = 9.52) and a modal income in the range from $50,000 to $74,999.

Design

This study employed a three (risk type) X three (message type) factorial design. Using the Adherence Estimator® (McHorney 2009), participants were classified into three groups based on their highest risk for nonadherence (commitment, concerns, and cost). Soft quotas were set in the recruiting process to ensure that all three risk dimensions would be adequately represented in the sample. Participants in each risk group were then randomly assigned to three message conditions: no message (control), positively framed messages, and negatively framed messages. The message library resulting from the Phase 1 study had nine messages addressing commitment, six messages addressing medication concerns, and eight messages addressing cost of prescription medications. For each message, a positive frame was created to emphasize the advantages and benefits individuals might gain by following message recommendations, and a negative frame was created to emphasize the disadvantages and losses individuals might suffer by not following message recommendations. The informational content of the pair of framed messages was otherwise identical. The study design and sample breakdown are summarized in Table 12.2.

According to this design, participants in noncontrol conditions were presented with messages appropriate to both their risk types and framing conditions. For example, a participant in the positive commitment condition would receive only messages addressing commitment issues that were positively framed. To reduce respondent burden, participants were each assigned three randomly selected mes-

Table 12.2

Phase 2 Study Design and Sample Allocation

	Control	Positive frame	Negative frame
Commitment	$n = 175$	$n = 175$	$n = 176$
Concerns	$n = 127$	$n = 124$	$n = 127$
Cost	$n = 123$	$n = 125$	$n = 123$

sages from the appropriate message set. Participants completed an evaluation instrument after receiving each of the three messages that assessed their future adherence intentions.

Measures

All measures in this study, unless otherwise noted, used a seven-point scale representing increasing order of favorable outcome. The evaluation measures were adopted from recent work on perceived argument strength in the persuasion literature (Zhao et al. in press). The measures included items assessing message quality (e.g., the statement said something about prescription medications that was convincing to me), message agreement (e.g., overall, how much do you agree or disagree with the statement?), message liking (e.g., how much do you like the statement?), and message engagement (e.g., how much did you feel interested/ inspired/informed when you were reading the statement). These items were averaged into an overall evaluation measure for each message (Cronbach's alpha range = 0.84 0.91).

A group of measures based on the integrative model of behavior prediction (Fishbein 2000) was used to assess participants' intention, attitude, subjective norm, and self-efficacy regarding adherence to future prescription medications. These measures were created following established norms in the behavioral literature (Fishbein et al. 2001). Intention was measured by asking how likely it was that the participants would take their new prescription medication for as long as their health care provider prescribed it ($M = 4.87$, $SD = 1.87$). Attitude toward taking new prescription medication as directed was measured with six semantic differentials (e.g., bad vs. good, Cronbach's alpha = 0.89, $M = 5.22$, $SD = 1.27$). Subjective norm was measured with five items asking whether important others in the participants' life would approve or disapprove of their taking new prescription medication as directed (e.g., spouse/partner, Cronbach's alpha = 0.88, $M = 5.75$, $SD = 1.23$). Self-efficacy was measured by a single item asking how confident participants were about taking new prescription medication as directed ($M = 3.64$, $SD = 2.02$).

Participants were also asked to rank order a number of sources (e.g., health-care provider, pharmacists) and channels (e.g., patient brochure, in-person conversation) through which they would like to receive the messages. These data were collected to guide eventual design of communication intervention strategies for delivering motivational messages to consumers via preferred channels that would be presented by credible sources of health information.

Analysis

Data analysis was carried out in four steps. First, we conducted a validation test of the evaluation measures used in this study. Although these measures were carefully crafted based on relevant persuasion theory and research, the extent to which they accurately captured message strength in this particular context remained a question. This question was answered by a regression analysis using message evaluations to predict intentions and cognitions about future adherence. The idea was that, if the message evaluation measures were good indicators of message strength, then participants who rated the messages they read as strong should be more likely to adhere to future prescription medications compared to those who rated the messages as weak.

Second, we calculated the average evaluation score for each motivational message. These scores were then used to rank messages in the library to inform future message selection and use. Third, we tested whether message framing mattered in motivational adherence messages. To that end, we conducted a series of analyses of variance (ANOVAs) to examine the effect of message framing on intention, attitude, subjective norm, and self-efficacy. Risk type and current adherence status were also included in the analysis as additional factors to control for their influences on the outcome variables. Finally, we ascertained participants' preferences for different message sources and channels. Ranking averages were used as the basis for ordering to determine the relative magnitude of message preferences for guiding eventual communication intervention strategies.

Results

Measurement Validation

To validate the evaluation measures, we averaged the overall evaluation scores across the three messages for each participant and used this aggregate evaluation measure to predict future adherence intention, attitude, subjective norm, and self-efficacy while controlling for gender, race, age, income, current health status, current adherence status, and current risk levels on commitment, concerns, and cost. The results of the regression analyses are summarized in Table 12.3. The aggregate evaluation measure emerged a strong and positive predictor in all regression models, and it accounted for 5 to 7 percent of the variance in the outcome measure even after extensive statistical control. These findings supported the validity of the message evaluation measures.

Table 12.3

Regression of Future Adherence Outcomes on Message Evaluation

	Intention	Attitude	Subjective norm	Self-efficacy
Block 1				
Female	−.08*	.00	−.06	−.10***
Age	.05	−.01	−.05	.01
White (vs. nonwhite)	.00	.04	.06	.04
Income	.04	−.03	.01	.08
Health status	.04	−.01	.03	.05*
Nonfulfiller (vs. nonpersister)	−.12***	−.11***	.01	−.08
Conviction risk	−.14***	−.18***	−.15***	−.09**
Concerns risk	−.16***	−.31***	−.15***	−.19***
Cost risk	−.07	.02	.00	−.25***
Block 2				
Aggregate message evaluation	.24***	.28***	.26***	.26***
Adj. R^2	.15	.32	.16	.18
ΔR^2	.05	.07	.06	.06

Note: Coefficients are standardized regressions weights. $*p < .05$, $**p < .01$, $***p < .001$.

Message Ranking

Each of the forty-six messages (twenty-three positively framed and twenty-three negatively framed) was evaluated by a sample of its target audience (e.g., commitment messages were only evaluated by patients with commitment issues; ns = 70 to 118). The average evaluation scores of the messages ranged from 3.07 to 4.46 ($M = 3.84$, $SD = .34$). The messages were then ranked based on their average evaluation scores within their respective risk categories based on the 3Cs, enabling refinement of targeted motivational message strategies.

Framing Effects

The effect of message framing on intention, attitude, subjective norm, and self-efficacy was examined via a series of ANOVAs. Framing had a significant effect on intention ($F(2, 1257) = 4.25, p = .015$), but its effect was not significant on attitude ($F(2, 1257) = 1.29, p = .276$), subjective norm ($F(2, 1257) = .25, p = .776$), and efficacy ($F(2, 1257) = 1.24, p = .291$). As is shown in Figure 12.1, both positively and negatively framed messages increased adherence intention compared to control. The negative frame showed greater impact than the positive frame, although the difference was not significant in post hoc comparisons. The same pattern largely held for the other three outcome measures, although none of the differences were significant.

Figure 12.1 **Framing Effects on Adherence Outcomes**

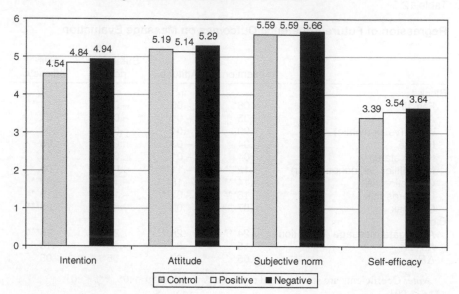

□ Control □ Positive ■ Negative

Source and Channel Preferences

Based on participants' average ranking, health care providers were clearly identified by respondents as their most preferred source for information about prescribed medications (M_{rank} = 1.69, SD = 1.27), followed by pharmacists (M_{rank} = 2.67, SD = 1.28), patient advocacy groups (M_{rank} = 3.95, SD = 1.63), government agencies (M_{rank} = 4.53, SD = 1.77), friends and family (M_{rank} = 4.81, SD = 1.67), pharmaceutical companies (M_{rank} = 5.10, SD = 1.73), and insurance companies (M_{rank} = 5.25, SD = 1.54). These data suggest the best sources for providing consumers with motivational messages about prescribed medications.

The most preferred channel for message delivery was in-person conversation (M_{rank} = 2.61, SD = 2.26), followed by patient brochure or handout (M_{rank} = 3.22, SD = 1.88), Internet website (M_{rank} = 3.73, SD = 2.00), mailing to home (M_{rank} = 4.56, SD = 2.06), email (M_{rank} = 4.64, SD = 2.09), video or DVD (M_{rank} = 5.79, SD = 1.94), telephone call (M_{rank} = 6.24, SD = 2.32), group presentation (M_{rank} = 6.34, SD = 2.04), and text message (M_{rank} = 7.87, SD = 1.57).

IMPLICATIONS

The multimethodological field research program was designed to develop and validate motivational messages and communication intervention strategies to encourage prescription medication adherence among chronically ill patients. Successful attempts to improve patient adherence depend upon establishing realistic assessments of patient knowledge and beliefs about recommended medication regimens and engaging in targeted motivating communication interventions to address impediments to adherence. The results of this research suggest that consumers have important information concerns about the appropriateness, safety, and expense of their medications that can be addressed through the provision of strategically targeted messages delivered via preferred communication channels by credible sources to provide needed information to motivate adherence with medication recommendations. This innovative research program should advance behavior-change theory and suggest specific communication strategies for improving medication adherence.

   Limitations to the quantitative testing of motivational messages include constraints in the sampling of respondents, which did not fully represent the diversity of consumers who do not adhere to medication recommendations. Follow-up intervention research should expand sample breadth and depth to test the influences of motivational messages on different health-care consumers. The delivery of messages via computer in our experimental tests did not adequately represent the situational factors that consumers experience when they are provided with and fill their medication prescriptions, limiting the ecological validity of the experimental conditions tested. Future research that builds upon this research should test the delivery of motivational messages about prescribed medication in realistic health settings, such as clinics, hospitals, pharmacies, and even in consumers' homes to test the effectiveness of communication interventions to promote medication adherence. Similarly, strategic decisions need to be made about the best sources for delivering motivational messages to consumers based on consumer preferences. It will also be important to build opportunities for feedback, interaction, and adjustment into the delivery of health information to consumers to increase the richness, specificity, appropriateness, and depth of information provided to specific consumers.

   The qualitative research suggested that perceived need for prescription medications (commitment) was the primary adherence issue (57 percent) for the fifty-eight participating patients with chronic disease, followed by concerns about side effects and the safety of prescribed medications (30 percent), and concerns about the costs of medications (13 percent). While the sample of consumers studied in this research program were patients with chronic diseases who have tremendous needs for adhering with ongoing medication recommendations, it will be important in future research to determine whether these results are similar or different for the general public of health-care consumers. These key issues were translated into draft motivational messages. Data from the experimental research showed that exposure to motivational messages (as opposed to receiving no messages) increased consumers' intention to adhere with medication recommendations in the future. The framing manipulation of the messages did not produce statistically significant effects, although mean differences across several outcome variables suggested a slight advantage for the loss-frame over the gain-frame messages, a finding found in previous message framing studies (O'Keefe and Jensen 2008). Moreover, the regression analysis validated the message evaluation measure used in this research.

The substantial associations between message evaluations and various behavioral antecedents (intention, attitude, subjective norm, and self-efficacy) also suggest that the motivational messages that are favorably received by consumers may have strong potential to motivate nonadherent chronically ill patients to adhere to future medication recommendations. Consumers exhibited preferences for receiving information about their medication prescriptions from health-care professionals. These findings and the messages developed through this research program are currently being used to guide a large-scale communication intervention to combat medical nonadherence.

A limitation to the qualitative results is that, by definition, participants in this study had to acknowledge having a chronic health condition. For this reason, patients who discounted a chronic diagnosis were not included in the study. If preliminary adherence decisions begin to occur at the moment of diagnosis, acceptance of a disease diagnosis could be enmeshed with the resulting nonadherence decision. Future research should consider whether nonacceptance of a diagnosis influences, and is influenced by, adherence judgments among nonadherent patients. Furthermore, future research should examine more fully whether consumers' concerns about prescribed medications differ significantly based upon the kinds of health-care problems they are confronting.

Follow-up intervention research using these motivational messages is needed to determine the level of influence of these messages on consumers' short-term and long-term decisions to adhere with medication recommendations. It will be important to develop strong exposure communication intervention strategies (including the strategic use of communication channels, sources, message repetition, and feedback) for delivering the motivational messages to patients in order to capture their attention, increase their understanding about the medication issues of concern to them, and reinforce the importance of their decisions to adhere with medication recommendations. To build upon this current research, future studies should evaluate the best delivery and implementation strategies for presenting motivational messages that support the information needs of nonadherent consumers and promote medication adherence.

This research program provides scaleable data for guiding strategic, evidence-based health communication interventions for improving prescription drug adherence that can be applied to a range of audiences and settings. The multimethodological field research program was designed to develop and validate motivational messages and communication intervention strategies to encourage prescription drug adherence in consumers with chronic health problems. Successful attempts to improve patient adherence depend upon establishing realistic assessments of consumer knowledge and attitudes about recommended drug regimens and engaging in targeted motivating communication interventions to address impediments to adherence. This innovative research program should advance behavior change theory and suggest specific strategies for improving medication adherence.

This research program can be applied to understanding and promoting adherence to other health behavior recommendations, such as exercise and nutrition recommendations, which are directly related to reducing obesity. Research that identifies the many complex, critical concerns influencing consumers' decisions about following exercise and nutrition recommendations can be used to design evidence-based communication interventions to address these concerns and promote behaviors that can reduce obesity.

REFERENCES

Ajzen, Icek, and Martin Fishbein. 1980. *Understanding Attitudes and Predicting Social Behavior.* Englewood Cliffs, NJ: Prentice-Hall.

Aladesanmi, Oluranti. 2007. "Medication Adherence and Physician Communication Skills." *Archives of Internal Medicine,* 167 (8), 859–860.

Ayalon, Liat, Patricia A. Arean, and Jennifer Alvidrez. 2005. "Adherence to Antidepressant Medications in Black and Latino Elderly Patients." *American Journal of Geriatric Psychiatry,* 13 (7), 572–580.

Bajcar, Jana. 2006. "Task Analysis of Patients' Medication-Taking Practice and the Role of Making Sense: A Grounded Theory Study." *Research in Social and Administrative Pharmacy,* 2 (1), 59–82.

Balkrishnan, Rajesh. 1998. "Predictors of Medication Adherence in the Elderly." *Clinical Therapeutics,* 20 (4), 764–771.

Bane, Catherine, Carmel M. Hughes, Margaret E. Cupples, and James C. McElnay. 2007. "The Journey to Concordance for Patients with Hypertension: A Qualitative Study in Primary Care." *Pharmacy World and Science,* 29 (5), 534–540.

Bangsberg, David.R., Sharon Perry, Edwin D. Charlebois, Richard A. Clark, Marjorie Roberston, Andrew R. Zolopa, and Andrew A. Moss. 2001. "Non-Adherence to Highly Active Antiretroviral Therapy Predicts Progression to AIDS." *AIDS,* 15, 1181–1183.

Barber, Nick, Jim Parsons, Sarah Clifford, Robert Darracott, and Rob Horne. 2004. "Patients' Problems with New Medication for Chronic Conditions." *Quality and Safety in Health Care,* 13 (3), 172–175.

Becker, Marshall H. 1974. "The Health Belief Model and Personal Health Behavior." *Health Education Monographs* 2, 324–473.

Belcher, Vernee N., Terri R. Fried, Joseph V. Agostini, and Mary E. Tinetti. 2006. "Views of Older Adults on Patient Participation in Medication-Related Decision Making." *Journal of General Internal Medicine,* 21 (4), 298–303.

Benson, John, and Nicky Britten. 2002. "Patients' Decisions About Whether or Not to Take Antihypertensive Drugs: Qualitative Study." *British Medical Journal,* 325 (7369), 873.

Berg, John S., James Dischler, Donald J. Wagner, John J. Raia, and Nancy Palmer-Shevlin. 1993. "Medication Compliance: A Healthcare Problem." *Annals of Pharmacotherapy,* 27 (9), S1–S24.

Blouin, Julie, Alice Dragomir, Yola Moride, Louis-Georges Ste-Marie, Julio Cesar Fernandez, and Sylvia Perreault. 2008. "Impact of Noncompliance with Alendronate and Risedronate on the Incidence of Nonvertebral Osteoporotic Fractures in Elderly Women." *British Journal of Clinical Pharmacology,* 66, 117–127.

Breekveldt-Postma, Nancy S., Fernie, Penning-van Beest, Satu J. Siiskonen, Jeroen Koerselman, Olaf H. Klungel, Heather Falvey, Gabor Vincze, and Ron M.C. Herrings. 2008. "Effect of Persistent Use of Antihypertensives on Blood Pressure Goal Attainment." *Current Medical Research and Opinion,* 24, 1025–1031.

Chang, Betty L., Gwen C. Uman, Lawrence S. Linn, John E. Ware, and Robert L. Kane.

1985. "Adherence to Medical Regimens Among Elderly Women." *Nursing Research*, 34 (1), 27–31.

Chia, Rebecca Lichun, Elizabeth A. Schlenk, and Jacqueline Dunbar-Jacob. 2006. "Effect of Personal and Cultural Beliefs on Medication Adherence in the Elderly." *Drugs and Aging*, 23 (3), 191–202.

DiMatteo, M. Robin. 1995. "Patient Adherence to Pharmacotherapy: The Importance of Effective Communication." *Formulary*, 30 (10), 596–602.

———. 2004. "Variations in Patients' Adherence to Medical Recommendations: A Quantitative Review of 50 Years of Research." *Medical Care*, 42, 200–209.

DiMatteo, M. Robin, Patrick J. Giordani, Heidi S. Lepper, and Thomas W. Croghan. 2002. "Patient Adherence and Medical Treatment Outcomes: A Meta-Analysis." *Medical Care*, 40 (9), 794–811.

Faught, Edward, Mei Sheng Duh, Jennifer R. Weiner, Annie Guerin, and Marianne C. Cunnington. 2008. "Nonadherence to Antiepileptic Drugs and Increased Mortality: Findings from the RANSOM Study." *Neurology*, 71, 1572–1578.

Fishbein, Martin. 2000. "The Role of Theory in HIV Prevention." *AIDS Care*, 12 (3), 273–278.

Fishbein, Martin, Harold C. Triandis, Frederic H. Kanfer, Marshall H. Becker, and Susan E. Middlestadt. 2001. "Factors Influencing Behavior and Behavior Change." In *Handbook of Health Psychology*, ed. Andrew S. Baum, Tracey A. Revenson, and Jerome E. Singer, 1–17. Mahwah, NJ: Lawrence Erlbaum.

Fogarty, Linda, Debra Roter, Susan Larson, Jessica Burke, Jeanne Gillespie, and Richard Levy. 2002. "Patient Adherence to HIV Medication Regimens: A Review of Published and Abstract Reports." *Patient Education and Counseling*, 46 (2), 93–108.

Gadkari, Abhijit, and Colleen McHorney. 2010. "Medication Non-Fulfillment Rates and Reasons for Non-Fulfillment: Narrative Systematic Review." *Clinical Therapeutics*, 26, 683–705.

Gardner, Marie E., Neil Rulien, William F. McGhan, and Robert A. Mead. 1988. "A Study of Patients' Perceived Importance of Medication Information Provided by Physicians in a Health Maintenance Organization." *Drug Intelligence and Clinical Pharmacy*, 22 (7–8), 596–598.

Glaser, Barney G. and Anselm L. Strauss. 1967. *The Discovery of Grounded Theory: Strategies for Qualitative Research*. Chicago: Aldine.

Haynes, R. Brian, Heather McDonald, and Amit X. Garg. 2002. "Helping Patients Follow Prescribed Treatment: Clinical Applications." *Journal of the American Medical Association*, 288, 2880–2883.

Haynes, R. Brian, Heather McDonald, Amit X. Garg, and Paul Montague. 2002. "Interventions for Helping Patients to Follow Prescriptions for Medications." *Cochrane Database System Review*, 2002 (2), CD000011.

Haynes, R. Brian, K. Ann McKibbon, and Ronak Kanani. 1996. "Systematic Review of Randomised Trials of Interventions to Assist Patients to Follow Prescriptions for Medications." *Lancet*, 348 (9024), 383–386.

Hays, Ron D., Richard L. Kravitz, Rebecca M. Mazel, Cathy Donald Sherbourne, M. Robin DiMatteo, William H. Rogers, and Sheldon Greenfield. 1994. "The Impact of Patient Adherence on Health Outcomes for Patients with Chronic Disease in the Medical Outcomes Study." *Journal of Behavioral Medicine*, 17, 347–360.

Ho, P. Michael, Chris L. Bryson, and John S. Rumsfeld. 2009. "Medication Adherence: Its Importance in Cardiovascular Outcomes." *Circulation*, 119, 3028–3035.

Ho, P. Michael, David J. Magid, Susan M. Shetterly, Kari L. Olson, Thomas M. Maddox, Pamela N. Peterson, Frederick A. Masoudi, and John S. Rumsfeld. 2008. "Medication Nonadherence Is Associated with a Broad Range of Adverse Outcomes in Patients with Coronary Artery Disease." *American Heart Journal*, 155 (4), 772–779.

Horne, Rob. 2006. "Compliance, Adherence, and Concordance: Implications for Asthma Treatment." *Chest*, 130 (1), 65S–72S.

Horne, Rob, David Price, Jen Cleland, Rui Costa, Donna Covey, Kevin Gruffy-Jones, John Haughney, Svein Hoegh Henrichsen, Alan Kaplan, Arnulf Langhammer, Anders Østrem, Mike Thomas, Thys van der Molen, J Christian Virchow, and Siân Williams. 2007. "Can Asthma Control Be Improved by Understanding the Patient's Perspective?" *BioMed Central Pulmonary Medicine*, 7, 8.

Hughes, Carmel M. 2004. "Medication Non-Adherence in the Elderly: How Big Is the Problem?" *Drugs and Aging*, 21 (12), 793–811.

Hulka, Barbara S., John C. Cassel, Lawrence L. Kupper, and James A. Burdette. 1976. "Communication, Compliance and Concordance Between Physicians and Patients with Prescribed Medications." *American Journal of Public Health*, 66 (9), 847–853.

Jackevicius, Cynthia A., Ping Li, and Jack V. Tu. 2008. "Prevalence, Predictors, and Outcomes of Primary Nonadherence After Acute Myocardial Infarction." *Circulation*, 117 (8), 1028–1036.

Kahneman, Daniel, and Amos Tversky. 1979. "Prospect Theory: An Analysis of Decision Under Risk." *Econometrica*, 47, 263–291.

Keller, Punam Anand, Isaac M. Lipkus, and Barbara K. Rimer. 2003. "Affect, Framing, and Persuasion." *Journal of Marketing Research*, 40 (1), 54–64.

Krapek, Kimberly, Kathleen King, Susan Warren, Karen G. George, Dorothy A. Caputo, Karen A. Mihelich, Elizabeth M. Holst, Michael B. Nichol, Sheng G. Shi, Kevin B. Livengood, Steve Walden, and Teresa J. Lubowski. 2004. "Medication Adherence and Associated Hemoglobin A1c in Type 2 Diabetes." *Annals of Pharmacotherapy*, 38, 1357–1362.

Kreps, Gary L. 2006. "One Size Does Not Fit All: Adapting Communication to the Needs and Literacy Levels of Individuals." *Annals of Family Medicine* (online commentary). www.annfammed.org/cgi/eletters/4/3/205.

———. 2008. "Strategic Use of Communication to Market Cancer Prevention and Control to Vulnerable Populations." *Health Marketing Quarterly*, 25 (1–2).

———. 2009. "Applying Weick's Model of Organizing to Health Care and Health Promotion: Highlighting the Central Role of Health Communication." *Patient Education and Counseling*, 74, 347–355.

Maibach, Edward W., and Roxane Parrott, eds. 1995. *Designing Health Messages: Approaches from Communication Theory and Public Health Practice*. Thousand Oaks, CA: Sage.

Martin, Leslie R., Summer L. Williams, Kelly B. Haskard, and M. Robin DiMatteo. 2005. "The Challenge of Patient Adherence." *Therapeutic Clinical Risk Management*, 1 (3), 189–199.

McDermott, Mary McGrae, Brian Schmitt, and Elisabeth Wallner. 1997. "Impact of Medication Nonadherence on Coronary Heart Disease Outcomes: A Critical Review." *Archives of Internal Medicine*, 157, 1921–1929.

McDonald, Heather P., Amit X. Garg, and R. Brian Haynes. 2002. "Interventions to Enhance Patient Adherence to Medication Prescriptions: Scientific Review." *Journal of the American Medical Association*, 288, 2868–2879.

McHorney, Colleen A. 2009. "The Adherence Estimator: A Brief, Proximal Screener for Patient Propensity to Adhere to Prescription Medications for Chronic Disease." *Current Medical Research and Opinion*, 25 (1), 215–238.

Mojtabai, Ramin, and Mark Olfson. 2003. "Medication Costs, Adherence, and Health Outcomes Among Medicare Beneficiaries." *Health Affairs*, 22 (4), 220–229.

Monohan, Patrick O., Kathleen A. Lane, Risa Hayes, Colleen A. McHorney, and David G. Marrero. 2009. "Reliability and Validity of an Instrument for Assessing Patients' Perceptions About Medications for Diabetes: The PAM-D." *Quality of Life Research*, 18 (7), 941–952.

O'Keefe, Daniel J., and Jacob D. Jensen. 2008. "Do Loss-Framed Persuasive Messages Engender Greater Message Processing than Do Gain-Framed Messages? A Meta-Analytic Review." *Communication Studies*, 39, 51–67.

Osterberg, Lars, and Terrence Blaschke. 2005. "Adherence to Medication." *New England Journal of Medicine*, 353, 487–497.

Stewart, Ronald B., and Leighton E. Cluff. 1972. "A Review of Medication Errors and Compliance in Ambulant Patients." *Clinical Pharmacology and Therapeutics*, 13 (4), 463–468.

Tversky, Amos., and Daniel Kahneman, 1981. "The Framing of Decisions and the Psychology of Choice. *Science*, 211, 453–458.

Vanelli, Mark, Marcelo Coca-Perraillon, and Amy Troxell-Dorgan. 2007. "Role of Patient Experience in Atypical Antipsychotic Adherence: A Retrospective Data Analysis." *Clinical Therapeutics*, 29, 2768–2773.

Weick, Karl. 1979. *The Social Psychology of Organizing*. Reading, MA: Addison-Wesley.

World Health Organization (WHO). 2003. *Adherence to Long-Term Therapies*. Geneva, Switzerland: World Health Organization.

Zhao, Xiaoquan, Andrew A. Strasser, Joseph N. Capella, Caryn Lerman, and Martin Fishbein. "A Measure of Perceived Argument Strength: Reliability and Validity." *Communication Methods and Measures*, in press.

PART IV

COMBATING OBESITY IN CHILDREN AND YOUNG ADULTS

CHAPTER 13

PREVENTING CHILDHOOD OBESITY BY PERSUADING MOTHERS TO BREASTFEED

Matching Appeal Type to Personality

JOHN J. SAILORS

That maintaining a healthy weight requires balancing caloric intake with caloric expenditure is well known, both to the general public and to researchers in a variety of disciplines whose interests concern obesity. Reflecting this, five of the six behaviors targeted by the U.S. Centers for Disease Control and Prevention are intended to achieve either a reduction in caloric intake or an increase in caloric expenditure (CDC 2009). But wait—five out of six? The sixth targeted behavior is breastfeeding—specifically, increasing the initiation, duration, and exclusivity of breastfeeding. It might come as a surprise to some that breastfeeding, in addition to its many other benefits to child and mother, also protects against obesity, not only in infancy, but also in childhood and adolescence and even into adulthood. Breastfeeding one's babies has an invaluable payback and its effective promotion should be a focal point in the struggle against obesity.

In this chapter, I will begin by briefly reviewing some of the research that establishes the protective benefit of breastfeeding against obesity. Next, I will discuss past and current efforts to promote breastfeeding, with an emphasis on attempts to use mass communication. Identification of certain characteristics of these efforts prompts the development of the hypothesis that is next presented and tested. Finally, the implications for future efforts at promoting breastfeeding beyond the specific context of the current research are presented.

BREASTFEEDING AND OBESITY: THE EVIDENCE

While debate on the protective effect of breastfeeding against obesity continues, the body of literature in support of its role is substantial. Three recent meta-analyses show that the preponderance of evidence supports the conclusion that breastfeeding offers protection against obesity in childhood, adolescence, and even into adulthood. These three meta-analyses will be reviewed in order of increasing selectivity of inclusion criteria employed by the authors.

Owen et al. (2005) is the least restrictive of the three meta-analyses reviewed here. The authors searched Medline and Embase databases, from 1966 and from 1980, respectively, to 2003 for articles that related breastfeeding to a measure of obesity later in life. Any definition of overweight or obesity was allowed and they included historical cohort, prospective cohort, cross-sectional, and case-control study designs. Their search initially yielded sixty-one such studies, subsequently filtered by whether the study included the unadjusted odds ratios of being over-weight or obese for formula-fed and breastfed babies. This one criterion left the researchers with twenty-eight studies, with a total sample size of 298,900. One of these studies included estimates for two different populations, bringing the total number of estimates included in the review to twenty-nine. The majority of these studies, twenty-three, involved children more than one year and less than sixteen years of age. Of the remaining studies, four included infants and two adults (defined as sixteen years of age and older).

Breastfeeding was related to lower odds of obesity in twenty-eight of these twenty-nine estimates. Owen et al. estimated a fixed-effects model including all studies, producing an odds ratio of 0.87 (95 percent confidence interval [CI]: 0.85 to 0.89). Smaller studies (with fewer than 500 subjects) showed a particularly strong protective effect of breastfeeding (odds ratio: 0.43; 95 percent CI: 0.33–0.55), but the effect was still present in what the authors termed medium-size studies (500 to 2,500 subjects; odds ratio: 0.78; 95 percent CI: 0.69–0.89) and in larger studies (with more than 2,500 subjects; odds ratio: 0.88; 95 percent CI: 0.85–0.90). There were six studies that adjusted for three major potential confounding factors: parental obesity, maternal smoking, and social class. In these six studies, controlling for confounds reduced the odds ratio from 0.86 to 0.93, but this reduced odds ratio was still significant at the .05 confidence level. Age at outcome measurement was not found to consistently affect results; across outcome age groups there was a protective effect of breastfeeding.

The second least restrictive study was by Harder et al. (2005). Studies were included that (1) used exclusively formula-fed subjects as the referent, (2) reported the duration of breastfeeding, and (3) reported the odds ratio and 95 percent CI (or the data to calculate them) of overweight associated with breastfeeding. The researchers permitted any definition of overweight or obesity and did not require an adjusted odds ratio or control for covariates. Sixteen studies met these inclusion criteria, one of which reported effects for two independent populations. Of the final seventeen estimates included, sixteen came from cohort studies, and one was from a case-control study. The total number of participants represented by these studies was 120,828.

Harder et al. applied a variety of statistical techniques to their data set, but the analyses all converged on the same finding: a dose-dependent association between longer duration of breastfeeding and decrease in risk of overweight. Specifically, they found that each month of breastfeeding reduced the risk of overweight by 4 percent, up to nine months when the effects plateau. The dose-response finding was independent of the definition of overweight and participant age at follow-up.

Finally, Arenz et al. (2004) was the most restrictive of these three meta-analyses. These researchers only included studies with adjustment for at least three of the following relevant confounding or interacting factors: birth weight, parental overweight, parental smoking, dietary factors, physical activity, and socioeconomic status. Additionally, age at the last follow-up had to be between five and eighteen years; feeding-mode had to be assessed and reported, and obesity as outcome had to be defined by body mass index (BMI) percentiles greater than or equal to specified threshold values, to allow for comparison of the studies. These criteria yielded nine studies with more than 69,000 participants to analyze.

Overall, Arenz et al. found breastfeeding to be inversely related to obesity; their analysis produced an odds ratio of 0.78 (95 percent CI: 0.71 to 0.85). This finding was not influenced by the type of study (cohort vs. cross-sectional), age at follow-up (younger than six years of age vs. six years of age and older), number of confounding factors adjusted for (fewer than seven vs. seven or more), and the threshold used in the definition of obesity (ninety-fifth percentile vs. ninety-seventh percentile). Four of eight studies that included information about the duration of breastfeeding showed a dose-response effect in both crude and adjusted odds ratios, one showed a dose-response effect only in the crude odds ratio, and the three remaining did not show a dose-response effect in either.

As stated earlier, while debate about the protective effect of breastfeeding on obesity is likely to continue, the preponderance of evidence, as seen in these three meta-analyses, supports the conclusion that breastfeeding provides a modest but relatively consistent protective benefit, not only in childhood, but also into adolescence and beyond. Furthermore, longer durations of breastfeeding are seen to increase this effect, at least through nine months. Given the truism that weight is maintained by balancing caloric intake and caloric expenditure, how does breastfeeding, which is typically ended in the West well before the end of the first year of life, combat obesity for years to come?

BREASTFEEDING AND OBESITY: POSSIBLE MECHANISMS

There are several possible mechanisms by which breastfeeding may reduce the risk of obesity (Bartok and Ventura 2009; Dewey 2003; Gillman et al. 2001), three of which will be briefly reviewed here: (1) self-regulation of energy intake, (2) early weight gain, and (3) leptin.

Regulation of Energy Intake

Ironically, it is one of the worries of a breastfeeding mother that turns out to be at least partially responsible for the protective benefit of breastfeeding against obesity.

Many, if not most or all, mothers who breastfeed experience concern at one point or another over whether their baby is getting enough milk. After all, one does not begin with a known quantity of milk in the breast, as one does with formula in the bottle, and this begs the question of how much milk the baby consumes. This worry is exasperated when the baby loses weight during the first few days back from the hospital (see relevant point in next section). However, in almost all cases, the answer is that the baby is getting exactly as much as she or he needs, judged by the output in wet and dirty diapers (La Leche League International 2006). Babies express a desire to nurse when hungry and leave the nipple when full; in other words, they learn to self-regulate and to respond to internal hunger and cues that they are full (Fisher et al. 2000).

In contrast, bottle-fed babies are often encouraged to eat beyond the point at which they feel full. Many parents define the meal as the amount that they put in the bottle, and if the child attempts to break away before emptying the bottle, the parent attempts to cajole the baby to continue to eat. Thus babies may learn that they do not have to stop eating when they are full, that it is okay and perhaps even desirable (after all, does not the parent look happy?) to eat beyond the point of being full.

Subsequently, as breastfed children age, they continue to exercise greater self-control over their eating than do their bottle-fed peers (Taveras et al. 2004). However, Taveras et al. (2006) showed that the beneficial impact of breastfeeding on obesity was only partially explained by decreased maternal feeding control, so additional mechanisms must be identified.

Early Weight Gain

Rolland-Cachera, Deheeger, and Bellisle (1999) report that an infant diet, through two years of age, that is too high in protein and too low in fat is positively related to adult obesity. They cite data indicating that the average percentage of energy from protein in the diets of one-year-old infants in five western European countries averages 16 percent, while energy from fat averages 28 percent. In contrast, human milk was described as providing only 7 percent of its energy from protein and 50 percent from fat. The higher levels of protein in formula lead to higher levels of plasma insulin and a more prolonged insulin response (Heinig et al. 1993; Lucas, Boyes, and Aynsley-Green 1981; Odeleye et al. 1997). Because higher insulin concentrations stimulate more development of fat tissue, formula-fed babies gain more weight more quickly than breastfed babies. This may itself be another causal factor related to obesity.

Singhal and Lanigan (2007) propose that the slower pattern of growth in breastfed compared to formula-fed infants, especially in the first few weeks of life (when breastfed babies tend to lose weight and formula-fed babies tend to gain weight), permanently programs a lower appetite. Rolland-Cachera, Deheeger, and Bellisle (1999) and Stettler et al. (2005) find that the very first week of life may be one of the critical periods where infant weight gain relates to adult obesity. In addition to programming a lower appetite, these effects may arise because of impact on development of certain areas of the brain, the development of adipose tissue, and by influencing the aforementioned production and concentrations of plasma insulin levels (Cottrell and Ozanne 2008; Stocker and Cawthorne 2008).

Leptin

Leptin is an an anorexigenic hormone that is found naturally in breast milk but, to date, is not in formula—but see final sentence in Palou and Picó (2009, 251). Several researchers (Miralles et al. 2006; Palou and Picó 2009; Savino et al. 2009; Singhal et al. 2002) find that leptin plays an important role in the central regulation of energy balance. The evidence is that infant body weight during the first two years may be influenced by milk leptin concentration during the first stages of lactation, with higher levels of leptin leading to lower risk of obesity. One study found that children who had the highest intake of breast milk early in life had more favorable leptin concentrations relative to their fat mass, even after controlling for confounding variables (Singhal et al. 2002).

While speculative, it seems likely that leptin is but one of many naturally occurring substances that make breast milk advantageous to the baby with respect to preventing future obesity and providing other benefits. As more of these are discovered, formula manufacturers will no doubt improve their products by making them more closely mimic human breast milk. But it would seem that they will forever be trying to catch up to nature.

PROMOTING BREASTFEEDING

Having seen that breastfeeding plays a positive role in combating obesity, one looks at breastfeeding rates in the United States and finds that, while there is some encouraging news, much remains to be done. The most recent data available suggest that although 77 percent of babies born in the United States are ever breastfed (surpassing established goals), an increase of 7 percent from 2003–2004, only about 35 percent are still breastfed at six months (McDowell, Wang, and Kennedy-Stephenson 2008). According to Li et al. (2003), less than 8 percent of U.S. babies are exclusively breastfed at six months. Effectively promoting breastfeeding should therefore remain a priority, as recognized by the CDC.

Breastfeeding is promoted through various means, including changing maternity-care practices, providing peer and professional support, making workplaces more breastfeeding-friendly, and staging education and media campaigns (Fairbank et al. 2000; Shealy et al. 2005). Obviously, the influence of physicians and hospitals is significant (Merewood et al. 2005; Thulier and Mercer 2009). As early as 1908 in Chicago and 1919 in Minneapolis, health officials demonstrated the power of home visits by public nurses to increases rates of breastfeeding (Wolf 2003).

Those interested in promoting breastfeeding have also long been interested in the power of mass media communications to achieve their purposes. Again, the earliest such efforts took place toward the beginning of the twentieth century, when the increasing popularity of bottle-feeding, coupled with the unsanitary supply of cow's milk, led to a marked rise in infant mortality. As described by Wolf (2003), these early advertising campaigns focused on the health risks to babies of not being breastfed. At the same time, public pressure resulted in cleaning up the supply of cow's milk through pasteurization and refrigeration; with cow's milk no longer unsanitary, the dramatic short-term outcome of infant death resulting from not breastfeeding was removed and pressure to promote breastfeeding abated.

Nearly a century later, as the health community identified the longer-term ill effects of not breastfeeding, including increased risk of obesity, a new mass media campaign to promote breastfeeding was planned. The campaign, developed by the U.S. Department of Health and Human Services (HHS) Office of Women's Health and the Ad Council, launched in February 2004. Conceived and developed to convince mothers that their babies faced substantial health risks if they were not breastfed, the ads originally featured photos of insulin syringes and asthma inhalers topped with rubber nipples. In spite of published data supporting the claims in the risk-based ads and in spite of the findings of focus groups that the approach was effective, the ads were toned down at the urging of formula company lobbyists. Instead of a campaign that stressed the risks of not breastfeeding, the ads eventually focused on the benefits of breastfeeding, even though the advertising company retained by HHS warned that this approach would be ineffective. The new ads featured images of dandelions, otoscopes, and ice cream, portrayed in a manner meant to be evocative of breasts, to illustrate the reduction in the likelihood of developing childhood respiratory infections, ear infections, and obesity, respectively, that one could expect from breastfeeding (Kaufman and Lee 2007).

Regardless of the relative merits of a risk-based versus benefit-based approach (see Chapter 8), the initially planned and ultimately run ad campaigns shared a single view of the consumer. They both implicitly regarded the consumer as strictly rational, basing the decision to breastfeed only on the health-related risks and rewards of doing so. This is striking because various HHS materials acknowledge that mothers are not homogeneous with regard to what might motivate a positive decision to breastfeed. For example, the CDC's publication *Segmenting Audiences to Promote Energy Balance*, which discusses the application of social marketing principles to health issues, states, "in the world of social marketing and communication, the 'general public' doesn't exist, and one approach or message does not fit all" (CDC 2009, 4). Another publication, *The CDC Guide to Breastfeeding Interventions*, contains the following: "Increasing the amount of positive images of breastfeeding to counteract advertising that markets infant formula should help to promote breastfeeding as a viable option for infant feeding. Normalizing the concept of breastfeeding makes it a more feasible choice for many women, who often see it as an unattainable ideal" (Shealy et al. 2005, 29). This same publication also notes that "social marketing campaigns are consumer driven and designed to address specific barriers identified during formative research" and that "promotion strategies should resonate with the target audience" (Shealy et al. 2005, 30). As a final example, the HHS *Blueprint for Action on Breastfeeding* calls for a media campaign that "contains images of breastfeeding as the normal way to feed infants in most places women and their infants go" (2000, 16).

Yet these government-created public service announcements (likewise the original versions) contained no positive images of breastfeeding, no images of breastfeeding as the normal way to feed infants, and were apparently targeted toward only one barrier women experience when deciding whether or not to breastfeed: lack of information. Certainly lack of accurate, detailed information about the benefits of breastfeeding (or the risks of not breastfeeding) hampers many women from choosing to breastfeed their babies. But as the CDC quote above says, one size is not likely to fit all: different women will respond strongly to different appeals. Germane to the statements about the importance of positive images of breastfeeding and portrayal of breastfeeding as the normal way to feed infants is the construct of self-monitoring (Snyder 1974, 1979, 1987).

SELF-MONITORING

Gangestad and Snyder offer a succinct summary of the self-monitoring construct:

> Some people, out of a concern for the situational appropriateness of their ex-pressive self-presentation, have come to monitor their expressive behavior and accordingly regulate their self-presentation for the sake of desired public appear-ances. Thus, the behavior of these high self-monitors may be highly responsive to social and interpersonal cues of situationally appropriate performances. By contrast, other people, those who (relatively speaking) do not engage in expressive control, have not acquired the same concern for the situational appropriateness of their expressive behavior. For these low self-monitors, expressive behaviors are not controlled by deliberate attempts to appear situationally appropriate; instead, their expressive behavior functionally reflects their own inner attitudes, emotions, and dispositions. (2000, 530–531)

One might therefore expect differences with respect to the type of appeal to which high versus low self-monitors would respond. High self-monitors have been found to be more responsive to ads focused on social imagery rather than product informa-tion; low self-monitors have been found to be more responsive to ads focused on the inherent qualities and benefits of the product advertised rather than its social status (DeBono and Packer 1991; Snyder and DeBono 1985, 1987; Shavitt, Lowrey, and Han 1992). One reason for this difference could be due to perceived self-relevance of the two types of ads to each group. DeBono and Packer (1991) found that high self-monitors classified image-oriented ads as more self-relevant than product information–oriented ads, while the opposite was true of low self-monitors.

In addition to high and low self-monitors differing in how self-relevant they perceive image- and information-oriented ads is the finding that high and low self-monitors hold product attitudes that serve different functional purposes. For products that can serve multiple attitudinal functions—for example, a pair of sunglasses that might be viewed as a fashion accessory or more narrowly construed according to its functional characteristics—the product attitudes of high-self monitors have been found to serve a social identity function (Smith, Bruner, and White 1956), helping them to mediate relationships with other people and to gain social acceptance. In contrast, the product attitudes of low-self monitors tend to serve a utilitarian function (Katz 1960), helping them to maximize the rewards and minimize the punishments obtained from products in their environment.

Such findings can be readily placed within the context of the theory of reasoned action (Ajzen and Fishbein 1980), where behavior is ultimately traced back to the influence of attitudes and social norms. The intentions and ultimately the behavior of high self-monitors are particularly guided by the social norms component, while low self-monitors are mostly guided by their own attitudes (Ajzen, Timko, and White 1982; Fazio 1990).

This suggests that high self-monitors are always on the lookout for information to help them learn how they should adjust their own behavior to fit a given situation, and therefore they find image ads relevant and informative; low self-monitors seek information that will help them obtain the benefits and functionality of objects in their environment—in other words, information that will help them reassess and update their attitudes, if need be—and therefore they find ads containing product quality information relevant and informative (DeBono 1987; DeBono and Harnish 1988; Gangestad and Snyder 2000; Shavitt, Lowrey, and Han 1992; Ziegler, Dobre, and Diehl 2007).

STUDY

The types of persuasive appeals made in the 2004 public service announcements (and in their original versions) would seem most suited to low self-monitors: those who would take in the benefit information and incorporate it into their internal attitudes. High self-monitors, looking for some clue as to the social acceptability of breastfeeding, would be less likely to have been influenced by the ads. To more formally test the interactive effect on persuasion of self-monitoring and ad type, a series of mock print ads was created and tested. Differences between ads constituted a manipulation of appeal type while self-monitoring was measured and participants were assigned to condition based on a median split of scores.

Materials

A total of eight mock print ads were created. Four were targeted toward low self-monitors and featured familiar information about the health benefits to mother and baby from breastfeeding, while the other four targeted high self-monitors and were designed to convey the impression that breastfeeding is socially desirable. In each set, three of the

Figure 13.1   **Low Self-Monitoring, Health Benefit Ad No. 1**

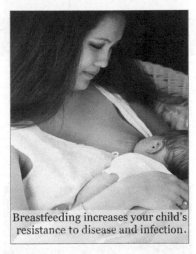

Breastfeeding increases your child's
resistance to disease and infection.

ads were predominantly graphic, and one was all text. In the low self-monitoring health benefit ads, the graphics depicted only a mother nursing her baby alone. In the high self-monitoring ads, one social image ad depicted a nursing mother surrounded by approving onlookers giving her a thumbs-up, another ad featured popular celebrity moms who had chosen to breastfeed their babies, and the third featured a collage of women breastfeeding their babies, to create a sense of popularity. The two text ads contained approximately the same amount of information across condition, but, of course, varied in that one reiterated health benefits and one conveyed facts relating to the social desirability of breastfeeding. Figure 13.1 exemplifies the graphic health benefit/rational ads, intended to appeal to low self-monitors, and Figure 13.2 exemplifies the graphic social imagery ads, intended to appeal to high self-monitors.

Participants

Because the hypotheses focused on the persuasive appeal of different types of ads to high and low self-monitors and not behavior, women actually facing the decision of whether or not to breastfeed were not required. However, for purposes of generalizability, participants from the same general population were deemed desirable. From the population of women of childbearing age attending classes at a Midwestern university, seventy-six women between the ages of nineteen and thirty-five were recruited in exchange for partial class credit.

Procedure

The study was conducted via the Internet, with participants located in a central location. Participants had volunteered for what was described to them as a survey

Figure 13.2   **High Self-Monitoring, Social Image Ad No. 1**

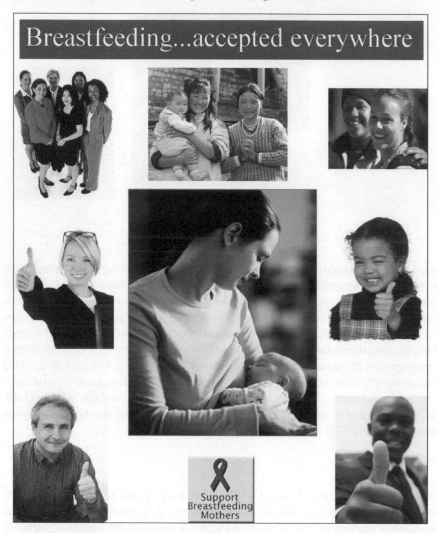

about marketing toward women. Consistent with this guise they began the session by filling out a questionnaire identifying their attitudes toward various consumer brands and various social and behavioral issues, such as equal pay for equal work, Title 9 (providing increased participation opportunities for women in collegiate sports), mandatory maternity and family medical leave, and breastfeeding. Responses were collected on a six-point scale that ranged from "very negative" to "very positive." Next, participants filled out the twelve-item O'Cass (2000) variation of the self-monitoring scale. This version differs from the Lennox and Wolfe (1984) revised self-monitoring scale in that it drops one item that had poor fit in O'Cass's confirmatory factor analysis. The participants responded to the twelve items using a six-point scale that ranged from "strongly disagree" to "strongly agree."

Participants were next randomly assigned by the survey software to either the health benefits/rational or the social desirability appeal condition. Across both conditions participants saw the following instructions accompanying each ad:

> Please click on the ONE area of the flier that makes the most impact on you.
> A cross-hair will appear where you click but that is the only change you will see.
> If you click an area and then change your mind, or accidentally click on more than one area, that's OK, as long as the LAST place you click on before leaving this screen is the area that is of MOST interest to you.

There were no hypotheses related to where in each ad participants would click; this merely served as a focusing instruction to help ensure that they actually attended to each ad. However, reaction times for clicking past each ad were recorded.

Postexposure attitudes toward breastfeeding were assessed via three questions. First was "What is your attitude toward breastfeeding?" responded to on a six-point scale ranging from "strongly negative" to "strongly positive." Second was "If you were to become a mother, how likely would you be to choose to breastfeed your baby?" responded to on a six-point scale ranging from "very unlikely" to "very likely." Next participants reacted to the statement "Breastfeeding is good" via a six-point scale ranging from "strongly disagree" to "strongly agree." Lastly, participants were asked if they were breastfed as a baby and whether or not they, siblings, or other close family or friends were mothers themselves. Following these questions they were debriefed and dismissed.

Results

The first step in the analysis required assigning participants to a self-monitoring condition. As this was a measured rather than manipulated variable, assignment to condition was achieved by calculating self-monitoring scores for all participants and performing a median split. While O'Cass (2000) found that a second-order factor model with two first-order factors fit the data better than did a single factor model, Cronbach's alpha for this data across the twelve items was 0.82; thus, for the present purposes, treating the items as arising from a single factor was deemed sufficient.

With a possible range from 12 to 72, the summed self-monitoring items in the present data ranged from 45 to 67 with a median of 54, indicating that the participants were generally high on self-monitoring. Participants with scores less than or equal to 54 were classified as low self-monitors, and participants with scores greater than 54 were classified as high self-monitors.

With participants randomly assigned to appeal type condition and classified into self-monitoring condition, the next step was to examine the postexposure attitudinal questions. These also correlated quite highly with each other, with a Cronbach's alpha of 0.87; thus, for analysis purposes, these items were averaged to create a single attitude measure.

This attitude measure was then analyzed via an ANOVA. It should be noted that the model was run both without covariates and with covariates; the covariates were initial attitudes toward breastfeeding, self-reported status as having been breastfed, and siblings, other close family, and friends being mothers (none of the participants themselves was a mother). Unless otherwise noted, the results did not change with the inclusion of covariates, so for simplicity's sake results discussed here will be from the model without covariates unless specified.

Neither main effect in the two-way ANOVA on attitudes was significant, but there was a significant appeal type X self-monitoring interaction, $F(1,72) = 9.45$, $p < .005$. As seen in Figure 13.3, attitudes toward breastfeeding within the health benefit/rational condition were more positive for low versus high self-monitors, $M = 5.6$ and $M = 5.1$, respectively, $F(1,72) = 5.91$, $p < .05$. In contrast, within the social imagery condition, attitudes toward breastfeeding were marginally more positive for high versus low self-monitors, $M = 5.6$ and $M = 5.2$, respectively, $F(1,72) = 3.68$, $p = .06$; this contrast was significant when the covariates were included in the model, $F(1,72) = 11.3$, $p < .01$. Thus the attitude data generally support the hypothesis that the type of appeal traditionally used, rationally stressing the health benefits of breastfeeding, works better for low self-monitors than for high self-monitors, with the reverse being supported for ads that feature positive social images of breastfeeding.

Additional support may be gleaned by examining the time spent by participants looking at the ads. Because the rational ads were hypothesized to be more appealing to low self-monitors, the expectation would be that they would spend more time with them. Conversely, because high self-monitors would find the social imagery appeal more appealing, they should spend more time with them. To examine these expectations, response times across the four ads that each participant saw were averaged and this average score was subjected to an ANOVA. There was a main effect of appeal type such that participants in the social imagery condition spent more time viewing their ads than did participants in the health benefits/rational condition, $M = 25.8$ seconds and $M = 21.8$ seconds, respectively, $F(1,72) = 4.52$, $p < .05$. However, this finding was qualified by a significant appeal type X self-monitoring interaction, $F (1,72) = 11.46$, $p < .001$. Low self-monitoring participants in the health benefit/rational condition did not spend significantly more time on the ads than did their high self-monitoring peers, though directionally that was the case, $M = 23.0$ seconds versus $M = 19.8$ seconds, respectively. However, as seen in Figure 13.4, high self-monitoring participants in the social imagery condition did spend significantly more time viewing their ads than did their low self-monitoring counterparts, $M = 30.0$ and $M = 23.8$, respectively, $F(1,72) = 10.75$, $p < .01$.

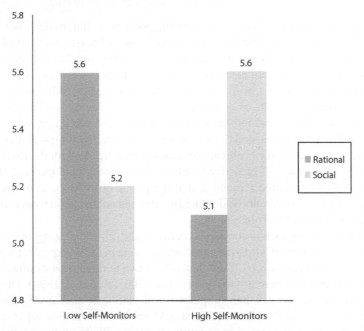

Figure 13.3 **Attitudes Toward Breastfeeding**

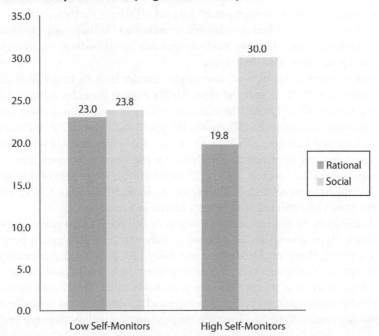

Figure 13.4 **Response Time (Log Transformed)**

DISCUSSION

The small study presented here illustrates the point made but, to date, not implemented by the CDC regarding the targeted marketing of breastfeeding, in this case
based on a specific personality characteristic, self-monitoring. This illustration has
several "close-in" implications as well as others that are broader in scope.

First, and most obvious, is that not all mothers will be persuaded to breastfeed
by communications that focus on the risks or rewards of breastfeeding. Although
this conclusion may sound too harsh, the data presented here suggest that some
women will be more persuaded by how they believe breastfeeding will make them
appear to others than by the health implications of breastfeeding for themselves and
their babies. Advocates of breastfeeding to combat obesity (and the host of other
benefits it accrues) should remember that the public needs to be communicated
with based on the public's motivations and desires and not based on what is deemed
important by the health professional.

Second, one of the factors considered in this study, self-monitoring, has implications for some current efforts to promote breastfeeding in the workplace. Data show
that breastfeeding rates drop off dramatically at two to three months after birth, a
time when many women return to work (Li et al. 2005; Roe et al. 1999). Therefore,
support for breastfeeding in the workplace is crucial (Shealy et al. 2005). However,
the sensitivities of high self-monitors should be considered. For these women,
anything that draws unwanted or negative attention to them will make them less
likely to continue to breastfeed upon returning to work. Even using language such
as "accommodation in the workplace" may set off alarms for these women. Before
high self-monitors will feel comfortable standing up for their rights to breastfeed
in the workplace, they must be made to feel that breastfeeding contributes to the
positive social image that they desire.

From a practical standpoint, one might wonder how to target high and low
self-monitors with the correct ad type. Media context provides a likely solution.
Among print media, high self-monitors are likely to read fashion magazines and
those focused on celebrities (Muzinich, Pecotich, and Putrevu 2003; Phau and Lo
2004). Low self-monitors might be more effectively reached via magazines that
focus on news and information. Similarly, for television advertisements, channel
will have some likely correlation to self-monitoring; it seems reasonable to expect
that E! will have more high self-monitors in its audience than CNN, while the
reverse would be expected with respect to low self-monitors.

Alternatively, recent research has begun to explore how to prime the desired
personality type among an ad's viewers, rather than target certain personality
types a priori. Wheeler, DeMarree, and Petty (2008) primed personality traits
(extroversion or introversion) prior to exposing study participants to an ad that
was varied in terms of its appeal to the personality traits. The results indicate that
a match between a primed personality type and a subsequent ad appeal enhanced
the persuasiveness of the ad. However, the priming manipulations employed in this

research seem ill-suited for use outside an experimentally controlled setting; that difficulty notwithstanding, Wheeler, DeMarree, and Petty indicate that priming of personality traits such as self-monitoring is possible.

A third route would be to create and run both types of ads and allow individuals to self-select which type they attend to. The risk here would be that viewing a mismatched ad (e.g., a low self-monitor seeing a social image ad) would have a negative effect on the viewer's attitudes. Certainly this risk should be guarded against, but the data presented here do not suggest it to be likely. Even when participants saw an ad that was a mismatch with respect to the level of self-monitoring the participants engaged in, participant attitudes were, on average, above five on a six-point scale. Taken outside of an experimental setting, where attention is less focused, it seems likely that people would simply ignore ads that were not targeted to their self-monitoring profile.

More broadly, self-monitoring is but one of many personality factors that might be useful for health advocates to consider when designing ads to promote breastfeeding. Indeed, marketing and communications researchers, including several contributors to this volume, have developed an abundance of knowledge that should be considered. For example, identity signaling (see Chapter 11) is a concept somewhat related to self-monitoring in that signaling is obviously a priority of high self-monitors; much more could be done to position breastfeeding as signaling one's identity, not just a generically positive identity, but some important identity to which the mother already belongs. Alternatively, undesirable out-groups could be used to cast a negative light on not breastfeeding (see Chapter 7).

Another example is temporal framing, which offers some interesting possibilities (see Chapter 3). Current guidelines call for babies to be breastfed for at least six months. For some mothers this might seem too long a time horizon; for these individuals, ads that suggest continuing breastfeeding for another day or week might frame the often-challenging task in a more manageable light.

CONCLUSION

Weight gain and obesity result from caloric intake exceeding caloric expenditure. Reducing weight requires that caloric expenditure exceeds caloric intake. However, as increasing numbers of people in the United States and around the world can attest, this simple truth can be exceedingly difficult to put into practice. Human nature being what it is, many people thus fall easy prey to weight loss fads and gimmicks. The truth is that nature provided its own gimmick to help people maintain a healthy weight. But there is a catch. It must occur during the first months of life and babies cannot do it themselves; it must be provided for them. Breastfeeding is nature's gimmick for lowering the risk of obesity as well as providing a variety of other health-related benefits.

June 2009 marked the twenty-fifth anniversary of the U.S. Surgeon General's Workshop on Breastfeeding and Human Lactation. Despite progress in many areas, more remains to be done. Initiation rates have met set goals, but duration and exclusivity rates are not what they should be. No mother should be made to feel guilty if she chooses not to breastfeed, but the societal benefits, including reduced risk of obesity, of reestablishing breastfeeding as the norm are too great not to do everything in our power to promote it.

Hopefully this chapter will serve to educate readers on the benefits of breast-feeding with respect to protection from obesity throughout life. In addition, it was intended to stimulate new thinking about how to promote breastfeeding beyond simply stating its benefits. Marketing and communications researchers and professionals have much to offer in this and other public health battles.

ACKNOWLEDGMENTS

With gratitude to Susan Sailors for helping to inspire this research through her passion for the topic and for helping to obtain the previously used breastfeeding promotional materials, and to Julie Kawecki and Luke Cahill, then MBA students at the University of St. Thomas Opus College of Business, for helping to create the stimuli used in this study.

REFERENCES

Ajzen, Icek, and Martin Fishbein. 1980. *Understanding Attitudes and Predicting Social Behavior*. Englewood Cliffs, NJ: Prentice-Hall.

Ajzen, Icek, Christine Timko, and John B. White. 1982. "Self-Monitoring and the Attitude-Behavior Relation." *Journal of Personality and Social Psychology*, 42 (3), 426–435.

Arenz, Stephan, Regina Ruckerl, Berthold Koletzko, and Rudiger von Kries. 2004. "Breast-Feeding and Childhood Obesity: A Systematic Review." *International Journal of Obesity Related Metabolic Disorders*, 28, 1247–1256.

Bartok, Cynthia J., and Alison K. Ventura. 2009. "Mechanisms Underlying the Association Between Breastfeeding and Obesity." *International Journal of Pediatric Obesity*, 4 (4), 196–204.

Centers for Disease Control and Prevention (CDC). 2000. "Segmenting Audiences to Promote Energy Balance." www.cdc.gov/nccdphp/DNPAO/socialmarketing/pdf/audience_segmentation.pdf.

———. 2009. "Overweight and Obesity: State-Based Programs." www.cdc.gov/obesity/stateprograms/index.html.

Cottrell, Elizabeth C., and Susan E. Ozanne. 2008. "Early Life Programming of Obesity and Metabolic Disease." *Physiology and Behavior*, 94 (1), 17–28.

DeBono, Kenneth G. 1987. "Investigating the Social Adjustive and Value Expressive Functions of Attitudes: Implications for Persuasion Processes." *Journal of Personality and Social Psychology*, 52, 279–287.

DeBono, Kenneth G., and Richard J. Harnish. 1988. "The Role of Source Expertise and Source Attractiveness in the Processing of Persuasive Messages: A Functional Approach." *Journal of Personality and Social Psychology*, 55, 541–546.

DeBono, Kenneth G., and Michelle Packer. 1991. "The Effects of Advertising Appeal on Perceptions of Product Quality." *Personality and Social Psychology Bulletin*, 17, 194–200.

Dewey, Kathryn G. 2003. "Is Breastfeeding Protective Against Child Obesity?" *Journal of Human Lactation*, 19 (1), 9–18.

Fairbank, L., S. O'Meara, M.J. Renfrew, M. Woolridge, A.J. Sowden, and D. Lister-Sharp. 2000. "A Systematic Review to Evaluate the Effectiveness of Interventions to Promote the Initiation of Breastfeeding." *Health Technology Assessment*, 4 (25), 1–171.

Fazio, Russell H. 1990. "Multiple Processes by Which Attitudes Guide Behavior: The MODE Model as an Integrative Framework." In *Advances in Experimental Social Psychology 23*, ed. Mark P. Zanna, 72–110. San Diego: Academic Press.

Fisher, Jennifer Orlet, Leann Lipps Birch, Helen Smiciklas-Wright, and Mary Frances Picciano. 2000. "Breast-Feeding Through the First Year Predicts Maternal Control in Feeding and Subsequent Toddler Energy Intakes." *Journal of the American Dietetic Association*, 100 (6), 641–646.

Gangestad, Steven W., and Mark Snyder. 2000. "Self-Monitoring: Appraisal and Reappraisal." *Psychological Bulletin*, 126 (4), 530–555.

Gillman, Matthew W., Sheryl L. Rifas-Shiman, Carlos A. Camargo Jr., Catherine S. Berkey, A. Lindsay Frazier, Helaine R.H. Rockett, Alison E. Field, and Graham A. Colditz. 2001. "Risk of Overweight Among Adolescents Who Were Breastfed as Infants." *Journal of the American Medical Association*, 285 (19), 2461–2467.

Harder, Thomas, Renate Bergmann, Gerd Kallischnigg, and Andreas Plagemann. 2005. "Duration of Breastfeeding and Risk of Overweight: A Meta-Analysis." *American Journal of Epidemiology*, 162, 397–403.

Heinig, M. Jane, Laurie A. Nommsen, Janet M. Peerson, Bo Lonnerdal, and Kathryn G. Dewey. 1993. "Energy and Protein Intakes of Breast-Fed and Formula-Fed Infants During the First Year of Life and Their Association with Growth Velocity: The DARLING Study." *American Journal of Clinical Nutrition*, 58 (2), 152–161.

Katz, Daniel. 1960. "The Functional Approach to the Study of Attitudes." *Public Opinion Quarterly*, 24, 163–204.

Kaufman, Marc, and Christopher Lee. 2007. "HHS Toned Down Breast-Feeding Ads: Formula Industry Urged Softer Campaign." *Washington Post*, August 31.

La Leche League International. 2006. "How Can I Tell If My Baby Is Getting Enough Milk?" www.llli.org/FAQ/enough.html.

Lennox, Richard D., and Raymond N. Wolfe. 1984. "Revision of the Self-Monitoring Scale." *Journal of Personality and Social Psychology*, 46 (6), 1349–1364.

Li, Ruowei, Natalie Darling, Emmanuel Maurice, Lawrence Barker, and Laurence M. Grummer-Strawn. 2005. "Breastfeeding Rates in the United States by Characteristics of the Child, Mother, or Family: The 2002 National Immunization Survey." *Pediatrics*, 115 (1), e31–e37.

Li, Ruowei, Zhen Zhao, Ali Mokdad, Lawrence Barker, and Laurence M. Grummer-Strawn. 2003. "Prevalence of Breastfeeding in the United States: The 2001 National Immunization Survey." *Pediatrics*, 111 (5, Part 2), 1198–1201.

Lucas, Alan, Sue Boyes, and Albert Aynsley-Green. 1981. "Metabolic and Endocrine Responses to a Milk Feed in Six-Day-Old Term Infants: Differences Between Breast and Cow's Milk Formula Feeding." *Acta Paediatrica*, 70 (2), 195–200.

McDowell, Margaret A., Chia-Yih Wang, and Jocelyn Kennedy-Stephenson. 2008. "Breastfeeding in the United States: Findings from the National Health and Nutrition Examination Surveys 1999–2006." *NCHS Data Briefs*, no 5. Hyattsville, MD: National Center for Health Statistics.

Merewood, Anne, Supriya D. Mehta, Laura Beth Chamberlain, Barbara L. Philipp, and Howard Bauchner. 2005. "Breastfeeding Rates in US Baby-Friendly Hospitals: Results of a National Survey." *Pediatrics*, 116, 628–634.

Miralles, Olga, Juana Sanchez, Andreu Palou, and Catalina Picó. 2006. "A Physiological Role of Breast Milk Leptin in Body Weight Control in Developing Infants." *Obesity*, 14, 1371–1377.

Muzinich, Natalie, Anthony Pecotich, and Sanjay Putrevu. 2003. "A Model of the Antecedents and Consequents of Female Fashion Innovativeness." *Journal of Retailing and Consumer Services*, 10 (5), 297–310.

O'Cass, Aron. 2000. "A Psychometric Evaluation of a Revised Version of the Lennox and Wolfe Revised Self-Monitoring Scale." *Psychology and Marketing*, 17 (5), 397–419.

Odeleye, Olalekan E., Maximilian de Courten, David J. Pettitt, and Eric Ravussin. 1997. "Fasting Hyperinsulinemia Is a Predictor of Increased Body Weight Gain and Obesity in Pima Indian Children." *Diabetes*, 46 (8), 1341–1345.

Owen, Christopher G., Richard M. Martin, Peter H. Whincup, George Davey-Smith, Matthew W. Gillman, and Derek G. Cook. 2005. "The Effect of Breastfeeding on Mean Body Mass Index Throughout Life: A Quantitative Review of Published and Unpublished Observational Evidence." *American Journal of Clinical Nutrition*, 82 (6), 1298–1307.

Palou, Andreu, and Catalina Picó. 2009. "Leptin Intake During Lactation Prevents Obesity and Affects Food Intake and Food Preferences in Later Life." *Appetite*, 52 (1), 249–252.

Phau, Ian, and Chang-Chin Lo. 2004. "A Study of Self-Concept, Impulse Buying and Internet Purchase Intent." *Journal of Fashion Marketing and Management*, 8 (4), 399–411.

Roe, Brian, Leslie A. Whittington, Sara Beck Fein, and Mario F. Teisl. 1999. "Is There Competition Between Breast-Feeding and Maternal Employment?" *Demography*, 36 (2), 157–171.

Rolland-Cachera, Marie-Francoise, Michele Deheeger, and France Bellisle. 1999. "Increasing Prevalence of Obesity Among 18-Year-Old Males in Sweden: Evidence for Early Determinants." *Acta Paediatrica*, 88 (4), 365.

Savino, Francesco, Maria F. Fissore, Stefania A. Liguori, and Roberto Oggero. 2009. "Can Hormones Contained in Mothers' Milk Account for the Beneficial Effect of Breast-Feeding on Obesity in Children?" *Clinical Endocrinology*, 71, 757–759.

Shavitt, Sharon, Tina M. Lowrey, and Sang-Pil Han. 1992. "Attitude Functions in Advertising: The Interactive Role of Products and Self-Monitoring." *Journal of Consumer Psychology*, 1 (4), 337–364.

Shealy, Katherine R., Ruowei Li, Sandra Benton-Davis, and Laurence M. Grummer-Strawn. 2005. *The CDC Guide to Breastfeeding Interventions*. Atlanta: U.S. Department of Health and Human Services, Centers for Disease Control and Prevention. Available at www.cdc.gov/breastfeeding/pdf/breastfeeding_interventions.pdf.

Singhal, Atul, Sadaf Farooqi, Stephen O'Rahilly, Tim J. Cole, Mary Fewtrell, and Alan Lucas. 2002. "Early Nutrition and Leptin Concentrations in Later Life." *American Journal of Clinical Nutrition*, 75, 993–999.

Singhal, Atul, and Julie Lanigan. 2007. "Breastfeeding, Early Growth and Later Obesity." *Obesity Reviews*, 8, 51–54.

Smith, M. Brewster, Jerome S. Bruner, and Robert W. White. 1956. *Opinions and Personality*. New York: Wiley.

Snyder, Mark. 1974. "Self-Monitoring of Expressive Behavior." *Journal of Personality and Social Psychology,* 30, 526–537.

———. 1979. "Self-Monitoring Processes." In *Advances in Experimental Social Psychology 12*, ed. Leonard Berkowitz, 85–128. New York: Academic Press.

———. 1987. *Public Appearances/Public Realities: The Psychology of Self-Monitoring*. New York: Freeman.

Snyder, Mark, and Kenneth G. DeBono. 1985. "Appeals to Image and Claims About Quality: Understanding the Psychology of Advertising." *Journal of Personality and Social Psychology*, 49 (3), 586–597.

———. 1987. "A Functional Approach to Attitudes and Persuasion." In *Social Influence*, ed. Mark P. Zanna, James M. Olson, and C. Peter Herman, 107–128. Hillsdale, NJ: Lawrence Erlbaum.

Stettler, Nicolas, Virginia A. Stallings, Andrea B. Troxel, Jing Zhao, Rita Schinnar, Steven E. Nelson, Ekhard E. Ziegler, and Brian L. Strom. 2005. "Weight Gain in the First Week of Life and Overweight in Adulthood: A Cohort Study of European American Subjects Fed Infant Formula." *Circulation*, 111 (15), 1897–1903.

Stocker, Claire J., and Michael A. Cawthorne. 2008. "The Influence of Leptin on Early Life Programming of Obesity." *Trends in Biotechnology*, 26 (10), 545–551.

Taveras, Elsie M., Sheryl L. Rifas-Shiman, Kelley S. Scanlon, Laurence M. Grummer-Strawn, Bettylou Sherry, and Matthew W. Gillman. 2006. "To What Extent Is the Protective Effect of Breastfeeding on Future Overweight Explained by Decreased Maternal Feeding Restriction?" *Pediatrics*, 118 (6), 2341–2348.

Taveras, Elsie M., Kelley S. Scanlon, Leann Birch, Sheryl L. Rifas-Shiman, Janet W. Rich-Edwards, and Matthew W. Gillman. 2004. "Association of Breastfeeding with Maternal Control of Infant Feeding at Age 1 Year." *Pediatrics*, 114 (5), e577–583.

Thulier, Diane, and Judith Mercer. 2009. "Variables Associated with Breastfeeding Duration." *Journal of Obstetric, Gynecologic, and Neonatal Nursing*, 38 (3), 259–268.

U.S. Department of Health and Human Services (HHS). 2000. *HHS Blueprint for Action on Breastfeeding.* October. www.womenshealth.gov/pub/hhs.cfm.

Wheeler, S. Christian, Kenneth G. DeMarree, and Richard E. Petty. 2008. "A Match Made in the Laboratory: Persuasion and Matches to Primed Traits and Stereotypes." *Journal of Experimental Social Psychology*, 44, 1035–1047.

Wolf, Jacqueline H. 2003. "Low Breastfeeding Rates and Public Health in the United States." *American Journal of Public Health*, 93 (12), 2000–2010.

Ziegler, Rene, Beatrice Dobre, and Michael Diehl. 2007. "Does Matching Versus Mismatching Message Content to Attitude Functions Lead to Biased Processing? The Role of Message Ambiguity." *Basic and Applied Social Psychology*, 29 (3), 269–278.

CHAPTER 14

ECOLOGICAL FACTORS AND CHILDHOOD OBESITY

A Structural Look

NANCY WONG AND MYOUNG KIM

The growth in obesity rates among American children is widely regarded as a leading public health concern. Since 1980, the prevalence of childhood obesity has tripled for both children aged six to eleven (from 6.5 percent to 18.8 percent) and adolescents aged twelve to nineteen (from 5 percent to 17.4 percent) based on the National Health and Nutrition Examination Survey (NHANES) (Ogden et al. 2006). If not addressed in a timely manner, this is a problem that will have dire consequences not only for the future health status and psychological well-being of individual children, but also for medical expenditures and welfare costs of society at large (Rippe and Aronne 1998).

There has been an increasing call for action from public health officials and policy scholars to combat this burgeoning health crisis. Segal and Gadola (2008) propose that in order to combat childhood obesity, scholars must identify and address the multiple contributing factors that have led to the current epidemic. Using Bronfenbrenner's (1986) ecological systems theory (EST), which conceptualizes that human development has to be understood within the context, or ecological niche, in which people are situated, Davison and Birch (2001) identified a multitude of factors associated with childhood obesity, roughly categorized as community and societal factors, parental factors and family characteristics, and child characteristics and behavioral risk factors. Community factors include characteristics such as neighborhood safety and school programs, parental factors include parental health status and frequency of family meals, and child characteristics include levels of physical activity and dietary patterns.

The ecological model of childhood obesity proposed by Davison and Birch (2001) provides a useful framework for incorporating and organizing both environmental and behavioral factors associated with childhood obesity (see Figure 14.1). However, the model is silent on the potential relationships among these factors on childhood obesity and how they would interact with each other. In order to gain sufficient insight for developing effective intervention programs, we must examine

Figure 14.1   **Ecological Model of Childhood Obesity**

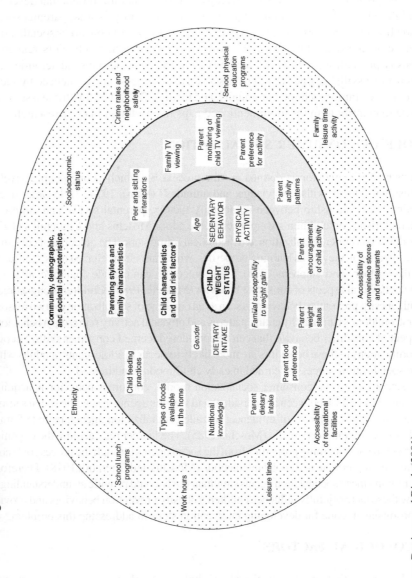

Source: Davison and Birch (2001).

the effects of these factors jointly. As Davison and Birch urge, "future research needs to move beyond bivariate relationships and develop a comprehensive model of the factors implicated in the development of childhood overweight" (2001, 160). The present study is an attempt to answer this call.

The goal of this study was to develop and test a structural model that describes childhood obesity by examining the impact of community factors, parental styles, and child characteristics jointly. By applying the theory of consumer socialization (Moschis and Churchill 1978), we postulate that children's behaviors related to obesity prevention, such as (un)healthy eating patterns and physical activities, are "consumer skills" learned through the socialization process and influenced by social agents (i.e., family, school, community, and media). By addressing these issues, we hope to contribute to the aforementioned gaps in childhood obesity research.

ROLE OF CONSUMER SOCIALIZATION

Consumer socialization is defined as "the process by which young people develop consumer-related skills, knowledge, and attitudes" (Ward, 1974, 2). In order to examine the relationship between community factors, parental styles, and children's characteristics on children's weight status, we adopt Moschis and Churchill's (1978) model of consumer socialization as a theoretical framework. The outcome of consumer socialization is viewed as learning properties, which are often referred to as "consumer skills" (Moore and Stephens 1975). These outcomes can include cognitive, affective, and behavioral aspects of consumer behavior (Moschis 1985). Children's engagement with obesity-prevention behaviors is seen as an outcome of socialization for two reasons. First, children's (un)healthy eating patterns and physical activity represent a behavioral aspect of consumer behavior that can be considered learned consumer skills. Second, modifications in these behaviors are more likely to occur in adolescents or adults when the socialization processes learned in early childhood are addressed.

According to the consumer socialization model, consumer behavior is acquired through interaction between an individual and various agents in specific social settings (Moschis 1985). Sources of influence, so-called socialization agents, include family, school, peers, and mass media (Moschis 1985). The learner may acquire the cognition and behavior of learning properties from the social agents through the process of "modeling, reinforcement, and social interaction" (Moschis and Churchill 1978). Therefore, examining these socialization agents simultaneously could provide an understanding of how these factors jointly influence children's obesity prevention behaviors and provide a promising avenue for developing intervention steps in addressing this problem.

ECOLOGICAL FACTORS

EST suggests that an ecological niche includes not only the immediate context in which a person is embedded, but also the larger environment in which the immediate context is situated. Therefore, for the child, the ecological niche includes the family and the school, which are in turn embedded in the larger social contexts of the community and society as a whole. Furthermore, characteristics unique to the child, such as gender and ethnicity, would interact with familial and community factors to influence development. Viewed from the perspective of the consumer socialization model, the ecological niche not only provides the contexts for understanding consumer behavior, but also serves as a source of influence as children acquire behavioral habits that contribute to their weight status. We now review the empirical relationships of these environmental and behavioral factors of childhood obesity in past research, which often examines a limited set of factors constrained by availability of data and, consequently, often produces inconsistent or inconclusive results.

Community and Societal Characteristics

At the broadest level, the larger community and societal characteristics such as the availability of convenience foods or the safety of the neighborhood often influence children's dietary behavior and leisure activities beyond the confines of their familial environment. In addition to the availability of time for food preparation, the type of foods parents feed children are also determined by their access (both physical and financial) to fresh foods rather than processed foods (Sturm and Datar 2005). Besides the availability of leisure time for parents, the level of children's activity is also influenced by the accessibility of recreational facilities, safe activity areas, and structure of school physical education programs.

Neighborhood Safety

Results from the Robert Wood Johnson Foundation's focus group indicate that obesity prevention programs are more effective when school changes are accompanied by environmental changes, as compared to school-based programs alone (Leviton 2008). A "built environment" where children live may play a central role in preventing childhood obesity by affecting energy expenditure as well as food consumption (Morill and Chinn 2004). The built environment's contribution to physical activity consists of safe neighborhoods, sidewalks, transportation systems, and land-use mix (Dearry 2004). In addition, food environments in the community such as healthy food availability, food marketing, and financial or tax incentives can encourage healthy food consumption.

H_1: Community factors such as safe neighborhoods where children can play outside have a positive impact on behavioral factors related to a child's weight status.

School Physical Education

School is an important avenue for exposing children to a variety of physical activities. Unfortunately, physical education is often a low priority in school budgets;

many schools no longer provide physical education during the school day (Hill et al. 2003). According to a Centers for Disease Control (CDC) report (1998), only 27.4 percent of children attended physical education class daily in 1997. This rate may be even lower today given the push for more academic programs and cancellation of recess breaks. Some evidence suggests that children who report no physical education class during school have lower physical activity in general (Sallis et al. 1988).

The lack of school physical education is particularly acute for children from impoverished backgrounds. In their study of the relationship between physical education in elementary school and children's body mass index (BMI), Datar and Sturm (2004) find a significant negative relationship between availability of physical education and the demographics of a community. For example, schools with no physical education in kindergarten have significantly fewer whites and more black children, a higher percentage of families with income under $15,000, and a lower percentage of children whose mothers attended college or have a bachelor's degree. In addition, small schools with a high percentage of minority students were also more likely to offer no physical education in kindergarten (Datar and Sturm 2004).

H_2:   The amount of physical education has a positive impact on behavioral factors related to a child's weight status.

School Vending Program

The significance of schools as a venue for preventing childhood obesity has been widely acknowledged since most children spend between six and eight hours per day in school [Institute of Medicine (IOM) 2006]. Some advocates suggest that policies dealing with childhood obesity prevention can be most readily monitored within schools (IOM 2006). U.S. schoolchildren consume a large portion (19 to 50 percent or higher) of their daily food while they are in school (Gleason and Suitor 2001). However, little research examines the relationships between the school food environment and changes in students' dietary outcomes or weight (Leviton 2008; Story, Kaphingst, and French 2006).

In general, there are two food environmental forces in schools: school meal programs partly funded by the U.S. Department of Agriculture (USDA) and "competitive foods" that compete with school lunch and breakfast. Foods sold in vending machines and à la carte offerings in the cafeteria and at snack bars, school stores, and fund-raisers are referred to as competitive foods (Trust for America's Health 2008).

Although nutrition standards exist for food available through school lunch and breakfast, competitive foods are of most concern due to the lack of nutrition standards. Story, Kaphingst, and French (2006) argue that competitive foods available in schools impede children's healthy food consumption. The authors also claim that unappetizing cafeteria food in schools encourages children's consumption of competitive foods. Despite the severity of problems caused by competitive foods, the availability of competitive foods in schools has been growing. The U.S. Department of Education reports that 94 percent of public elementary schools offer food for sale outside school lunch and breakfast (Parsad and Lewis 2006). Furthermore, nearly 40 percent of all schools have vending machines near the cafeteria and about 70 percent fail to restrict the types of food sold in vending machines (Frost and McKinney 2006).

H_3: School factors (accessibility of sweets, salty snacks, and soda pop at school) have a negative impact on behavioral factors related to a child's weight status.

Parental Factors and Family Characteristics

It is well established that children's dietary patterns are shaped within the confines of the family, and consistent similarities have been found between the eating habits of children and their parents (Brown and Ogden 2004; Bruss et al. 2005). Children's diets are affected by the types of food eaten by their parents, showing a transmission of eating-related attitudes; furthermore, dietary habits acquired in childhood persist to adulthood (Borah-Giddens and Falciglia 1993). While these studies indicate the considerable influence of parents on their child's eating habits, it is not clear how these patterns and preferences contribute to childhood obesity. Within the context of this inquiry, we are more interested in exploring the specific roles of parental health status, maternal work hours, and family meals eaten together in influencing childhood obesity.

Parental Health Status and Parents' Education

Although parents represent only one of many socialization agents (e.g., peers, schools), socialization of health-related behavior occurs within the family, with parents' beliefs, attitudes, and behaviors substantially affecting children's health behaviors (Pugliese and Tinsley 2007). With respect to genetically determined parental impact on children's weight status, several studies have examined the relationship between parents' BMI compared to their children's BMI level (Locard et al. 1992). Consistently, maternal obesity has been shown to have a positive impact on children's excessive weight. However, according to Crossman, Sullivan, and Benin (2006, 2256), the dramatic increase in the prevalence of childhood obesity "signals that biology is not the primary force behind this epidemic"; the authors emphasize that children's predisposition to so-called obesigenic physical, social, economic, and cultural environments plays a more significant role in the obesity epidemic than children's genetic and metabolic conditions. Davison, Cutting, and Birch (2003) define an obesigenic family as a family in which parents have high dietary intake and low physical activity. Studies have shown that the family environment created by parents with their own pattern of diet and physical activity has a lasting effect on children's weight status. While previous studies have focused on the association between parents' BMI and children's weight status, it is important to consider a possible impact of parents' overall health since the obesigenic family environment can be shaped by parents' health status rather than weight status. More recently, Perez-Pastor et al. (2009) find significant and stronger correlations between same-sex parent and child pairs than opposite-sex correlations.

With respect to the association between physical activity and children's weight status, past research has found that children from high socioeconomic status (SES) families engage in higher levels of physical activity (Gottlieb and Chen 1985). The higher physical activity in high SES families may be explained by more financial resources to support children's sporting activities (Davison and Birch 2001) as well as parental characteristics such as more leisure time and more knowledge of the benefits of exercise due to higher levels of education (Sobal and Stunkard 1989). Furthermore, family SES influences children's dietary patterns (Davison and Birch 2001). Wolfe and Campbell (1993) find that children from lower SES families have a less diverse diet compared to those from higher SES families. Similarly, Guillaume, Lapidus, and Lambert's (1998) study shows that fat intake is higher for children whose fathers have a low education status. Children also play outside significantly less as their parents' income and education level decrease (Burdett and Whitaker 2005).

H_4: Parental health status has a positive impact on behavioral factors related to a child's weight status.

H_5: Parents' education has a positive impact on behavioral factors related to a child's weight status.

Maternal Work Hours

The rise in the number of women working outside the home coincides with the rise in childhood weight problems. In the United States, employment rates for married women with children under six rose from 19 percent in 1960 to 60 percent in 2005 (U.S. Bureau of Census, www.bls.gov/cps/cpsaat2.pdf). There are several potential mechanisms through which children's eating patterns and level of physical activity may be affected by having parents who work outside the home. For example, childcare providers may be more likely than parents to give children food that is highly caloric and of poor nutritional value. Unsupervised children may spend a great deal of time indoors, perhaps due to their parents' safety concerns, watching television or playing video games rather than engaging in more active outdoor activities (Anderson, Butcher, and Levine 2003). In general, there is a positive correlation between maternal work intensity and the probability that the child is overweight (Anderson, Butcher, and Levine 2003). Mothers who work more intensively in the form of more hours per week over the child's life are significantly more likely to have an overweight child. Furthermore, this relationship is dominated by families of higher socioeconomic status, despite the fact that these children are the least likely to have weight problems (Anderson, Butcher, and Levine 2003).

In a longitudinal study of the relationship between maternal employment and children's weight status (at age seven, eleven, and sixteen), the proportion of overweight children generally increased with age for all employment categories (Von Hinke Kessler Scholder 2008). Furthermore, a mother's full-time work is associated with the highest proportion of overweight children at all ages and also the steepest increases over age categories. When controlling for all observed employment spells of the mother, it is a woman's full-time work during her offspring's mid-childhood years (age seven to eleven) that is positively and significantly associated with the probability that the child is overweight. Miller and Han (2008) also find significant association between maternal nonstandard shifts and child overweight, particularly for those who worked two to four years or continuously from two-parent families or those with income near the poverty line. It is possible that their income level places them out of the eligibility range for a number of public programs and the mothers are forced into nonstandard work that could interfere with family meal preparation and activity routines.

H_6: Mothers' working hours has a negative impact on behavioral factors related to a child's weight status.

Family Meals/Breakfast Together

The more often families eat together the healthier are the children's dietary habits (Gillman et al. 2000). Eating family dinner together was associated with healthful dietary intake patterns, which included consuming more fruits and vegetables, less fried food and soda; consuming food with less saturated and trans fat, lower glycemic load, more fiber and micronutrients, but there were no significant differences in red meat or snack food consumption (Gillman et al. 2000). Because eating family dinners together would lead to fewer ready-made dinners, the result is a better-quality diet.

While it would seem that the frequency of eating family meals together should positively influence children's eating behavior, findings on the relationship between family meals and childhood obesity have been inconsistent (Utter et al. 2008). For example, Taveras et al. (2005) find no association between the frequency of family meals and young adolescents' self-reported body weight. However, another longitudinal study (Gable, Chang, and Krull 2007) suggests that fewer family meals are a significant predictor of children's overweight status. These inconsistent findings may be due to the nature of the data (i.e., either cross-sectional or longitudinal), type of BMI measure (i.e., self-report or actual measurement of height and weight), or selection of confounding variables included in the model (Utter et al. 2008). Furthermore, the definition of family meals used in past studies was limited to the frequency of family dinners eaten together, without specifying whether dinners were consumed at home or in restaurants.

Past research on the impact of skipping breakfast on children's weight status has also shown mixed findings (Dialektakou and Vranas 2008). While a number of studies have documented a negative relationship between skipping breakfast and weight status (Dubois, Girard, and Kent 2006; Dwyer et al. 2001), other studies find no association (Fujiwara 2003; Resnicow 1991). Recent consumer research suggests that the strength of eating habits varies over the time of day (i.e., breakfast, lunch, and dinner) and that within-meal effects are stronger than across-meal effects (Khare and Inman 2006). Because consumers have fewer cognitive resources available to think about food choices in the morning, carryover habit is stronger at breakfast than at lunch and dinner. Breakfast foods also seem more dominated by positive nutrients and dinner foods by negative nutrients. While carryover habit highlights temporal stability in food consumption behavior, baseline habit highlights contextual stability in food consumption behavior (Khare and Inman 2006). Therefore, it seems that frequency of breakfasts eaten together should exert a negative influence on a child's weight status.

H_7:   The frequency of having breakfast together has a negative impact on behavioral factors related to a child's weight status.

Child Characteristics, Demographics, and Behavioral Risk Factors

The relationship between community and parental factors and a child's dietary patterns and weight status is also likely to differ as a function of a child's socioeconomic background, gender, and ethnicity. For example, even though food has become relatively inexpensive, the price structure of the food supply is such that the least expensive foods are those with the highest energy density. This means that people with limited discretionary incomes or unstable incomes may rely on foods with high energy density, and these foods increase the likelihood of passive overconsumption and, therefore, weight gain (Kumanyika 2008).

Children's energy needs also differ as a function of their rate of growth; also, the timing of growth spurts differs between boys and girls. Therefore, study results that combine data for boys and girls become difficult to interpret in terms of the relationship between energy intake and weight status (Davison, Cutting, and Birch 2003; Perez-Pastor et al. 2009). Finally, racial and ethnic minorities in the United States are more likely than whites to live in poverty and to be undereducated and underemployed (Kumanyika 2008). Single-mother households are more prevalent among African Americans and, to a lesser extent, Hispanics. Low birth weight is more frequent in African Americans, and teen pregnancy is more common among both blacks and Hispanics. Together, these characteristics combine to put children from such ethnic backgrounds at higher risk of obesity (Ashiabi and O'Neal 2007).

Socioeconomic Status

Research has shown that low household income in the earliest period of life had a significant association with eventual weight measures (Ashiabi and O'Neal 2007; Ziol-Guest, Duncan, and Kalil 2009). The negative relationship between income during the prenatal and birth years in relation to adult BMI is consistent with the hypothesis that fetal programming induced by early stimulants and insults increases long-term physiology and disease risks. Ashiabi and O'Neal (2007) find that poverty significantly affects children's health status; however, it is mediated by parental factors. Therefore, the impact of poverty is really an outcome of parental factors. However, these are often correlated factors. For example, being from an ethnic minority group and a low socioeconomic household often jointly influence the family environment, such as higher proportions of female-headed households, lower parental education levels, and higher rates of teen parenting.

H_8:   Family income has a positive impact on behavioral factors related to a child's weight status.

Ethnicity

Public health statistics have consistently shown a higher prevalence of overweight in ethnic minority groups, compared to whites, in this country. Fifteen percent of black boys were overweight in 1988–1994 (National Center for Health Statistics 1998), while 18.8 percent of Mexican-American boys, 17.4 percent of black girls, and 11.7 percent of white girls were overweight. Children from ethnic minority backgrounds are also more likely to be exposed to urban violence when outdoors and have less access to supervised recreational facilities, which combine to reduce their physical activity. Also, studies of the frequency and content of food advertisements have shown that television markets with a high viewership of African American children have higher than average occurrence of food ads and a higher proportion of ads for high-calorie snack foods, soft drinks, and candy in comparison to ads in predominantly white markets (Grier et al. 2007; Kumanyika 2008).

In addition to these environmental factors, there are also sociocultural factors that combine to influence child obesity. For example, parental concern about children's weight may be one element of feeding style; for example, a parent's lack of perception that a child is overweight or a perception that a normal-weight child is underweight may predispose to overfeeding. Studies have shown that African American mothers often do not accept growth charts as the basis for determining their children's weight and that having a large body size is culturally acceptable as long as the children are healthy and active, have good self-esteem, and are not teased by their peers (Kumanyika 2008). In addition, the excess of obesity among women in ethnic minority populations creates a sociocultural milieu in which obesity is normative in children's female role models. While ethnicity is likely to have a significant influence on children's weight status, it is often correlated with other factors such as education and income status. Consequently, its effect is not hypothesized here.

Gender

Although past research provides vast evidence for gender difference in physical activity, research addressing gender difference in links among environmental factors, behavioral factors, and children's weight status is scarce. Many studies find that boys are more physically active than girls (Antshel and Andermann 2000; Sallis, Prochaska, and Taylor 2000). Furthermore, this gender difference appears to increase as children grow from early childhood to adolescence (Myers et al. 1996). With respect to the gender difference in sedentary behaviors, Myers et al. (1996) report that girls spend more time watching TV than boys. As Davison and Birch (2001) point out, gender difference in the influence of TV viewing time on weight status is not clear. A study by Gortmaker et al. (1999) provides evidence that the positive relationship between TV viewing time and weight status is only significant for girls, but not for boys. Gortmaker et al.'s study is based on reduction of TV viewing time using a school-based obesity prevention program. On the other hand, girls are more responsive to the benefit of physical activity, given the right context. For example, physical education has a strong negative effect on BMI change for girls who are overweight or at risk for overweight. On the other hand, the effect of physical education for boys who are overweight or at risk for overweight is not significant (Datar and Sturm 2004). Since it is more beneficial to examine the effects of gender with respect to different ecological and behavioral factors rather than its direct effect, the effect of gender is not hypothesized here.

Dietary Intake

Studies have shown that Americans eat non-nutritious food more than ever before. On average, Americans consume about 300 calories more per day compared to the 1980s (Putnam, Allshouse, and Kantor 2002). Nielsen and Popkin (2003) find that the increased energy intake is attributable to food eaten away from home as well as increased portion size. In terms of healthy food intake, only 19 percent of adult men and 27 percent of adult women meet the recommended consumption level of five servings per day of fruits and vegetables (CDC 2004).

The increased calorie intake in adults seems to lead to increased consumption of "junk" food (i.e., food with high calories and minimal nutrition) in children as well. Over 60 percent of children consume too much fat, and less than 20 percent of children eat the recommended number of fruit and vegetable servings per day (CDC 2004). Several studies have examined a relationship between soft drink consumption and children's weight status (Nielsen and Popkin 2004). Ludwig, Peterson, and Gortmaker (2001) find that the risk of being obese increases by 50 percent due to consumption of each additional serving of soft drinks per day. Likewise, Mrdjenovic and Levitsky (2003) report that there is a significant difference in weight gain between children who drink more than twelve ounces of sweetened drinks a day and those who consume less than six ounces a day. In addition, the authors find that there is no reduction of food and other beverage (except for milk) consumption as children consume more sweetened drinks.

H_9: Behavioral factors such as frequency of healthy food consumption has a negative impact on a child's weight status.

H_{10}: Behavioral factors such as frequency of unhealthy food consumption has a positive impact on a child's weight status.

Sedentary Behavior and TV Viewing Time

Although there have been mixed findings, causal mechanisms linking children's TV viewing and weight gain can be summarized as follows. First, TV viewing decreases resting energy expenditure. While some experimental studies (Klesges, Shelton, and Klesges 1993) find lower resting energy expenditure due to TV watching, other studies (Dietz et al. 1994) fail to demonstrate a significant difference in metabolic rate between TV viewing and reading. Second, TV viewing creates a more sedentary lifestyle and reduces children's physical activity level. While some ecological studies (Andersen, Crespo, and Bartlett 1998) support the link between TV viewing time and physical activity, most studies (Neumark-Sztainer et al. 2003; Robinson 2001) report either a weak negative or no significant association between TV viewing time and physical activity level. Results from experimental research (Epstein et al. 2002) also find no impact of increased TV viewing time on reduced physical activity.

Third, mindless eating while watching TV increases energy intake because people, regardless of age, tend to forget how much they are eating when they are distracted by various types of media such as TV viewing (Wansink 2005). Physiologically speaking, this distraction leads people to ignore sensory signals of satiation received by the brain, thus making them eat more. In addition, some epidemiological and experimental studies report that schoolchildren consume about 17 to 35 percent of their total calories while watching TV (Matheson et al. 2004). Children in households that consume their family meals with the TV on report eating more red meat, pizza, snack foods, and soft drinks, and fewer fruits and vegetables (Jordan and Robinson 2008).

Lastly, exposure to food advertising during TV viewing also leads to increased energy intake. Studies have consistently shown a positive relationship between children's unhealthy food choices (i.e., foods high in calories and low in nutritional content) and increased TV viewing time (Gorn and Goldberg 1982). Researchers have also illustrated children's misperception about the health benefits of certain foods due to TV advertisements (Signorielli and Staples 1997).

H_{11}: Behavioral factors such as TV viewing time have a positive impact on a child's weight status.

Physical Activity

Adequate physical activity not only reduces the risk for many health complications, but also leads to obesity prevention (Leviton 2008). Using both experimental and quasi-experimental studies, Strong et al. (2005) show the negative relationship between physical activity and children's BMI. The percentage of body fat in overweight children and youth decreases significantly as they engage in moderately intense activity between thirty and sixty minutes per day. However, there is no change in the percentage of body fat for normal-weight children as a result of comparable physical activity.

Only about one-half of U.S. children engage in some form of vigorous physical activity despite mandated physical education programs in many states; furthermore, the level of physical activity decreases as children's age and grade in school increase (Grunbaum et al. 2002). Grunbaum et al. also find that students' daily attendance in physical education classes has declined even though enrollment in physical education has increased. This suggests that simply increasing children's enrollment in physical education does not necessarily lead to increased physical activity. In order to combat childhood obesity, there is an urgent need to better understand factors contributing to children's physical activity.

H_{12}: Behavioral factors such as amount of physical activity have a negative impact on a child's weight status.

RESULTS

Using data from the Early Childhood Longitudinal Survey-Kindergarten (ECLS-K), we estimated a multiple-indicator multiple-cause (MIMIC) model combined with a second-order confirmatory factor analysis. LISREL 8.5 (Joreskog and Sorbom 1993) is used for evaluating both measurement and structural models. The ECLS-K was conducted by the National Center for Educational Statistics to provide information on children's status and progression from kindergarten through eighth grade. Despite the longitudinal nature of the ECLS-K data, this study used only the data collected about fifth graders in 2004. We focused on the fifth-grade data because the ECLS-K started to include information on children's food consumption since fifth grade; however, the seventh-grade data are not yet available to the public (when this analysis was conducted). Among a total of 11,820 students from the fifth-grade data, our sample was limited to 9,019 students who attended public schools and provided information on BMI. About 22 percent of the children in our final sample were obese; nearly 18 percent of them were overweight. The mean age of the sample was 11.2, ranging from 9.8 to 12.9, and 51 percent were boys.

Figure 14.2   **Ecological Model of Environmental and Behavioral Factors Affecting Children's Weight Status**

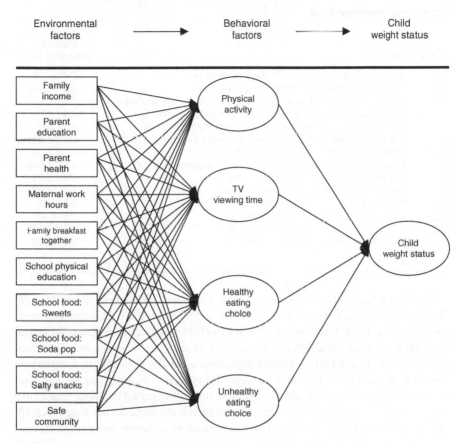

Almost 55 percent of the children were white, 12 percent were African American, 20 percent were Hispanic, and 7 percent were Asian. Average household income was approximately $54,300; 32.6 percent of parents had earned a bachelor's or higher degree.

Weight status is classified based on BMI, which is defined as weight in kilograms divided by height in meters squared (kg/m^2). With respect to children's weight status, the CDC has endorsed an age- and gender-specific BMI distribution in order to account for children's growth patterns. The CDC defines "obese" children as having a BMI above the 95th percentile given their gender and age group and classifies children as "overweight" if their BMI is between the 85th and 95th percentile. The hypothesized ecological model in Figure 14.2 shows the influence of environmental factors on the behavioral factors that directly impact children's weight status.

Table 14.1

Structural Relationships

Hypothesized path		Estimate (standard error)
H_1	Neighborhood safety → Physical activity (+)	.04* (.02)
H_2	Physical education → Physical activity (+)	.03** (.01)
H_3	School factors (selling salty snacks) → Unhealthy eating (+)	.02 (.03)
	School factors (selling sweets) → Unhealthy eating (+)	−.03 (.03)
	School factors (selling soda) → Unhealthy eating (+)	−.06 (.03)
H_4	Parental health status → Physical activity (+)	.05** (.01)
H_5	Parents' education → TV viewing time (−)	−.11** (.01)
H_6	Maternal work hours > 35 hours → TV viewing time (+)	.18** (.04)
H_7	Breakfast together → Healthy eating (+)	.02** (.01)
H_8	Family income → Physical activity (+)	.01** (.00)
H_9	Healthy eating → Weight status (−)	.02 (.02)
H_{10}	Unhealthy eating → Weight status (+)	.05* (.02)
H_{11}	TV viewing time → Weight status (+)	.06** (.01)
H_{12}	Physical activity → Weight status (−)	−.39** (.02)

$*p < .05, **p < .01.$

Results of structural relationships suggest that parents' education, parents' health, family income, and family eating breakfast together have a significant and positive impact on behavioral factors related to a child's obesity-prevention. Maternal working hours exceeding thirty-five hours per week have a negative and significant effect on behavioral factors related to a child's obesity-prevention. Contrary to expectations, school factors such as accessibility to sweets, salty snacks, and soda pop at school are not significant in predicting unhealthy eating behavior related to a child's weight status. However, frequency of physical education has a significantly positive effect on behavioral factors related to a child's obesity-prevention. Having a safe neighborhood where children can play outside, a community factor, leads to higher physical activity. Time spent watching TV has a negative and significant impact on behavioral factors in reduced physical activity and increased unhealthy food choice. Significant and negative paths are observed between weight status and a child's healthy eating and physical activity, whereas TV viewing and unhealthy eating have a significant and positive impact on a child's weight status. The results of the structural model are listed in Table 14.1.

DISCUSSION AND IMPLICATIONS

The results from this study provide empirical support for identifying the relative importance among multiple factors contributing to childhood obesity. Here are the major findings from our study: (1) When family, school, community, and media factors are considered jointly, the family factors appear to be the most significant determinants of a child's involvement with (un)healthy eating patterns and physical activities; (2) especially, maternal working hours exceeding thirty-five hours per week have a significant and direct impact on a child's weight status; (3) school factors (such as types of food in vending machines) do not have a significant impact on a child's behaviors related to obesity-prevention; and (4) media factors such as time spent viewing TV have a significant impact on a child's weight status.

The findings from our study are important in several ways. First, it might be one of the first studies to look at the relationship between childhood obesity and multiple factors, including both environmental and behavioral factors, simultaneously. In doing so, it provides some insight on inconsistent past findings based on largely bivariate relationships. Second, the relative importance of family or parental factors contributing to childhood obesity leads to a reexamination of the current intervention programs. More effective education materials and health communication tools targeting parents are urgently needed to improve children's healthy eating and increased physical activities. Third, political support that aids systematic intervention programs is needed. For example, income transfers, especially investments in early childhood, that influence children's eventual health, especially those who are the most economically disadvantaged, should have the biggest impact in addressing this problem early on.

Finally, given the four mechanisms (Robinson 2001) linking television viewing to childhood overweight (lower resting energy expenditure, displacement of physical activity, food advertising leading to greater energy intake, and eating while viewing leading to greater energy intake), the following intervention strategies may be useful: (1) eliminating televisions from children's bedrooms, (2) encouraging mindful viewing, (3) budgeting TV time, (4) turning off the TV while eating, (5) using school-based curricula to reduce children's screen time, and (6) providing training for health care professionals to counsel parents on reducing children's media use (Jordan and Robinson 2008).

While findings from this study may offer vital implications on the prevention of childhood obesity, we acknowledge several limitations of this study and offer possible directions for future research: (1) performing a longitudinal analysis of the models developed in this study, (2) including other potential environmental variables from the comprehensive model, (3) improving the measurements used in our study, and (4) incorporating qualitative insights from parents and children.

REFERENCES

Andersen, Ross E., Carlos J. Crespo, and Susan J. Bartlett. 1998. "Relationship of Physical Activity and Television Watching With Body Weight and Level of Fatness Among Children: Results From the Third National Health and Nutrition Examination Survey." *Journal of the American Medical Association*, 279 (12), 938–942.

Anderson, Patricia M., Kristin F. Butcher, and Philip B. Levine. 2003. "Maternal Employment and Overweight Children." *Journal of Health Economics*, 22 (3), 477–504.

Antshel, Kevin M., and Eric M. Andermann. 2000. "Social Influences on Sports Participation During Adolescence." *Journal of Research and Development in Education*, 33, 85–94.

Ashiabi, Godwin S., and Keri K. O'Neal. 2007. "Children's Health Status: Examining the Associations Among Income Poverty, Material Hardship, and Parental Factors." *PLoS One*, 2 (9), 1–9.

Borah-Giddens, Jacqueline, and Grace Falciglia. 1993. "A Meta-Analysis of the Relationship in Food Preferences Between Parents and Children." *Journal of Nutritional Education*, 25, 102–107.

Bronfenbrenner, Urie. 1986. "Ecology of the Family as a Context for Human Development: Research Perspectives." *Developmental Psychology*, 22, 723–742.

Brown, Rachel, and Jane Ogden. 2004. "Children's Eating Attitudes and Behavior: A Study of the Modeling and Control Theories of Parental Influence." *Health Education Research*, 19 (3), 261–271.

Bruss, Mozhdeh B., Joseph R. Morris, Linda L. Dannison, Mark Orbe, Jackie A. Quitugua, and Rosa T. Palacios. 2005. "Food, Culture, and Family: Exploring the Coordinated Management of Meaning Regarding Childhood Obesity." *Health Communication*, 18 (2), 155–175.

Burdett, H., and R. Whitaker. 2005. "A National Study of Neighborhood Safety, Outdoor Play, Television Viewing, and Obesity in Preschool Children." *Pediatrics*, 116, 657–662.

Centers for Disease Control and Prevention (CDC). 1998. "Youth Behavior Risk Surveillance—United States." *Morbidity and Mortality Weekly Report*, 47, SS-03.

———. 2004. "Trends in Intake of Energy and Macronutrients—United States, 1971-2000." *Morbidity and Mortality Weekly Report*, 53, SS-04, 80-82.

Crossman, Ashley, Deborah Anne Sullivan, and Mary Benin. 2006. "The Family Environment and American Adolescents' Risk of Obesity as Young Adults." *Social Science and Medicine*, 63, 2255–2267.

Datar, Ashlesha, and Roland Sturm. 2004. "Physical Education in Elementary School and Body Mass Index: Evidence from the Early Childhood Longitudinal Study." *American Journal of Public Health*, 94 (9), 1501–1506.

Davison, Kirsten K., and Leann L. Birch. 2001. "Childhood Overweight: A Contextual Model and Recommendations for Future Research." *Obesity Review*, 2 (3), 159–171.

Davison, Kirsten K., Tanja Cutting, and Leann L. Birch. 2003. "Parents' Activity-Related Parenting Practices Predict Girls' Physical Activity." *Medicine and Science in Sports and Exercise*, 35 (9), 1589–1595.

Dearry, Allen. 2004. "Editorial: Impacts of Our Built Environment on Public Health." *Environmental Health Perspectives*, 112 (1), A600–601.

Dialektakou, Kiranni D., and Peter B. Vranas. 2008. "Breakfast Skipping and Body Mass Index Among Adolescents in Greece: Whether an Association Exists Depends on How Breakfast Skipping Is Defined." *Journal of the American Dietetic Association*, 108, 1517–1525.

Dietz, William H., Linda G. Bandini, Julie A. Morelli, Kristen F. Peers, and Pamela L.Y.H. Ching. 1994. "Effect of Sedentary Activities on Resting Metabolic Rate." *American Journal of Clinical Nutrition*, 59 (3), 556–559.

Dubois, Lise, Manon Girard, and Monique P. Kent. 2006. "Breakfast Eating and Overweight in a Pre-School Population: Is There a Link?" *Public Health Nutrition*, 9 (4), 436–442.

Dwyer, Johanna T., Marguerite Evans, Elaine J. Stone, Henry A. Feldman, Leslie Lytle, Deanna Hoelscher, Carolyn Johnson, Michelle Zive, and Minhua Yang. 2001. "Adolescents' Eating Patterns Influence Their Nutrient Intakes." *Journal of the American Dietetic Association*, 101 (7), 798–802.

Epstein, Leonard, Rocco A. Paluch, Angela Consalvi, Kristy Riordan, and Tammy Scholl. 2002. "Effects of Manipulating Sedentary Behavior on Physical Activity and Food Intake." *Journal of Pediatrics*, 140, 334–339.

Frost, Alberta, and Patricia McKinney. 2006. "FNS School Meals . . . Do They Measure Up?" ANC06, Los Angeles. July 16. USDA Food and Nutrition Service. www.fns.usda. gov/oane/MENU/Presentations/SNA-ANC2006.pdf.

Fujiwara, Tomoko. 2003. "Skipping Breakfast Is Associated with Dysmenorrhea in Young Women in Japan." *International Journal of Food Sciences and Nutrition*, 54 (6), 505–509.

Gable, Sara, Yiting Chang, and Jennifer L. Krull. 2007. "Television Watching and Frequency of Family Meals Are Predictive of Overweight Onset and Persistence in a National Sample of School-Aged Children." *Journal of the American Dietetic Association*, 107, 53–61.

Gillman, Matthew W., Sheryl L. Rifas-Shiman, A. Lindsay Frazier, and Helaine R.H. Rockett. 2000. "Family Dinner and Diet Quality Among Older Children and Adolescents." *Archives of Family Medicine*, 9 (3), 235–240.

Gleason, Philip, and Carol Suitor. 2001. "Children's Diets in the Mid-1990s: Dietary Intake and Its Relationship with School Meal Participation." Nutrition Assistance Program Report Series, Report No. CN-01-CD1. USDA Food and Nutrition Service, January.

Gorn, Gerald, and Marvin Goldberg. 1982. "Behavioral Evidence of the Effects of Televised Food Messages on Children." *Journal of Consumer Research*, 9, 200–205.

Gortmaker, Steven L., Karen Peterson, Jean Wiecha, Arthur M. Sobol, Sujata Dixit, Mary Kay Fox, and Nan Laird. 1999. "Reducing Obesity via a School-Based Interdisciplinary Intervention Among Youth." *Archives of Pediatrics and Adolescent Medicine*, 153 (4), 409–418.

Gottlieb, Nell H., and Meei-Shia Chen. 1985. "Sociocultural Correlates of Childhood Sporting Activities: Their Implications for Heart Health." *Social Science and Medicine*, 21 (5), 533–539.

Grier, Sonya A., Janell Mensinger, Shirley H. Huang, Shiriki K. Kumanyika, and Nicolas Stettler. 2007. "Fast-Food Marketing and Children's Fast-Food Consumption: Exploring Parents' Influences in an Ethnically Diverse Sample." *Journal of Public Policy and Marketing*, 26 (2), 221–235.

Grunbaum, Jo Anne, Laura Kann, Steven A. Kinchen, Barbara Williams, James G. Ross, Richard Lowry, and Lloyd Kolbe. 2002. "Youth Risk Behavior Surveillance—United States, 2001." *Morbidity and Mortality Weekly Report*, 51 (SS-4), 1–64.

Guillaume, M., L. Lapidus, and A. Lambert. 1998. "Obesity and Nutrition in Children. The Belgium Luxembourg Child Study IV." *European Journal of Clinical Nutrition*, 52, 323–328.

Hill, James O., Holly R. Wyatt, George W. Reed, and John C. Peters. 2003. "Obesity and the Environment: Where Do We Go from Here?" *Science*, February 7, 853–855.

Institute of Medicine (IOM). 2006. *Progress in Preventing Childhood Obesity: Health in the Balance*. Washington, DC: National Academy Press.

Jordan, Amy B., and Thomas N. Robinson. 2008. "Children, Television Viewing, and Weight Status: Summary and Recommendations from an Expert Panel Meeting." *Annals of the American Academy of Political and Social Science*, 615, 119–132.

Joreskog, Karl, and Dag Sorbom. 1993. *LISREL 8 User's Reference Guide*. Chicago: Scientific Software International.

Khare, Adwait, and J. Jeffrey Inman. 2006. "Habitual Behavior in American Eating Patterns: The Role of Meal Occasions." *Journal of Consumer Research*, 32 (March), 567–575.

Klesges, Robert C., Mary L. Shelton, and Lisa M. Klesges. 1993. "Effects of Television on Metabolic Rate: Potential Implications for Child Obesity." *Pediatrics*, 91, 281–286.

Kumanyika, Shiriki K. 2008. "Environmental Influences on Childhood Obesity: Ethnic and Cultural Influences in Context." *Psychology and Behavior*, 94, 61–70.

Leviton, Laura C. 2008. "Children's Healthy Weight and the School Environment." *Annals of the American Academy of Political and Social Science*, 615 (1), 38–55.

Locard, Elisabeth, Nicole Mamelle, Agathe Billette, Michell Migniac, Francoise Munoz, and Sylvie Rey. 1992. "Risk Factors of Obesity in Five Years Old Population: Parental Versus Environmental Factors." *International Journal of Obesity*, 16 (10), 721–729.

Ludwig, David S., Karen Peterson, and Steven L. Gortmaker. 2001. "Relation Between Consumption of Sugar-Sweetened Drinks and Childhood Obesity: A Prospective, Observational Analysis." *Lancet*, 357, 505–508.

Matheson, Donna M., Joel D. Killen, Yun Wang, Ann Varady, and Thomas N. Robinson. 2004. "Children's Food Consumption During Television Viewing." *American Journal of Clinical Nutrition*, 79, 1088–1094.

Miller, Daniel P., and Wen-Jui Han. 2008. "Maternal Nonstandard Work Schedules and Adolescent Overweight." *American Journal of Public Health*, 98 (8), 1495–1502.

Moore, Roy L., and Lowndes F. Stephens. 1975. "Some Communication and Demographic Determinants of Adolescent Consumer Learning." *Journal of Consumer Research*, 2 (September), 80–92.

Morill, Allison C., and Christopher D. Chinn. 2004. "The Obesity Epidemic in the United States." *Journal of Public Health Policy*, 25 (3–4), 353–366.

Moschis, George P. 1985. "The Role of Family Communication in Consumer Socialization of Children and Adolescents." *Journal of Consumer Research*, 11 (March), 898–913.

Moschis, George P., and Gilbert A. Churchill. 1978. "Consumer Socialization: A Theoretical and Empirical Analysis." *Journal of Marketing Research*, 15 (November), 599–609.

Mrdjenovic, Gordana, and David A. Levitsky. 2003. "Nutritional and Energetic Consequences of Sweetened Drink Consumption in 6- to 13-Year-Old Children." *Journal of Pediatrics*, 142 (6), 604–610.

Myers, Leann, Patricia K. Strikmiller, Larry S. Webber, and Gerald S. Berenson. 1996. "Physical and Sedentary Activity in School Children Grades 5–8: The Bogalusa Heart Study." *Medicine and Science in Sports and Exercise*, 28 (7), 852–859.

Neumark-Sztainer, Dianne, Mary Story, Peter J. Hannan, Terri Tharp, and Jeanna Rex. 2003. "Factors Associated with Changes in Physical Activity: A Cohort Study of Inactive Adolescent Girls." *Archives of Pediatrics and Adolescent Medicine*, 157, 803–810.

Nielsen, Samara Joy, and Barry M. Popkin. 2003. "Patterns and Trends in Food Portion Sizes, 1977–1998." *Journal of the American Medical Association*, 289, 450–453.

———. 2004. "Changes in Beverage Intake Between 1977 and 2001." *American Journal of Preventive Medicine*, 27 (3), 205–210.

Ogden, Cynthia L., Margaret D. Carroll, Lester R. Curtin, Margaret A. McDowell, Carolyn J. Tabak, and Katherine M. Flegal. 2006. "Prevalence of Overweight and Obesity in the United States, 1999–2004." *Journal of the American Medical Association*, 295 (13), 1539–1577.

Parsad, Basmat, and Laurie Lewis. 2006. "Calories In, Calories Out: Food and Exercise in Public Elementary Schools, 2005." http://nces.ed.gov/Pubs2006/nutrition/ack.asp.

Perez-Pastor, Elena M., Brad S. Metcalf, Joanne Hosking, Alison N. Jeffery, Linda D. Voss, and Terry J. Wilkin. 2009. "Associative Weight Gain in Mother-Daughter and Father-Son Pairs: An Emerging Source of Childhood Obesity. Longitudinal Study of Trios (EarlyBird 43)." *International Journal of Obesity*, 33, 727–735.

Pugliese, John, and Barbara Tinsley. 2007. "Parental Socialization of Child and Adolescent Physical Activity: A Meta-Analysis." *Journal of Family Psychology*, 21 (3), 331–343.

Putnam, Judy, Jane Allshouse, and Linda Scott Kantor. 2002. "U.S. Per Capita Food Supply Trends." *Food Review*, 25 (3), 2–15.

Resnicow, Ken. 1991. "The Relationship Between Breakfast Habits and Plasma Cholesterol Levels in Schoolchildren." *Journal of School Health*, 61 (2), 81–85.

Rippe, James, and Lou Aronne. 1998. "Public Policy Statement on Obesity and Health from the Interdisciplinary Council on Lifestyle and Obesity Management." *Nutrition in Clinical Care*, 1, 34–37.

Robinson, Thomas N. 2001. "Television Viewing and Childhood Obesity." *Pediatric Clinics of North America*, 48, 1017–1025.

Sallis, James F., Thomas L. Patterson, Thomas L. McKenzie, and Philip R. Nader. 1988. "Family Variables and Physical Activity in Preschool Children." *Journal of Developmental Behavioral Pediatrics*, 2 (April), 57–61.

Sallis, James F., Judith J. Prochaska, and Wendell C. Taylor. 2000. "A Review of Correlates of Physical Activity of Children and Adolescents." *Medicine and Science in Sports and Exercise*, 32 (5), 963–975.

Segal, Laura M., and Emily A. Gadola. 2008. "Generation O: Addressing Childhood Overweight Before It's Too Late." *Annals of the American Academy of Political and Social Science*, 615, 195–213.

Signorielli, Nancy, and Jessica Staples. 1997. "Television and Children's Conceptions of Nutrition." *Health Communication*, 9 (4), 291–301.

Sobal, J., and A. Stunkard. 1989. "Socioeconomic Status and Obesity: A Review of the Literature." *Psychological Bulletin*, 105 (2), 260–275.

Story, Mary, Karen M. Kaphingst, and Simone French. 2006. "The Role of Schools in Obesity Prevention." *Future of Children*, 16 (1), 109–142.

Strong, William B., Robert M. Malina, Cameron J.R. Blimkle, Stephen R. Daniels, Rodney K. Dishman, Bernard Gutin, Albert C. Hergenroeder, Aviva Must, Patricia A. Nixon, James M. Pivarnik, Thomas Rowland, Stewart Trost, and François Trudeau. 2005. "Evidence Based Physical Activity for School-Age Youth." *Journal of Pediatrics*, 146 (6), 732–737.

Sturm, Roland, and Ashlesha Datar. 2005. "Body Mass Index in Elementary School Children, Metropolitan Area Food Prices and Food Outlet Density." *Public Health*, 119, 1059–1068.

Taveras, Elsie M., Sheryl L. Rifas-Shiman, Catherine S. Berkey, Helaine R.H. Rockett, Alison E. Field, A. Lindsay Frazier, Graham A. Colditz, and Matthew W. Gillman. 2005. "Family Dinner and Adolescent Overweight." *Obesity Research*, 13 (May), 900–906.

Trust for America's Health. 2008. "F as in Fat 2008: How Obesity Policies Are Failing America." October. http://healthyamericans.org/reports/obesity2008.

Utter, Jennifer, Robert Scragg, David Schaaf, and Cliona Mhurchu. 2008. "Relationship Between Frequency of Family Meals, BMI, and Nutritional Aspects of the Home Environment Among New Zealand Adolescents." *International Journal of Behavioral Nutrition and Physical Activity*, 5, 1–7.

Von Hinke Kessler Scholder, Stephanie. 2008. "Maternal Employment and Overweight Children: Does Timing Matter?" *Health Economics*, 17, 889–906.

Wansink, Brian. 2005. *Mindless Eating: Why We Eat More Than We Think*. New York: Bantam Dell.

Ward, Scott. 1974. "Consumer Socialization." *Journal of Consumer Research*, 1 (September), 1–14.

Wolfe, W. and C. Campbell. 1993. "Food Pattern, Diet Quality, and Related Characteristics of School Children in New York State." *Journal of American Dietetic Association*, 93, 1280–1284.

Ziol-Guest, Kathleen M., Greg J. Duncan, and Ariel Kalil. 2009. "Early Childhood Poverty and Adult Body Mass Index." *American Journal of Public Health*, 99 (3), 527–532.

CHAPTER 15

THE IMPACT OF HEALTH GAMES ON CONSUMERS' PHYSICAL ACTIVITY AND HEALTHY EATING INTENTIONS

SEUNG-A ANNIE JIN

Obesity and excessive food consumption have recently become a major public health concern. Health professionals are actively promoting sensible eating and physical activity in order to reduce the health risks of obesity. As exergames (combination of "exercise" and "games") are increasingly being used as an interventional tool to fight the obesity epidemic in clinical studies, society is feeling their impact to a more intense degree (Jin 2009a). The current chapter introduces a recent research stream that leverages avatar-based interactive health games for effective health communication about improving consumers' physical activity and promoting healthy dietary habits.

The structure of this chapter is as follows. First, the chapter starts with the concept of *physical self* and its relevance to the obesity epidemic, consumers' body image perception or (dis)satisfaction, and the key features of health games (e.g., avatars) that can prime consumers' physical self. Second, the chapter provides an extensive literature review on recent health games research streams and theoretical frameworks, including entertainment-education (Singhal and Rogers 2002), regulatory focus theory (T. Higgins 1997), self-concept discrepancy theory (E. Higgins 1987), and objective self-awareness theory (Duval and Wicklund 1972). Third, the key findings of experimental studies conducted by the author are summarized. Lastly, the chapter concludes with action-oriented implications for public health communications with regard to obesity.

The *physical* dimension of the *self* is particularly relevant to consumers' body image perceptions and food consumption behaviors. Given the high profile afforded by society to issues such as fitness, body image, physical attractiveness, obesity, dieting, and eating disorders (Fox 1997), the physical self is a critical concept in exploring consumers' health attitudes and behaviors. An examination of the physical self can provide helpful insights into consumers' self-esteem, self-view confidence, and their subsequent health behaviors, including physical activity, exercise, food choice, dieting, plastic surgery, and so forth. Recently, a burgeoning body of research on obesity, physical activity, and nutrition education examines the "physical self" as a key construct (e.g., Annesi 2007; Chiang, Huang, and Fu 2006; Marsh et al. 2007).

Avatar-based health games can be used as an innovative and effective apparatus to prime consumers' various aspects of the physical self (e.g., ideal self vs. actual self, attractive self vs. less attractive self, thin body image vs. obese body image). Key features that distinguish exergames from conventional sports games are the utilization of consumers' actual physical activity and the use of avatars that reflect or represent consumers' physical attributes, especially their body images. This chapter investigates the role of marketing and consumer psychology in testing the effects of avatar-based health games on consumers' physical exercise and healthy eating intentions.

Every day consumers see ideal body images of celebrities and models in a wide variety of media, ranging from advertisements, movies, and fashion magazines to promotional health messages about diet programs and fitness products. Considerable research has demonstrated a trend over the last forty years toward thinness as the ideal standard of female attractiveness (Davis 1997; Groesz, Levine, and Murnen 2002; Willinge, Touyz, and Charles 2006). At the same time, consumers are exposed to rather realistic body images by looking into the mirror or observing the many obese people around them. What are the effects of being exposed to either actual or ideal body images of oneself on the low-calorie dieting intention of an individual? Does priming one's actual self versus ideal self significantly affect an individual's view of the self? Scholars and practitioners from a wide range of disciplines (e.g., health communication, media studies, consumer psychology, social psychology, preventive medicine, and nutrition education) have approached these research topics from diverse theoretical angles and empirically examined these problems with various methodologies. This chapter presents an innovative approach using interactive media and a fresh perspective on relevant theories. To this end, the following section contains a literature review about avatar-based interactive video and computer games and the theoretical underpinnings of the author's experiments.

REVIEW OF RESEARCH STREAMS

Health Games Research

A video game is any game played on a digital device. The term encompasses a wide range of games played at arcades, over the Internet on personal computers, on dedicated game consoles (e.g., Nintendo GameCube, Sony PlayStation, or Microsoft Xbox), or on handheld units (e.g., Nintendo Wii, Nintendo Game Boy, Sony PSP).

Psycho-educational multimedia games have the potential to change dietary behavior substantially. For example, Baranowski et al. (2003) found that children participating in health games called Squire's Quest! increased their fruit, juice, and vegetable consumption by 1.0 serving more than the children not receiving the program. S.J. Brown et al. (1997) evaluated Packy & Marlon®, an interactive video game designed to improve self-care among children and adolescents with diabetes, in a six-month, randomized, controlled trial and indicated that well-designed, educational video games can be effective tools for health promotion and interventions. Lieberman (2001) demonstrated that children and adolescents improved their self-care and reduced their use of emergency clinics after playing health education and disease management video games in randomized clinical trials. Positive impacts were also found in clinical trials of games for asthma self-management (Lieberman 2001) and smoking prevention (Tingen et al. 1997). Funk and Buchman (1995) argued for the use of video games and discussed their potential benefits in healthcare education. The authors also proposed that the interactive, story-telling, and repetitive nature of playing a video game might result in an amplified impact of the information contained in the game.

A new generation of active video games (exergames), such as Sony EyeToy and Dance Dance Revolution, provide a novel strategy for increasing physical activity levels in the younger generations. Mhurchu et al. (2008) evaluated the effect of active video games on children's physical activity levels and suggested that playing active video games on a regular basis may have positive effects on children's overall physical activity levels. However, a longitudinal field experiment over a sustained period of time is needed to further confirm the long-term positive effects of these games on people's body weight and body mass index (BMI) (Mhurchu et al. 2008).

One key feature of electronic games that attracts consumers is *interactivity*. Interactivity can involve feedback and help messages tailored to the individual player and adapted to players' changing abilities. These interactive elements can be educationally effective (Lieberman 2006). Interactivity is also defined as "the degree to which users of a medium can influence the form and content of the media environment" (Steuer 1995, 41). A recent experimental study found that the self-priming apparatus in interactive health games such as Wii Fit has effects on consumers' perceived interactivity in media environments (Jin 2009a).

Another key feature of video and computer games is consumers' motivation for goal achievement. In Squire's Quest!, for example, the consumer plays a squire earning his or her way to knighthood. To become a knight, the consumer must do different tasks to help the kingdom, such as create fruit, juice, and vegetable recipes in a virtual kitchen to make sure that the king and court are strong enough to battle invaders (D. Brown 2006). A game is a physical or mental contest with a goal or objective, played according to a framework or rules that determine what a player can and cannot do inside the game world (Huizinga 1970). In this regard, health games can be used as an apparatus to prime consumers with certain health-related goals (e.g., promotion goals, prevention goals).

Interactive Health Games

Sport video games like simulations of basketball, tennis, or football, which allow consumers to participate virtually in athletic activities, are very popular among young people (Papastergiou 2009). In recent years, a new type of electronic game called the exergame, which involves physical activity as a means of interacting with the game, has emerged (Lieberman 2006). Exergames use the electronic game format to promote exercise and body movement to control the game (Khoo, Merritt, and Cheok 2009; White, Lehmann, and Trent 2007). These games use a USB camera or motion-tracking sensor placed on top of a television screen to track players' motion and place the players onscreen in the center of the games. Players physically interact with images onscreen in games that range from sport-based activities like football and boxing to dancing and kung fu (Mhurchu et al. 2008). The game is dependent on player movement in front of the camera, for both control and actual gaming (Jin and Park 2009).

Wii Fit is an avatar-based physical activity exergame. Wii Fit consists of two parts: training sessions and body test. Wii Fit provides a variety of easy-to-accomplish training sessions. Training exercises can be modified to fit game players' goals and needs. The body test in Wii Fit is a short, simple set of activities used to gauge players' body performance. Game players use the Wii balance board to measure center of balance, BMI, and body control. Based on these results, the game indicates the players' fitness age at the end of the body test session.

Second Life, an avatar-based online role-playing game in 3D virtual environments, can be utilized as a self-care game. Avatar-based 3D virtual reality computer games such as Second Life are a promising communication channel for e-health interventions and health education. A number of medical and health education projects (the Nutrition Game proposed by Ohio University; the Second Life Virtual Hallucinations Lab; the Virtual Neurological Education Center, and so on) are currently conducted inside Second Life. In addition, HealthInfo Island, funded by the U.S. National Library of Medicine, provides game players with health information services. In an effort to extend the lab experiment with video games to reach diverse populations, health practitioners and researchers can conduct a field experiment using a virtual-reality-based networked game. In order to reach diverse populations with a wide variety of ethnicities, cultural backgrounds, and socioeconomic status, researchers can recruit participants from social networking game users in Second Life. Conducting a field experiment across a diverse population beyond undergraduate student samples can increase the generalizability, ecological validity, and social impact of interactive self-care health games.

Entertainment-Education

Entertainment-education refers to the use of entertainment media as a means of educating people about important health and social issues. Singhal and Rogers define entertainment-education as "the intentional placement of educational content in entertainment messages" (2002, 117). It is the process of designing and implementing media messages for the purpose of increasing people's knowledge about educational issues and encouraging attitudinal and behavioral changes. Thus, entertainment-education is a strategic intervention that disseminates ideas to bring about attitudinal, behavioral, and social growth and improvement (Singhal and Rogers 2002).

Entertainment-education paradigm-based learning can be more enjoyable, more interesting, more motivating, and ultimately more effective than traditional learning modes (Gee 2003). People enjoy interactive, experiential learning that gives them a great deal of control, involves them in active decision-making, and provides continuous feedback (Lieberman 2006). Therefore, interactive games are powerful environments for learning (Ritterfeld and Weber 2006) and health communication (Lieberman 1997). Video games provide extensive player involvement for large numbers of consumers, thereby serving as a channel for delivering health behavior change experiences and messages in an engaging and entertaining format. Using video games to promote behavior change can capitalize on consumers' enjoyment of them (Baranowski et al. 2008). The impact of interactive health games as entertainment media on educational outcomes (e.g., physical activity improvement, healthy eating intentions, low-calorie dieting intentions) and the mediating role of entertainment on health attitudinal and behavioral changes via avatar-based exergames can be examined drawing from the entertainment-education paradigm.

Regulatory Focus Theory

Regulatory focus is defined as "the extension of the basic hedonic principle of approach and avoidance to allow for distinct self-regulatory strategies and needs" (Lee, Aaker, and Gardner 2000, 1122). There are two types of desired goals that make people feel good or bad about the target object or behavior. One type of goal is to achieve positive outcomes by focusing on "promotion." Individuals with such a promotion focus are concerned with obtaining the presence of positive outcomes. The other type of goal is to fulfill desired consequences by avoiding losses with a focus on "prevention." Individuals with the prevention focus pay close attention to obtain the absence of negative outcomes.

Specific strategic orientations and types of goal pursuit can be differentiated reflecting self-regulation guided by two distinct motivational systems—promotion focus and prevention focus (T. Higgins 1997, 2000). Self-regulation toward any specific goal may be focused on promotion, such as the pursuit of gains and ideal goals, or alternatively may be focused on prevention, like the avoidance of losses (Lee, Aaker, and Gardner 2000). Self-regulation with a prevention focus entails the motivation to attain security and avoid negative outcomes. Prevention-focused health messages can be designed in a way to emphasize security needs, the absence of negative outcomes, and means of goal pursuit that ensure the absence of poor consequences (e.g., Exercise to "avoid" aging!). People experience regulatory fit when they employ means of goal pursuit that match their regulatory focus (T. Higgins 2000). Promoters motivated by advancement and accomplishment use means of goal pursuit that ensure the presence of positive outcomes. Preventers, on the other hand, use means of goal pursuit that ensure the absence of negative outcomes.

Social psychology and consumer behavior research have empirically verified that individuals' self-construal is an important moderator in studying regulatory focus. Self-construal is a person's view of self and the structure of self-schema (Cross, Morris, and Gore 2002). Regulatory focus differs as a function of self-construal patterns that encourage different strategies for goal pursuit. For example, the independent self-construal of being positively distinct, with its emphasis on goals of personal achievement and autonomy, is consistent with a promotion focus. In contrast, the interdependent self-construal of getting along harmoniously with others, with its emphasis on goals of maintaining connections with others, is consistent with a prevention focus (Lee, Aaker, and Gardner 2000). Research shows that individuals with a dominant interdependent self-construal prefer to focus on the absence of negative outcomes (prevention).

Goal-setting and goal achievement are integral components of physical activity and weight management. Drawing upon regulatory focus theory, consumer behavior and media scholars can examine the interactive effects of priming different types of goals (prevention vs. promotion), using health games and individual difference in regulatory focus and/or self-construals, on people's exercise intentions and healthy eating intentions. Driven by this theoretical thinking, Experiment 1 presented in this chapter examined the effect of interdependent self-construal and independent self-construal in individuals' cognitive processing of prevention versus promotion goals embedded in health games on these consumers' physical exercise intentions.

Avatars, Self-Concept Discrepancy Theory, and Objective Self-Awareness Theory

Avatars in video games are visual representations of game players' selves. Avatars are increasingly being used in interactive media environments, including e-commerce (Jin 2009b), console-based video games (e.g., Wii and Xbox), and 3D virtual environment-based, massively multiplayer online role-playing games (MMORPG) (e.g., World of Warcraft, Second Life, V-Side, Sims). In avatar-based interactive media environments, users can customize a wide range of their avatars' physical features (Jin 2009a, 2009b). For example, in Second Life, users can change their avatars' facial features, skin color, hair color and length, general body shape (height, thinness, amount of muscle), and specific body parts, including neck, torso, arms, shoulders, breasts, belly, and so on. Second Life offers sophisticated and technologically advanced avatar-creating features. The avatar-based video game console Wii offers similar avatar-creating features. In Wii, users are encouraged to choose an avatar (Mii) before actually playing the game. They can either choose from the ready-made avatars or create a new avatar by customizing various physical attributes to express individual identity. After the avatar selection or creation, users can play the game using their personalized avatar. Therefore, game players can relate the prior avatar-creation activity (Mii Channel) to the subsequent physical exercise (Wii Fit) using the same product (Wii). The benefit of relating one's own body image perception to fitness activity in a sequential manner within an ecologically valid setting was the key impetus for deploying the Wii in Experiment 2 and Experiment 3 in the present chapter.

Using avatars and controlling them via a motion-sensitive remote, which are the newly added functions of avatar-based interactive video games, have blurred the clear dividing line between the authentic (real) self and the para-authentic (virtual) self. In a third-person perspective avatar-based exergame like Wii, players can see and control their embodied avatars physically manifested in real time. Empirical evidence supporting the impact of avatar creation on consumers' self-image perception and self-esteem will advance current knowledge about how to design and implement avatar-based health games for health promotion and education about physical and mental health.

According to E. Higgins's self-concept discrepancy theory (1987), the actual self is a representation of the attributes an individual actually possesses, whereas the ideal self is a representation of the attributes an individual would ideally like to possess. Self-concept discrepancy theory posits that people are motivated to reach a condition in which their self-concept matches their personally relevant self-directive standards or ideals (E. Higgins 1987). Discrepancy between the actual self and the ideal self involves people's belief that their attributes do not match their personal needs, goals, or hopes and consequently results in the individual's dissatisfaction (E. Higgins, Klein, and Strauman 1985). Similarly, Duval and Wicklund's (1972) objective self-awareness theory claims that increasing self-focused attention intensifies a person's awareness of discrepancies between the real self and ideal self and subsequently induces motivation to reduce this incongruity.

Objective self-awareness and self-focused attention are fundamental constructs in a host of health phenomena, especially to the obesity epidemic. Projecting one's physical appearance can provide helpful insight into an individual's self-focused attention and its impact on body image perception, body satisfaction, general self-esteem, and subsequent health behaviors, including healthy eating, low-calorie dieting, physical activity, and so on. Objective self-awareness is particularly relevant to Experiment 2 in two aspects: (1) the increase in self-awareness in avatar-based games; and (2) the relationship between self-awareness and self-esteem and the impact of self-concept perception on exercise intentions.

Prior research has examined the influence of objective self-awareness in self-focusing situations on people's self-evaluations of physical attractiveness, exercise self-efficacy, social comparison of physical appearance, body dysmorphic disorder, muscle dysmorphia, and consumption of fatty food. Body dissatisfaction is strongly related to dietary restraint after statistically controlling body mass, physical activity levels, and certain salient personality characteristics (Davis et al. 1993). Driven by objective self-awareness theory, the interactive effects of priming the actual self versus ideal self and individuals' body satisfaction on health-related intentions, attitudes, and behaviors can be examined.

Drawing upon these three streams of theoretical thinking, series of experimental studies introduced in this chapter (1) investigated entertainment-education in health games, (2) examined the roles of regulatory focus and regulatory fit in persuasive health communications, and (3) delved into the fundamental psychological mechanism by which objective self-awareness brings about consumers' attitudinal and behavioral changes, including body satisfaction, healthy eating, and physical exercise.

KEY FINDINGS

Results from the proposed research projects produced data consistent with the theoretical propositions. First, Experiment 1 had the following hypothesis: People with a high interdependent self-construal in the prevention goal condition will show greater exercise intentions than those with a high interdependent self-construal in the no-goal condition, whereas people with a low interdependent self-construal in the no-goal condition will show greater exercise intentions than those with a low interdependent self-construal in the prevention goal condition. Experiment 1 employed a 2 (goal manipulation: no goal vs. priming a prevention goal [lower your fitness age]) × 2 (interdependent self-construal: low vs. high) between-subjects full factorial design. Participants were randomly assigned to either the control condition (no goal) or the treatment condition (prevention goal) and asked to complete a pre-experimental questionnaire that measured their interdependent self-construal. As manipulation stimuli, participants randomly assigned to the treatment condition were given a prevention goal ("Use the Wii Fitness to *decrease* your fitness age") and asked to play Wii Fitness. In contrast, participants randomly assigned to the control condition were simply asked to play Wii Fitness without any manipulation. Results from Experiment 1 indicated that regulatory fit (vs. mismatch) between the nature of the goal and the individual's self-construal increases exercise intentions (Jin 2010). The imposition of a prevention goal significantly improves the exercise intentions of those with a high interdependent self-construal, whereas offering no goal improves the exercise intentions of those with a low interdependent self-construal. This finding suggests the applicability of regulatory focus findings in consumer research to health games research from a communication perspective.

Second, Experiment 2 had the following hypothesis: Individuals with a high BMI who are primed to create the ideal self will perceive their actual body image less thin (more obese) than those with a high BMI primed to create the actual self, whereas individuals with a low BMI primed to create the ideal self will perceive their actual body image thinner (less obese) than those with a low BMI primed to create the actual self. Experiment 2 employed a 2 (self-priming: ideal self vs.

actual self manipulated between-subjects) × 2 (BMI: high vs. low BMI measured) between-subjects factorial deign. Results from Experiment 2 demonstrated that consumers with a high BMI primed to create their ideal self perceive themselves as less thin (more obese) than those with a high BMI primed to create their actual self. In contrast, consumers with a low BMI primed to create their ideal self perceive themselves as thinner (less obese) than those with a low BMI primed to create their actual self. Priming actual versus ideal self and BMI covaried, and BMI played a significant moderating role in shaping game players' body image perception and subsequent health behaviors.

Lastly, Experiment 3 had the following hypothesis: The persuasive impact of a primed physical self on low-calorie dieting intentions varies based on the consumer's perception of negative physical self. Consumers maintaining a highly negative perception of physical self (who score high on the Negative Physical Self Scale) will show greater low-calorie dieting intentions when primed to create an ideal physical self. Consumers maintaining a highly positive perception of physical self (who score low on the Negative Physical Self Scale) will show greater low-calorie dieting intentions when primed to create the actual physical self. Experiment 3 examined the interactive effects of self-priming and consumers' score on the Negative Physical Self Scale (subjective body dissatisfaction as supplementary measure of objective BMI). Results from Experiment 3 demonstrated that the persuasive impact of a primed physical self on low-calorie dieting intentions varies based on the consumer's perception of negative physical self. Consumers maintaining a highly negative perception of physical self (who score high on the Negative Physical Self Scale) demonstrate greater low-calorie dieting intentions when primed to create an ideal physical self. In contrast, consumers maintaining a highly positive perception of physical self (who score low on the Negative Physical Self Scale) show greater low-calorie dieting intentions when primed to create the actual physical self.

IMPLICATIONS FOR PUBLIC HEALTH COMMUNICATIONS

Consumers encounter an overwhelming number of promotional messages about diet products, fitness programs, and even liposuction surgery. One of the most common strategies used by marketers is providing a short narrative (e.g., "I lost twenty-five pounds of stomach fat in only one month!" "I cut out two pounds of stomach fat per week by obeying one golden rule!" or "Get rid of fat and cellulite! Feel sexy and sculpted this summer!"), accompanied by pictures of health consumers taken before (actual self) and after (ideal self) using the advertised diet product or participating in the advocated weight loss program. Some advertisements prime both ideal and actual selves, while others prime only one. Experiments presented in this chapter provide helpful insights into how managers can identify consumers with different self-construals (e.g., through a personality quiz or filter questions) and different views of the physical self (e.g., through measurement of subjective body satisfaction or the objective BMI) and then strategically segment the market based on these consumer characteristics. Marketers can design health messages by taking advantage of regulatory fit and objective self-awareness, as described in this chapter.

Findings from the studies addressed in this chapter also have important managerial and practical implications for video game designers and the general interactive media industry. Game developers are leveraging the exergame trend. A variety of exergames are compatible with Microsoft Xbox, Sony Playstation, and Nintendo Wii. Priori stimuli (e.g., priming a player's body image perception, instigating objective awareness of the discrepancy between the actual self and the ideal self) to which game players are exposed before playing a game cause and influence changes in their affective responses. Measuring players' current height, weight, and BMI in the body test phase in Wii Fit is a clever use of body measures to prime people's goals or motivations for physical activity in the exergame.

In the IMPACT (Increasing and Maintaining Physical Activity by Connecting and Tracking participants) project, Cholewa and Irwin (2008) report that the greatest increase in obesity prevalence was among eighteen- to twenty-nine-year-olds and those with some college education. Prior research shows that 21 percent of college students are obese. This is a significant statistic given that nearly 25 percent of all eighteen- to twenty-four-year-olds attend colleges or universities and 50 percent of all students are not meeting physical activity guidelines (Irwin 2004). Clearly, entertainment-education interventions present enormous potential for targeting the young generation.

Entertainment and recreation companies offer innovative products to promote people's physical activity. Exergames can be used for experimentation with interactive media to promote physical activity and weight management. For example, Konami pioneered the exergame market and has sold more than 3 million copies of Dance Dance Revolution (DDR) in North America. Middle schools in West Virginia now use DDR in physical education classes (Berry, Seiders, and Hergenroeder 2006). Findings from this line of research support the use of interactive health games as an intervention method in practice and contribute to the physical activity intervention literature. The exergame trend represents both the private (e.g., industry) and public (e.g., education) sectors' increased interest in leveraging video games as an entertainment-education tool, as well as their valuable effort to promote the public's physical health in light of the recent obesity epidemic.

REFERENCES

Annesi, James J. 2007. "Relations of Changes in Physical Self-Appraisal and Perceived Energy with Weight Change in Obese Women Beginning a Supported Exercise and Nutrition Information Program." *Social Behavior and Personality*, 35, 1295–1300.
Baranowski, Tom, Janice Baranowski, Karen W. Cullen, Tara Marsh, Noemi Islam, Issa Zakeri, Lauren Honess-Morreale, and Carl Demoor. 2003. "Squire's Quest! Dietary Outcome Evaluation of a Multimedia Game." *American Journal of Preventive Medicine*, 24, 52–61.

Baranowski, Tom, Richard Buday, Debbe I. Thompson, and Janice Baranowski. 2008. "Playing for Real: Video Games and Stories for Health-Related Behavior Change." *American Journal of Preventive Medicine*, 34, 74–82.

Berry, Leonard L., Kathleen Seiders, and Albert C. Hergenroeder. 2006. "Regaining the Health of a Nation: What Business Can Do About Obesity." *Organizational Dynamics*, 34, 341–356.

Brown, Damon. 2006. "Playing to Win: Video Games and the Fight Against Obesity." *Journal of American Dietetic Association*, 106 (February), 188–189.

Brown, Stephen. J., Debra A. Lieberman, B.A. Gemeny, Y.C. Fan, D.M. Wilson, and David. J. Pasta. 1997. "Educational Video Game for Juvenile Diabetes: Results of a Controlled Trial." *Medical Informatics*, 22, 77–89.

Chiang, Li-Chi, Jing-Long Huang, and Lin-Shien Fu. 2006. "Physical Activity and Physical Self-Concept: Comparison Between Children with and Without Asthma." *Journal of Advanced Nursing*, 54 (June), 653–662.

Cholewa, Scott, and Jennifer D. Irwin. 2008. "Project IMPACT: Brief Report on a Pilot Programme Promoting Physical Activity Among University Students." *Journal of Health Psychology*, 13, 1207–1212.

Cross, Susan, W, Michael L. Morris, and Jonathan S. Gore. 2002. "Thinking About Oneself and Others: The Relational-Interdependent Self-Construal and Social Cognition." *Journal of Personality and Social Psychology*, 82, 399–418.

Davis, Caroline. 1997. "Body Image, Exercise, and Eating Behaviors." In *The Physical Self: From Motivation to Well-Being*, ed. Kenneth R. Fox, 143–174. Champaign, IL: Human Kinetics.

Davis, Caroline, Colin M. Shapiro, Stuart Elliott, and Michelle Dionne. 1993. "Personality and Other Correlates of Dietary Restraint: An Age by Sex Comparison." *Personality and Individual Difference*, 14 (February), 297–305.

Duval, Thomas S., and Robert A. Wicklund. 1972. *A Theory of Objective Self-Awareness*. New York: Academic Press.

Fox, Kenneth R. 1997. *The Physical Self: From Motivation to Well-Being*. Champaign, IL: Human Kinetics.

Funk, Jeanne B., and Debra D. Buchman. 1995. "Video Game Controversies." *Pediatric Annals*, 24 (February), 91–94.

Gee, James P. 2003. *What Video Games Have to Teach Us About Learning and Literacy*. New York: Palgrave Macmillan.

Groesz, Lisa M., Michael P. Levine, and Sarah K. Murnen. 2002. "The Effect of Experimental Presentation of Thin Media Images on Body Satisfaction: A Meta-Analytic Review." *International Journal of Eating Disorders*, 31 (January), 1–16.

Higgins, Edward T. 1987. "Self-Discrepancy: A Theory Relating Self and Affect." *Psychological Review*, 94, 319–340.

Higgins, Edward T., Ruth Klein, and Timothy Strauman. 1985. "Self-Concept Discrepancy Theory: A Psychological Model for Distinguishing Among Different Aspects of Depression and Anxiety." *Social Cognition*, 3, 51–76.

Higgins, Tory E. 1997. "Beyond Pleasure and Pain." *American Psychologist*, 52 (December), 1280–1300.

———. 2000. "Making a Good Decision: Value From Fit." *American Psychologist*, 55 (November), 1217–1230.

Huizinga, Johan. 1970. *Homo Ludens: A Study of the Play Element in Culture*. New York: J. & J. Harper.

Irwin, Jennifer D. 2004. "Prevalence of University Students' Sufficient Physical Activity: A Systematic Review." *Perceptual and Motor Skills*, 98, 927–943.

Jin, Seung-A Annie. 2009a. "Avatars Mirroring the Actual Self Versus Projecting the Ideal Self: The Effects of Self-Priming on Interactivity and Immersion in an Exergame, Wii Fit." *CyberPsychology & Behavior*, 12 (6), 761–765.

————. 2009b. "The Modes of Modality Richness and Involvement in Shopping Behavior in 3D Virtual Stores." *Journal of Interactive Marketing*, 23 (3), 234–246.

————. 2010. "Does Imposing a Goal Always Improve Exercise Intentions in Avatar-Based Exergames? The Moderating Role of Interdependent Self-Construal on Exercise Intentions and Self-Presence." *CyberPsychology & Behavior*, 13 (3), 335–339.

Jin, Seung-A Annie, and Namkee Park. 2009. "Parasocial Interaction with My Avatar: Effects of Interdependent Self-Construal and the Mediating Role of Self-Presence in an Avatar-Based Console Game, Wii." *CyberPsychology & Behavior*, 12 (6), 723–727.

Khoo, Eng Tat, Tim Merritt, and Adrian David Cheok. 2009. "Designing Physical and Social Intergenerational Family Entertainment." *Interacting with Computers*, 21 (January), 76–87.

Lee, Angela Y., Jennifer L. Aaker, and Wendi L. Gardner. 2000. "The Pleasures and Pains of Distinct Self-Construals: The Role of Interdependence in Regulatory Focus." *Journal of Personality and Social Psychology*, 78 (6), 1122–1134.

Lieberman, Debra A. 1997. "Interactive Video Games for Health Promotion: Effects on Knowledge, Self-Efficacy, Social Support, and Health." In *Health Promotion and Interactive Technology: Theoretical Applications and Future Direction*, ed. Richard L. Street, William R. Gold, and Timothy Manning, 103–120. Mahwah, NJ: Lawrence Erlbaum.

————. 2001. "Management of Chronic Pediatric Diseases with Interactive Health Games: Theory and Research Findings." *Journal of Ambulatory Care Management*, 24 (1), 26–38.

————. 2006. "What Can We Learn From Playing Interactive Games?" In *Playing Video Games: Motives, Responses, and Consequences*, ed. Peter Vorderer and Jennings Bryant, 379–397. Mahwah, NJ: Lawrence Erlbaum.

Marsh, Herbert, Kit-Tai Hau, Rita Y.T. Sung, and Chung-Wah Yu. 2007. "Childhood Obesity, Gender, Actual-Ideal Body Image Discrepancies, and Physical Self-Concept in Hong Kong Children: Cultural Differences in the Value of Moderation." *Developmental Psychology*, 43 (May), 647–662.

Mhurchu, Cliona Ni, Ralph Maddison, Yannan Jang, Andrew Jull, Harry Prapvessis, and Anthony Rodgers. 2008. "Couch Potatoes to Jumping Beans: A Pilot Study of the Effect of Active Video Games on Physical Activity in Children." *International Journal of Behavioral Nutrition and Physical Activity*, 5 (February), 1–5.

Papastergiou, Marina. 2009. "Exploring the Potential of Computer and Video Games for Health and Physical Education: A Literature Review." *Computers & Education*, 53 (November), 603–622.

Ritterfeld, Ute, and Rene Weber. 2006. "Video Games for Entertainment and Education." In *Playing Video Games: Motives, Responses, and Consequences*, ed. Peter Vorderer and Jennings Bryant, 399–413. Mahwah, NJ: Lawrence Erlbaum.

Singhal, Arvind, and Everett M. Rogers, 2002. "A Theoretical Agenda for Entertainment-Education." *Communication Theory*, 12, 117–135.

Steuer, Jonathon. 1995. "Defining Virtual Reality: Dimensions Determining Telepresence." In *Communication in the Age of Virtual Reality*, ed. Frank Biocca and Mark R. Levy, 33–56. Hillsdale, NJ: Lawrence Erlbaum.

Tingen, Martha S., Lou F. Gramling, Gerald Bennett, Ethlyn M. Gibson, and Margaret M. Renew. 1997. "A Pilot Study of Preadolescents Using Focus Groups to Evaluate Appeal of a Video-Based Smoking Prevention Strategy." *Journal of Addictions Nursing*, 9, 118–124.

White, Mary, Harold Lehmann, and Maria Trent. 2007. "Disco Dance Video Game-Based Interventional Study on Childhood Obesity." *Journal of Adolescent Health*, 40 (February), 32.

Willinge, Amy, Stephen Touyz, and Margaret Charles. 2006. "How Do Body-Dissatisfied and Body-Satisfied Males and Females Judge the Size of Thin Female Celebrities?" *International Journal of Eating Disorders*, 397, 576–582.

PART V

ENVIRONMENTAL AND POLICY PERSPECTIVES

CHAPTER 16

BRINGING A BIT OF SOCIAL MARKETING TO THE PROBLEM OF OBESITY

MICHAEL L. ROTHSCHILD

Dear Reader: Do you eat at least five servings of produce each day and exercise at least five times per week? If you are like the people who work in, or close to, public health and who have heard this question, there is about a .25 probability that you answered "yes." If you are in the general population, the probability is closer to .1 (King et al. 2009).

Why don't you behave in these ways? Are you unaware that these are important health behaviors? Do you feel that these are silly behaviors? Are you unmotivated to behave? If we, who are professionally close to the problem, do not behave properly, who will? We generally know what to do, we generally are motivated to behave, and yet we do not do so. Why is that? This chapter considers the difficulties in behaving as desired, even when we are aware and are motivated.

This book is about advertising and consumer psychology as they relate to obesity, but I was invited to give a social marketing perspective on changing public health behaviors. The level of obesity in the United States (and most other industrialized nations) has been increasing annually for at least twenty-five years, and over 65 percent of the U.S. population is now overweight or obese (CDC 2009). Recently, Hornik and colleagues (2008) completed an analysis of $1 billion worth of anti–drug abuse advertising from 1998 to 2004. They found no effect. The British government did a similar analysis of advertising expenditures across many public health problems and found no impact. Clearly, advertising, the dominant class of behavior change strategies, has not had an overwhelming impact.

The Institute of Medicine estimates that 60 percent of all premature deaths are preventable by changes in individual behavior and social and environmental conditions (Leonhardt 2009). Of the roughly $2.2 trillion spent on all forms of health-related activities each year in the United States, about 3 percent is spent on public health activities (Kaiser Family Foundation 2009). Relatively little is spent on prevention and much of what is spent is ineffective. Woolf writes that prevention is necessary if we are to improve the public's health (2008).

Hastings (2007) titled his recent text *Social Marketing: Why Should the Devil Have All the Best Tunes?* That is, why are commercial firms using marketing while public health organizations ignore these powerful tools? In Chapter 1 of this book, Keller observes that commercial marketing is a key driver of obesity. These tools have a long track record of success in the private sector, yet most are ignored in dealing with public health projects. The result, too often, is little or no success.

In this chapter, I will present some of the basic concepts of social marketing, show how they have been successfully applied in a project to reduce alcohol-impaired driving, and then suggest how social marketing might help reduce obesity.

A CONCEPTUAL BASE FOR SOCIAL MARKETING

There are three major classes of tools available for managing behavior. These are the 3 Es: education, enforcement, and environment (Hastings and Elliott 1993). Education consists of sending messages that can inform and/or persuade, but these do not reinforce behavior. Enforcement uses the force of law to punish, or threaten to punish, undesired behavior. Environment creates a context for behavior. Social marketing fits here and provides tools to lessen the barriers that keep people from behaving, to increase the benefits of behaving, and to reinforce the desired behavior.

All three classes are useful, but are differently appropriate for different issues, population segments, and times. In the past, public health seems to have overrelied on education while public safety has overrelied on education and enforcement. Environmental change, too often, is ignored.

Perhaps this skew comes from an underlying assumption about the targets being served. If managers assume that their target is proactive and that the classical economic model of rational man holds (Madden 2000), there might be an overreliance on message strategy. That is, if people only knew what to do, they would do the right thing. This perspective often leads managers to top-down strategies and messages that tell people how to behave.

Another view, closer to that used in commercial marketing, is that people react within their environments and that they are not too thoughtful about most of the decisions they need to make every day. With that view, messages would be less likely to be used because they would not be carefully considered, and behavior change would be more likely to happen in response to environmental change. Bottom-up, market-based strategies would consider the problems that people have in behaving as desired, from the perspective of the target.

This chapter continues by considering some of the key concepts that underlie marketing (Rothschild 1999).

Self-Interest

The basis of modern marketing is accommodating customer self-interest. This can be seen in the marketing concept that posits that organizational success comes through meeting customer needs (Perrault and McCarthy 1996). Too often, public health campaigns ask for a behavior that is the opposite of self-interest and the opposite of current behavior.

Exchanges

Marketers meet needs by offering exchanges that are explicit and where both parts of the transaction occur together. An exchange occurs when a customer takes a product off the store shelf and then pays for it. Too often, public health campaigns offer a vague payback in the distant future in exchange for today's behavior. The exchange is weak when the citizen is asked to start exercising and eat more produce now in order to postpone or avoid, in twenty years, a stroke, heart attack, or onset of cancer that may never occur.

Competition, Power, and Free Choice

Marketers understand that they work in a competitive environment, wherein they can succeed only if their offer is better than that of all other brands. Because of this demand, brands continuously improve. Since consumers have free choice between brands, they have power. The only power held by the firm is to create a better brand than what is offered by competitors. Too often, public health campaigns only offer information and do not attempt to offer a better deal than what the competition offers. In a free choice society, there always is competition. Consumers have a choice between an apple and a jelly donut, between safe sex and risky sex, between watching television and taking a walk. In order to change behavior, public health campaigns need to create a better offer.

Fun, Easy, Popular

Marketers succeed by positioning their brands as offering more fun, less work, and/ or the promise of popularity. Part of "easy" is reducing the hassles of life and the barriers that keep customers from acting appropriately. Some barriers to be over-come are price, availability, convenient size, and the risk of trying a new product. Too often public health campaigns tell people to stop doing what they previously had decided is fun, easy, and/or popular. Next, people are asked to make their lives more difficult and less enjoyable by going through withdrawal, learning to cook, or starting to exercise.

Segmentation

Marketers rarely pursue an entire market, but rather seek out those individuals who are most likely to behave. While public health managers also segment, they are more likely to do so on the basis of epidemiologic variables such as demographics, psychographics, and geographics. These variables describe people, but do not yield strong insights into the relationship between the person and the issue. The following segmentation variables might assist in creating a better understanding of the individual:

Prone/Resistant to the Desired Behavior

For any issue, a population can be placed along a continuum starting with "prone to behave as desired," going through "unable to behave as desired," and ending with "resistant to behaving as desired." Those who are prone can easily see the value of the desired behavior. Education is appropriate here, for these people would change their behavior if they only knew what to do. Those who are resistant will not change, no matter what the message or the offered exchange. If it is important to change their behavior, then enforcement will be needed. Those who are unable need assistance. The environment needs to be changed by increasing the benefits of the desired behavior and/or reducing the barriers that keep them from the desired behavior. Social marketing is most appropriately used for segments that are unable to behave.

Stages of Change

There are many stages of change models, but in general they suggest that people go from unawareness to awareness to positive attitude to trial behavior to repeat behavior.

Combining Prone/Resistant With Stages of Change

For people who are prone, messages will help them move through all stages of change. For people who are unable or resistant, education is necessary to create awareness and to develop positive attitudes for the desired behavior. Marketers are most concerned with those who are aware but unable to behave. In too many cases, managers assume a prone target and only use a message strategy. As a result, in too many issues there is a disconnect between the high level of awareness that has been achieved and the low level of behavior that is desired.

Motivation, Opportunity, and Ability

Information processing models of consumer behavior have long suggested that behavior is a result of the individual's motivation, opportunity, and ability (MacInnis, Moorman, and Jaworski 1991). Motivation is, in large part, a reflection of the self-interest described earlier, plus group norms. Opportunity reflects the environment, its barriers, its benefits, and its incentives. Ability reflects the skills and proficiencies of the individual. Creating a 2 × 2 × 2 matrix of the presence or absence of each variable leads to eight segments for any issue. When there is motivation, opportunity, and ability, then education will be sufficient to take this segment to behavior. If there is motivation but opportunity or ability or both are missing, then social marketing is needed to change the environment. If motivation is missing in the presence of opportunity and ability, then perhaps enforcement is required.

Marketing is defined as "the activity, set of institutions, and processes for creating, communicating, delivering, and exchanging offerings that have value for customers, clients, partners, and society at large" (American Marketing Association 2007). "Creating value" means creating opportunities and increasing benefits. "Delivering value" means decreasing barriers, fitting into the daily hassles of life, and being available. "Communicating value" means informing, persuading, and motivating through messages. "Exchanging value" means that each party in the transaction must receive perceived benefit. Too often, those claiming to practice social marketing focus exclusively on "communicating." Marketing requires "creating," "delivering," and "exchanging"; without these components, there may be an excellent communications plan, but it is not marketing and should not be referred to as such.

Alexander Hamilton is reputed to have said that the role of government is to create opportunity while the role of the citizen is to seize opportunity. Social marketing creates opportunity and then motivates people to seize that opportunity. Margo Wootan has said, "We need to create an environment where it is as easy to eat well as it is to eat poorly" (2009). For many issues, the opportunity to make the "bad" choice is easy, while there are barriers that keep people from making "good" choices.

A PUBLIC SAFETY EXAMPLE

The Road Crew project (Rothschild, Mastin, and Miller 2006) was designed to reduce alcohol-impaired driving in Wisconsin. It began when program managers in the Department of Transportation, frustrated with their inability to reduce crashes through either education or enforcement, discovered social marketing as a way to change the environment.

The goals were to decrease alcohol-related crashes by 5 percent in targeted communities by the end of the first year of operation and to have programs that were self-sufficient and independent of government funds by the end of that year. The goal was to change driving behavior; changing drinking behavior never was a goal of this highway safety project.

The work began with qualitative new product development research. To that end, the research needed to develop a detailed understanding of the primary target, the major competition in the marketplace, and the characteristics of a new product that would take market share away from the major competitor.

Epidemiologic and existing studies showed that the primary target consisted of twenty-one- to thirty-four-year-old single men living in rural areas, who drove after excessive drinking and then crashed (Karsten and Rothschild 2003).

Seven focus groups were then held with "expert observers" of this target. These experts were from the hospitality industry, law enforcement, the judicial system, health care, and relevant other fields. Another eleven focus groups were held with the target, and these were conducted in the back rooms of local taverns in rural areas of the state. The focus groups discussed the following topics:

• How can the target be described beyond demographics and geographics?
• What are they looking for out of life (beyond drinking)?
• Why do they drink?
• Why do they drive after excessive drinking?
• Why don't they drive after drinking?
• What are the processes and hassles of life that lead them to be drunk at the end of the evening with their car at the bar?
• What are their motivations, opportunities, and abilities?

Detailed information on the research as well as other facets of this project can be found in Rothschild, Mastin, and Miller (2006). The complete National Highway Traffic Safety Administration report can be seen in Karsten and Rothschild (2003). A few key insights follow.

It was important to know why the target drove after drinking. This would shed light on the question of why they were buying the competitive product, a brand called "I can drive myself home no matter how drunk I am." What were the benefits of the major competitive brand (which often had a monopoly position in rural communities that had no taxi or bus service), and what were the barriers that would keep the target from purchasing our brand?

There were several key reasons why people drove after drinking excessively:

• They did not want to leave their vehicle behind, as they needed it the next morning. In addition, some other drunk might smash into it if it were parked near the bar.
• Generally there were no available alternative ways to get home.
• There was strong pressure from group norms to drive. After all, what sort of real man would not be able to drive home after only eight or nine beers?
• The more inebriated they became, the more confident they were that they could safely drive themselves home.
• There was a low risk of crashing or of being stopped by law enforcement. While those in government had data to support this view, the target knew it from nightly anecdotal observations showing that almost everybody made it home without incident.

Before beginning the new product-development research, the goal had been to create the best possible ride home at the end of the evening. As focus groups were conducted, a new understanding of the processes and hassles of life suggested a different sort of program. The participants stated that if a ride were offered at the end of the evening, it would be rejected because they did not want to leave their vehicles behind. They thought that in order to keep them from driving home, a ride service should pick them up at home, take them to the bars, and then take them home. If they got their first ride of the evening with the program, their vehicles would be at home and they would not be able to make the wrong decision at the end of the evening.

The respondents also felt that any vehicle used would need to be at least as nice as their own vehicles. In addition, they felt that since they smoked and drank while they drove, they should be allowed to do the same in the developing program.

The research led to Road Crew, a program that uses older limousines to pick up drinkers at home and drive them to bars, between bars, and home at the end of the evening. They would be allowed to smoke and drink in the vehicles. Research showed that the target would be willing to pay $20 per night for this service so that the goal of self-sustainability could be achieved. As opposed to earlier programs that were not successful, Road Crew listened to the target and developed a service that could compete with the alternative choice, reduce barriers to behavior, and become viable.

The implementation of Road Crew began in June 2002 with a field experiment pilot test consisting of three treatment counties (each consisted of several towns) and five control counties, with pre- and posttests in each. Each community developed a coalition of bar owners, law enforcement, community leaders, local media, and public health practitioners for the purpose of creating a locally oriented ride program. Each coalition was required to have an advisory board of twenty-one- to thirty-four-year-old men who regularly drove while intoxicated. Anything the coalition wanted to do had to be approved by the advisory board. In addition, before beginning a community's plan, there was a session where the men in the target talked about how they spent their evenings and what they thought they might like and dislike about the proposed program. Each community then developed a program based on the Road Crew model, but tailored it to its own opportunities and constraints.

Awareness developed quickly with the appearance in the small towns of large limousines with the Road Crew logo on the side. Advertising consisted mainly of posters placed in bars and above the urinals in men's bathrooms. These posters never told people not to drive drunk and did not point out the hazards of this behavior. The posters showed the advantages of purchasing the desired brand. By using Road Crew, people would have more fun and have less to worry about. Promotional specialty items such as key fobs, beer can cozies, coasters, and refrigerator magnets also were created with the Road Crew logo and local phone number.

The pilot test was successfully completed (Rothschild, Mastin, and Miller

2006) and was expanded into other communities over several years. By July 2007 the program was in parts of six rural counties covering about 2 percent of Wisconsin. Over 85,000 rides had been given, avoiding about 140 crashes and six deaths (Rothschild 2010). The pilot test showed that while driving behavior was changed, there was no increase in drinking. All communities were self-sufficient by the end of their first year of operation. The cost of an alcohol-related crash was about $231,000 (National Safety Council 2005), but the cost to avoid a crash (all project costs amortized across crashes avoided) was about $6,200 (Rothschild 2010). Savings to Wisconsin were about $31 million (Rothschild, in process) over the five years of observation.

CONSIDERING THE CONCEPTS AND AN APPLICATION WITH REGARD TO REDUCING OBESITY

Reducing alcohol-impaired driving is an issue where all the costs and benefits of any event occur immediately and the events are independent. Much more complex are issues where costs and benefits accumulate over time so that a series of insignificant, short-run decisions can have large, long-run implications. Obesity is such an issue.

There are basically two choices that can be made. "Bad" choices, such as eating too much pizza or watching too much television, yield immediate benefits, while the accumulation of costs (of poor health) does not occur until the distant future. "Good" choices, such as eating fresh vegetables and exercising, yield immediate costs (learning to cook, preparing vegetables, exercising that is risky and will hurt), but the benefits of good health cannot be seen for some time into the future.

"Good" is at a severe disadvantage, for while people claim to seek long-run good health, their actions show that they generally maximize short-run gain. In behavioral economics, the work on preference reversals predicts that this will happen. When the choice point is not immediate, people choose the long-run option over the short, but as the choice point becomes more immediate, they choose the short-run option over the long (Simonson and Tversky 1992).

This research finding predicts much diet and exercise behavior. For example, as people prepare for work they often tell themselves that they will exercise after work, but as the workday ends, these same people reflect on their busy day and decide to go home to watch television and relax. Tomorrow, they promise, will be better. There are hundreds of small opportunities each day to choose the long- or short-run benefit. It is too easy to choose the short-run benefit and promise to be better tomorrow. This "tyranny of small decisions" (Kahn 1966) explains much of why so many people are overweight or obese.

In general, people are aware of how they should behave and have positive attitudes toward this behavior, but the environment makes it too difficult to behave properly and too easy to choose the short-run benefit. Public health message strategies (education) will only provide marginal help here. Environmental change is necessary.

For most public health issues, the targets most likely to suffer from poor health have low education and low income and come from underserved communities of disparities. They are more likely to have a short-run view because their difficult lives will not allow them to plan for the future. As a result, they tend to discount the future at a higher rate than would most readers of this chapter. The choice of long-run health is remote and elusive compared to the immediate needs of feeding their family today. While public health message strategies advocate behaving with the goal of long-run behavior, the target is struggling to get through today. This disconnect cannot be overcome with messages.

Marketers do not just send out messages; they change environments. What is needed are ways to overcome the barriers that do not allow long-run behavior. Long-run good health needs to compete against the "tyranny of small decisions." Strategies need to increase the immediate benefits of the desired behavior, to decrease the immediate barriers to the desired behavior, and to accommodate the daily hassles of life that keep people's focus on the short run.

How can such strategies be developed and who would want to invest in their implementation? Who cares if obesity is reduced? In the United States (at the time of this writing), the organizations with the greatest stake in increasing the number of healthy people of normal weight are employers who pay health insurance premiums. Their workforces are becoming heavier and less healthy, leading to increased insurance costs. Wellness strategies can be developed at the workplace to increase the immediate benefits of desired behavior and to reduce the immediate barriers that impede this behavior.

Increasing Immediate Benefits of the Desired Behavior

Immediate rewards for desired behavior: Offer to pay a larger share of health insurance premiums in return for proof that the employee is exercising regularly. Conversely, impose a higher premium on employees not engaged in regular exercise.

Social events based on exercising: Develop walking clubs to encourage employees to walk before work, at lunch, and/or after work. Develop sports teams to compete across departments or against other firms.

Incentives for purchasing "good" food: Change the pricing in vending machines and cafeterias so that "good" food is more favorably priced.

Incentives for using stairs and remote parking: Encourage employees to walk more by placing card readers on the stairs or in remote areas of parking lots. Employees can swipe their ID cards when they are passing the readers. Swipes yield points that can be redeemed for health-oriented merchandise at local retailers.

Reducing Immediate Barriers That Impede the Desired Behavior

No skill or ability: Have a nutritionist, personal trainer, cooking classes, and exercise classes at the work site.

No availability or access to healthy food: In addition to changing offerings in the vending machines and cafeteria, work with a grocer to have a produce truck come to the work site several times per week.

No time or energy to cook healthy meals: Keep the cafeteria open at the end of the workday so employees can purchase healthy meals to take home for the family dinner.

No money to pay for exercise classes or healthy food: Subsidize these programs. Price food in vending machines and cafeterias to favor healthy purchases.

Unsafe neighborhood for exercising: Create exercise space at work or have lighted paths at the work site.

Freudenheim (2008) recently has written about ten small firms in Michigan that worked together to create plans to help their employees achieve and maintain healthy weights. After the first year of operation, the firms were saving about $2,000 per employee in health-care costs. This easily covered the costs incurred in developing the above set of ideas. There are many examples of firms adopting similar plans and reducing their health-care costs.

DISCUSSION

Public health and obesity have primarily focused on using messages to change behaviors. Public safety has focused on messages plus laws. While these sets of strategies can have an impact, merely focusing on these tools is too limiting. The health of the public has been deteriorating for several decades and a rising level of obesity is the main determinant. Messages are appropriate to gain awareness and positive attitudes, but are weak in actually changing behaviors. In order to impact on behavior, we need to reduce barriers that inhibit behavior, make the immediate benefits of behaviors more desirable, and understand why long-run good health options lose to short-run bad health options. This chapter has outlined issues that need to be considered so that social marketing can have an impact. As social marketers, we need to

- accommodate the self-interest of our targets;
- respond to the conditions of a competitive marketplace where alternative choices have great immediate appeal;

- recognize that we have limited power to change behavior through messages; we can only win by offering the target a better self-interested deal than that offered by the competition;
- create immediate benefits and make them easily accessible;
- reduce the barriers that make it difficult for targets to behave as they would like to behave;
- fit the desired behavior into the daily processes and hassles of life so it makes life easier and not more difficult;
- overcome the "tyranny of small decisions"; and
- develop strong partnerships outside of traditional governmental and nonprofit agencies.

We need to "organize policy and strategy until self-interest does what community requires" (adapted from LeGrand 2003). We need to change our approach to public health issues because "If you always do what you've always done, you'll always get what you've always gotten."

ACKNOWLEDGMENTS

The Road Crew project was supported by grants from the Wisconsin Department of Transportation, the National Highway Traffic Safety Administration, and Miller Brewing. The author thanks Beth Mastin, Tom Miller, and Karen Hodgkiss for their contributions.

REFERENCES

American Marketing Association. 2007. "Definition of Marketing." www.marketingpower.com/AboutAMA/Pages/DefinitionofMarketing.aspx.

Centers for Disease Control and Prevention (CDC). 2009. "Overweight and Obesity Trends Among Adults." www.cdc.gov/obesity/data/index.html.

Freudenheim, Milt. 2008. "Building Better Bodies." *New York Times*, October 1.

Hastings, Gerard B. 2007. *Social Marketing: Why Should the Devil Have All the Best Tunes?* Oxford, UK: Butterworth-Heinemann.

Hastings, Gerard B., and B. Elliott. 1993. "Social Marketing Practice and Traffic Safety." In *Marketing of Traffic Safety*, 35–53. Paris: OECD.

Hornik, Robert L., Lela Jacobsohn, Robert Orwin, Andrea Piesse, and Graham Kalton. 2008. "Effects of the National Youth Anti-Drug Media Campaign on Youths." *American Journal of Public Health*, 98 (12), 2229–2236.

Kahn, Alfred E. 1966. "The Tyranny of Small Decisions: Market Failures, Imperfections, and the Limits of Economics." *Kyklos*, 19, 23–47.

Kaiser Family Foundation. 2009. "U.S. Health Care Costs." www.kaiseredu.org/topics_im.asp?imID=1&parentID=61&id=358.

Karsten, Carol, and Michael L. Rothschild. 2003. "The Road Crew Project." www.dot.wisconsin.gov/library/publications/topic/safety.htm.

King, Dana E., Arch G. Mainous, Mark Carnemolla, and Charlers J. Everett. 2009. "Adherence to Healthy Lifestyle Habits in U.S. Adults, 1988–2006." *American Journal of Medicine*, 122, 528–534.

LeGrand, Julian. 2003. *Motivation, Agency and Public Policy: Of Knights and Knaves, Pawns and Queens*. New York: Oxford University Press.

Leonhardt, David. 2009. "Fat Tax." *New York Times Magazine*, August 16, 9–10.

MacInnis, Deborah L., Christine Moorman, and Bernard J. Jaworski. 1991. "Enhancing and Measuring Consumers' Motivation, Opportunity and Ability to Process Brand Information from Ads." *Journal of Marketing*, 55, 32–53.

Madden, Gregory J. 2000. "A Behavioral Economics Primer." In *Reframing Health Behavior Change with Behavioral Economics*, ed. Warren Bickel and Rudolph E. Vuchinich, 115–144. Mahwah, NJ: Lawrence Erlbaum.

National Safety Council. 2005. "Estimating the Costs of Unintentional Injuries, 2005." www.nsc.org/lrs/statinfo/estcost.htm.

Perrault, William D., and Edmund J. McCarthy. 1996. *Basic Marketing: A Global Managerial Approach*. Chicago: Irwin.

Rothschild, Michael L. 1999. "Carrots, Sticks, and Promises: A Conceptual Framework for the Management of Public Health and Social Issue Behaviors." *Journal of Marketing*, 63 (October), 24–37.

———. 2010. "The Impact of Road Crew on Crashes, Fatalities, and Costs."

Rothschild, Michael L., Beth Mastin, and Thomas W. Miller. 2006. "Reducing Alcohol Related Crashes Through the Use of Social Marketing." *Accident Analysis and Prevention*, 38 (6), 1218–1230.

Simonson, Itamar, and Amos Tversky. 1992. "Choice in Context: Tradeoff Contrasts and Extremeness Aversion." *Journal of Marketing Research*, 29 (3), 281–295.

Woolf, Steven H. 2008. "The Power of Prevention and What It Requires." *Journal of the American Medical Association*, 299 (May 28), 2437–2439.

Wootan, Margo. 2009. Personal communication.

CHAPTER 17

MARKETING MYPYRAMID

Taking the Dietary Guidelines Home

BRIAN WANSINK

No country has a more comprehensive, research-based set of dietary guidelines than the United States. It is revised every five years, and its "logo"—the food guide pyramid—was recognized by 61 percent of the population in 2007, according to a 2008 IFIC Study. Yet knowing is not doing. Most people know an apple is better for them than a cookie, but cookies outsell apples 3 to 1. Most people know salads are better for them than French fries, but Burger King fries outsell salads 30 to 1 (Wansink 2006a).

How can people know so much and do so little when it comes to healthy eating? Certainly, the wide availability and variety of tempting, convenient, inexpensive foods are a formidable match for willpower (Cutler, Glaeser, and Shapiro 2003). Yet three overlooked factors can help explain why past efforts to promote the dietary guidelines have been less effective than hoped. Past efforts were too diffuse, used inappropriate media, and relied on an ineffective model of information processing.

These mistakes can be changed. Although everyone eats, the nutritional gatekeeper—the person who purchases and prepares the food—disproportionately influences many of these decisions. Focusing disproportionate efforts on this person will have a ripple influence on others. Since people make 200 or more decisions about food every day (Wansink and Sobel 2007)—many of them mindless and impulsive—it is important to give them reminders, guidance, or nudges whenever and wherever they might be making these decisions.

By changing the focus, the media, and the message, the website for the U.S. Dietary Guidelines became the most accessed federal government (.gov) website, increasing 44 percent to 5.6 million hits a day (Bouchoux 2008). This chapter examines how this shift occurred and what lessons it has for consumer behavior and for public policy research.

A BRIEF HISTORY OF THE DIETARY GUIDELINES

The U.S. Dietary Guidelines are a formalized, federally approved set of science-based recommendations on how a generalized population should eat to be in good

319

Figure 17.1   **Periodic Samples of Evolution of U.S. Dietary Guidelines**

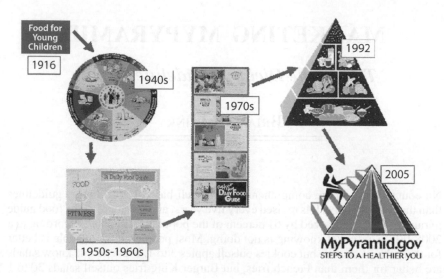

health. Using the latest peer-reviewed nutrition research, the dietary guidelines are revised every five years by a publicly nominated, federally appointed group of thirteen top experts spanning the field of nutrition.

The culmination of their eighteen-month collaboration is published in the form of a 250- to 300-page analysis and recommendations. This, in turn, is summarized into a thirty-two-page booklet for educators and health professionals, which is summarized in a wide range of printed materials and electronic materials (at My-Pyramid.gov), including posters and brochures. Lastly, the basic concept of the guidelines is encapsulated into a logo. For the past twenty years, this logo has been in the form of a pyramid.

Over the years there has been a wide variety of food guidance systems. These systems were originally developed with expert advice and are currently based upon generally accepted scientific evidence, as is found in peer-reviewed journal articles. The early food guidance systems were summarized in the form of wheels or checklists (see Figure 17.1). In the 1980s, this image changed to a pyramid shape. Although modified over the past fifteen years, the familiar image has kept the same basic triangular or pyramid shape.

The Dietary Guidelines are housed in the U.S. Department of Agriculture (USDA), in the mission area of Food, Nutrition and Consumer Services. The agency in charge of the Dietary Guidelines is the Center for Nutrition Policy and Promotion (CNPP), an agency of approximately forty people, one-third PhDs and one-third master's level nutritionists or marketing experts.

The executive director of CNPP is a political appointee with White House approval. Over the years, executive directors have typically been PhDs in nutrition with both research and administrative experience. In 2007, the White House did something unexpected. It appointed a marketing professor who focuses on eating behavior and change.

After being invited to interview for the position, I was told I would receive the appointment if I received security approval. Because such approvals can take upward of four months, I began planning what to do when I arrived in Washington. To leverage the intervening time, I had discussions with staff, dietitians, consumers, food companies, and politicians, and I developed a three-point plan that we began implementing my first week with the agency:

1. Target the nutritional gatekeeper
2. Launch new tools to increase relevance and usability
3. Employ 360° marketing: partnering with MyPyramid

These three steps constitute the sections of this chapter. While academic research informed much of my vision, the value of this chapter may be viewed in terms of how theory is implemented and how the governmental gap between great ideas and great policy can be spanned.

1. TARGET THE NUTRITIONAL GATEKEEPER

The notion of a nutritional gatekeeper has its roots in World War II, when the United States faced a nutrition crisis. Because much of the country's meat was being sent overseas to feed troops and allies, there was concern that Americans would face a protein-related nutrition crisis on the home front. The solution was to educate people about alternative forms of protein (such as organ meats—liver, kidneys, beef tongue).

Under the direction of anthropologist Margaret Mead, the Committee on Food Habits of the National Research Council assembled leading dietitians, food researchers, and social scientists to determine how to encourage families to eat organ meats as nutritious alternative sources of protein (Mead 1943). While some experts believed that the education effort should be focused on the traditionally bread-winning husband, others believed it should focus on the traditionally bread-baking wife. Still others believed attention should be spread across the entire family, with special attention paid to educating and developing nutritious habits in the children.

The early research of the committee showed a surprising twist. Wives conservatively believed that their husbands and children had de facto gatekeeping control based on their approval or disapproval of what food was served. To avoid disapproval, wives were often hesitant to stray too far from conventional recipes. The twist was that husbands and children did not share this perception. They instead indicated that they would eat almost anything that the wife served. They also believed that most if not all of the food they ate was either knowingly or unknowingly controlled by the wife. It was food she had purchased, grown, baked, or bartered (Bowers 2000).

This was a tremendous insight for the Committee on Food Habits (Polegoto and Zaichlowsky 1999). With limited resources and limited time, the committee did not need to concern itself with educating the entire American population, but could focus on the specific people who acquired the food and prepared it—the "nutritional gatekeepers" (Bowers 2000). During these war years, the majority of these gatekeepers were women. The first task was to convince a woman that she had much more latitude and food influence than she believed. The food decisions were not being made and ratified by her family. The foods that the family ate were determined by her, acquired by her, and prepared by her. The rest of the family then accepted them.

The 72 Percent Solution

Much has changed in seventy years. Yet with all that has changed in who does the cooking, ordering, or carryout, every home still has a nutritional gatekeeper (Wansink 2003). While the person who purchases most of the food is not always the person who does most of the cooking or serving, 92 percent of the time it is— whether male or female, young or old, parent or relative.

The question is this: In today's distracting and cluttered media environment, how much influence does the nutritional gatekeeper still have over the children's food intake and nutrition?

To estimate this, three different groups of people were approached in three different ways (in person, by phone, and over the Internet) at three different time intervals over eight years (Wansink 2006b). In total, 1,784 parents were asked, "Of the total amount of food your children consume (in home and away), what percent do you think you directly or indirectly influence?" Many of these respondents were registered dietitians, nurses, and physicians who watched patients and their families eat day in and day out. On average, these experts estimated that the nutritional gatekeeper of a household controlled—for better or worse—72 percent of the food that was eaten by the children both inside and outside the home.

The experts commented that nutritional gatekeepers bought most of what was eaten at home, but also they emphasized that these gatekeepers had a direct and an indirect impact on what their children ate outside the home. They exerted this influence every time they made their children's lunches and every time they gave them enough money to afford whatever lunch or snack they wanted. They also did this whenever they influenced the restaurant orders of their family by what they recommended or ordered themselves.

Today the nutritional gatekeeper may be a stay-at-home father, grandparent, housekeeper, or older sibling. Yet despite a record level of women in the workforce and despite their record level of education, the responsibility of being a nutritional gatekeeper still disproportionately falls on mothers.

Figure 17.2 **Project MOM: Mothers, Others, and MyPyramid**

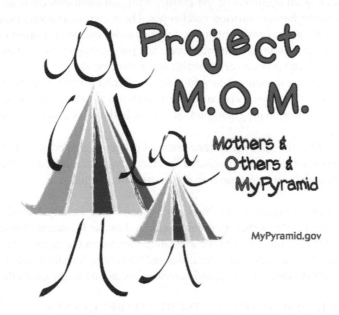

There are many potential courses of action to improve child nutrition. As the Committee on Food Habits did in 1943, the USDA Center for Nutrition Policy and Promotion will be focusing its efforts on making it easier for these nutritional gatekeepers—regardless of their sex or age—to feed the children in their families as nutritiously as possible and to set them on the path to a better nutritional future. The CNPP's messages, education efforts, and new tools will be sharpened and focused on opinion-leading nutritional gatekeepers. This is "Project M.O.M.: Mothers & Others & MyPyramid" (Figure 17.2).

The President's Council for Family Nutrition

Consistent with this focus on the nutritional gatekeeper, I proposed and wrote a charter to form the President's Council for Family Nutrition. As a counterpart to the President's Council for Physical Fitness and Sports, its objective is to provide an influential platform for change-making institutions to coordinate efforts to change family nutrition.

The council is to have four functions:

1. advise the president, through the secretary of agriculture, on the progress made in carrying out the provisions of the national program and recommend actions to accelerate progress;

2. advise the secretary on ways to encourage improved dietary behavior among all segments of the public, with particular emphasis on children and the family nutrition gatekeeper. The recommendations may include public awareness campaigns, federal, state, and local improved dietary guidance and nutrition initiatives, and partnership opportunities between public and private sector health promotion entities;

3. serve as a liaison to relevant state, local, and private entities in order to advise the secretary regarding opportunities to extend and improve nutrition education programs and services at both the local and national levels; and

4. monitor the need for enhancement of programs and educational and promotional materials sponsored, overseen, or disseminated by the council, and advise the secretary, as necessary, concerning such need.

In the proposed charter, the President's Council for Family Nutrition would be composed of up to twenty members appointed by the President. The executive director of CNPP would also be the executive director of the council, responsible for managing program and staff operations and for serving as liaison to the secretary and the White House on matters and activities pertaining to the council.

2. LAUNCH NEW TOOLS TO INCREASE RELEVANCE AND USABILITY

Between November 2007 and January 2009, CNPP launched four tools to help nutritional gatekeepers. The tools were designed to be useful to nutritional gatekeepers and dietitians, as well as consumer science teachers and students in middle schools and high schools.

MyPyramid Menu Planner

Although many people may be able to identify which of two foods is healthier or even more nutrient-dense (an orange versus a cinnamon roll), the concept of a nutritious diet is more elusive. While many parents hope that they offer their family a nutritious diet, they are probably not very certain about it.

The MyPyramid Menu Planner (MyPyramid.gov) translates foods (even mixed foods, such as a club sandwich or pasta primavera) into food groups found in MyPyramid, interactively noting how well the diet met MyPyramid recommendations on that day. Because it also asks for each family member's age, gender, height, weight, and activity level, it can also estimate calorie requirements. Last, if there is an area in which a family continually falls short—say fruit intake—the Menu Planner suggests easy changes to try, and it can track dietary changes over a week.

The MyPyramid Menu Planner provides the opportunity to (1) determine whether a person's diet for up to seven days meets MyPyramid recommendations, (2) determine small changes that would improve diet quality, and (3) understand whether the calorie level recorded would lead to weight gain or weight loss if consumed over a long period of time. In the future, it may even offer a shopping list.

Dietitians often ask clients to keep a food record to help them become more aware of what they eat. The MyPyramid Menu Planner has a number of advantages over paper-and-pencil food records. It is easy and interactive, it does the necessary calculations, it shows a broad picture of diet quality in terms of food groups (not only calories or a few nutrients), and it gives real-time suggestions for improvement. In 2008 it received 750,000 page views every day.

MyPyramid for Pregnant and Breastfeeding Moms

Regardless of how accomplished or educated a person is, once a woman learns that she is pregnant, her interest in nutrition—not just calories—often reaches a new high. Whereas many physicians prescribe prenatal vitamins and periodically check weight gain, they may not allow as much time for nutrition advice as their patients need. For some women, their understanding of nutrition may not improve much even after delivery.

MyPyramid for Pregnant and Breastfeeding Mothers ("MyPyramid for Moms") gives these gatekeepers critical advice on what and how much to eat. In addition to seeing MyPyramid for Moms posters in thousands of physicians' offices and WIC clinics across the country, new mothers can use the MyPyramid Menu Planner to guide them through the trimesters and through their breastfeeding months.

MyPyramid for Preschoolers

It is challenging for parents to know what to do when faced with eating jags, picky eaters, and conflicting advice from well-meaning relatives. MyPyramid for Preschoolers helps parents better understand food intake patterns, growth patterns, and to determine whether their preschooler is overweight or not. In addition, it helps them set reasonable expectations for food-related behaviors and behavioral eating issues. This tool is available on the CNPP website, and related posters were sent to the offices of pediatricians and family physicians.

The Cost of Raising a Child Calculator

Since 1960, the USDA has been providing estimates of how much it costs to raise a child from birth to seventeen years of age. These estimates can be used to determine how much money should be allocated to ensure that a child is provided for.

This "child cost calculator" is an interactive tool that enables parents—or advising dietitians or educators—to estimate how much it will cost to raise a child by determining how much other families are spending on food and other necessities (including housing, clothing, transportation, education, and child care) according to household income, number of children in the family, and region of the country. The power of this tool is in helping families manage their household budget in a way that ensures there is enough money for good nutrition and enough left over for the other necessities of life.

As summarized in Table 17.1, these four tools solved many of the most vexing problems related to putting nutritional advice into action. They made it specific, they addressed real behavior problems with a wide range of tailored advice, they enabled users to easily assess whether they and their families were eating in balance, they helped parents determine exactly how much money to set aside for a healthy food budget for their children across the month, they advised pregnant and breastfeeding mothers what to do and what to expect, and they advised parents how to feed difficult children who are going through unhealthy food patterns. What was missing was a means to promote these tools.

3. EMPLOY 360° MARKETING: PARTNERING WITH MYPYRAMID

It is estimated that people make over 200 decisions about food every day (Wansink and Sobel 2007)—not simply what to have for breakf\ast, but how much to eat and when to stop. These decisions are made not only at mealtime and snack time, but anytime someone purchases and prepares food at work and at play.

Suppose we each had our own 24/7 personal dietitian shadowing us who could read our thoughts before we acted on them. If that person could gently remind us to think again each time we were likely to make a less than healthy decision, it is almost certain that a few of these decisions would be made in a healthier direction than originally planned. Such dietitians do not exist. Without vigilant reminders around us to think twice, we have to rely on our willpower and mindfulness.

There is not one entity that touches people wherever they purchase and prepare food and wherever they work and play—there are thousands: They include food companies, schools, grocery stores, trade associations, and not-for-profit organizations. They touch people through food labels, websites, text reminders, downloadable games, commercials, posters, tray liners, and so on.

These entities have the potential to be "information multipliers" for the U.S. Dietary Guidelines. Imagine quickly selecting foods in the grocery store with key nutrition information on the front of the package. Imagine that it is easier to prepare dinner than to order out. Imagine that every day at 11:44 A.M. you get a lunch tip on your cell phone. Or even imagine having an avatar on your computer who helps you choose a better diet.

Partnering With MyPyramid

Partnering with MyPyramid is a program initiated by CNPP that encourages organizations to use MyPyramid messages in promoting healthy food and lifestyle

Table 17.1

Education Tools From the USDA's Center for Nutritional Policy and Promotion

Tool (launch date)	Questions addressed	Important features
MyPyramid Menu Planner (March 2008)	• How do you know if you and your family are eating a balanced diet? • Where can you get personalized advice on how to improve the quality of your diet? • How do you know if you are on track to gain or lose weight?	• Determines the percentage of each food group a person or family member has consumed. Also tracks calorie intake and compares it to what is needed for energy balance • Uses a colorful interactive feature to input the type and quantity of food consumed • Breaks foods (such as pizza or a club sandwich) into their daily contribution to the basic food groups • Provides stylized ways to change behavior to achieve balance
MyPyramid for Pregnant and Breastfeeding Mothers (June 2008)	• How should your diet change once you become pregnant? • How can you track how many calories you should be consuming during the different trimesters? • What dietary changes should you make when breastfeeding?	• By linking to MyPyramid Menu Planner, "My Pyramid for Moms" shows whether a woman is eating in balance and consuming too few or too many calories. • Offers a wide range of small steps that pregnant and breastfeeding mothers can take to balance their unique nutrition requirements
MyPyramid for Preschoolers (October 2008)	• Should you feed a four-year-old like a mini-adult? What changes are needed? • How do you know whether your child is eating a good diet?	• Uses research-based guidance of an expert committee to lead preschoolers to eat a more balanced diet • Links to the MyPyramid Menu Planner and is featured in waiting room posters sent to pediatricians and family physicians
The Cost of Raising a Child Calculator (January 2009)	• How much money needs to be allocated each month to ensure that your children are fed a nutritious diet?	• An interactive interface calculates tailored food cost estimates for children depending on their age, gender, and family size

Source: MyPyramid.gov.

Figure 17.3 **The 200 Daily Food Decisions People Make**

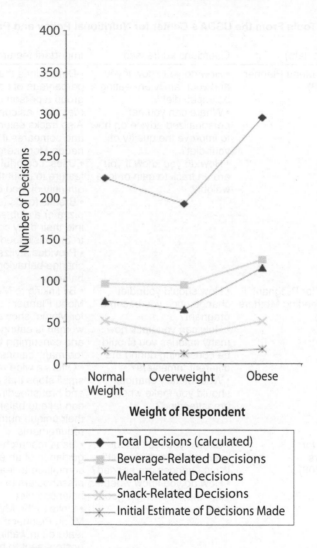

choices. It focuses on helping a family's nutrition gatekeeper make choices that are consistent with the Dietary Guidelines for Americans (2005) and MyPyramid.

By signing a simple memorandum of intent and planning an initiative, organizations can join CNPP in the partnership initiative. Partnering with MyPyramid members are diverse in scope, with community-based programs, professional societies, and food industry, food service, communications, and medical groups participating.

This is an opportunity to think differently about connecting with families and helping them make healthy food and lifestyle choices. For example, a company could provide MyPyramid food group information on packaging, develop a new product, create a website that shows easy and fun ways to be more physically active, or give a free MyPyramid Menu Planner CD to customers. Perhaps another group could bundle the MyPyramid Menu Planner software with their video game systems, make it easy for consumers to download the Menu Planner, or send MyPyramid messages to consumers' cell phones. Organizations that sign on as partners and promote messages consistent with the 2005 Dietary Guidelines for Americans and MyPyramid will

- be identified on the Partnering with MyPyramid web page;
- be invited to participate in in-person partnership meetings;
- have partner-to-partner networking opportunities; and
- receive periodic "e-post" updates of accomplishments.

To sign up to Partner with MyPyramid, organizations need to complete three web-downloadable documents—an application, a memorandum of intent, and a proposed project description—and return them to the USDA. The project description should include project goals, a project synopsis (limited to 100 words), a project timeline, and the target audience. To facilitate sign-up, a Partnering with MyPyramid Action Kit provides a wide range of examples and answers to frequently asked questions.

When this program was officially launched in June 2008, thirty-two organizations had signed letters of intent and had been acknowledged by the USDA as Partnering with MyPyramid. Since then, over 200 companies, trade associations, and nonprofit organizations have Partnered with MyPyramid to multiply the behavior-based message of the U.S. Dietary Guidelines. This program has resulted in websites, new products, billboards, games, tray liners, reformulations, and the distribution of more than 1,000 products around the globe with Dietary Guidelines information on them. Here are some of the results:

- By Summer 2009, MyPyramid food group information has been included on the labels of about 700 ConAgra food products in grocery stores.
- 500,000 MyPyramid posters and tear pads have been printed and over 950,000 brochures, toolkits, and tear pads distributed by the National Cattleman's Beef Association.
- Posters and brochures have been distributed to over 7,000 Burger King restaurants.
- General Mills is reaching 10,000 Latinas with a ten-lesson nutrition plan. The Box Tops for Education newsletter on MyPyramid has been sent to 2 million coordinators and 1.3 million consumers; 482,000 unique visitors went to the MyPyramid website article.

Table 17.2

Partnering With MyPyramid: Sample Project Ideas

General area of focus	A sample of possible project ideas
Product formulation and packaging	• Include information about the MyPyramid food group content of a product on the front of package labeling • Develop a new packaging initiative that assists consumers in following MyPyramid recommendations and monitoring portion sizes • Formulate a new food product to be consistent with U.S. Dietary Guidelines recommendations (e.g., a frozen meal or side dish made with a large proportion of whole grains or additional vegetables)
Computer applications and websites	• Develop computer games and other software for children that include MyPyramid nutrition and physical activity messages for use on the organization's website • Set up a website for parents that gives great ideas for healthy snacking based on MyPyramid, with links to MyPyramid.gov • Develop and place MyPyramid pop-ups on the organization's web pages and advertising to point parents to the MyPyramid Menu Planner
Promotions and advertisements	• Integrate MyPyramid messaging into product advertising and promotions • Encourage physical activity through a product promotion or consumer education campaign • Distribute a CD-ROM of the MyPyramid Menu Planner in food packages such as cereal boxes (e.g., "Buy 3, get a free CD!") • Include a MyPyramid message and promotion with product ads in the weekend newspaper coupon inserts • Run and/or use MyPyramid PodCasts in promotion activities
Contests and games	• Design a MyPyramid-related contest for consumers to enter • Develop computer games and other software for kids that include MyPyramid nutrition and physical activity messages
On-site promotions	• Develop placemats with MyPyramid messages and information for use in restaurants
Professional outreach	• Send a targeted mailing to nutrition education professionals (e.g., members of the American Dietetic Association or the Society for Nutrition Education) with the CD-ROM of the MyPyramid Menu Planner, to assist them in using the Menu Planner with clients • Reprint a MyPyramid poster (e.g., MyPyramid for Kids, MyPyramid for Moms, or MyPyramid for Preschoolers) and send to professionals who work with these audiences

- Over 800,000 people have viewed the "Eat Learn Live" animated videos that promote MyPyramid. Links to MyPyramid on www.eatlearnlive.com website. Digital signage by the Compass Group in cafes and dining rooms promotes MyPyramid.
- MyPyramid-related booklets reached a total of 956,787 consumers from July to December 2008 via the California Dairy Council.

- Aramark has distributed 176,900 educational materials highlighting MyPyramid to more than 200 school districts and 940 elementary schools and has supplied newsletters incorporating MyPyramid to all food service directors to distribute to more than 400 middle schools and 350 high schools.
- Within one year of the start of the program, U.S. Dietary Guidelines behavior-related information was distributed on 1 million brochures by Taco Bell, 1,344,700 brochures and 6,882 posters by KFC, 300 million brochures printed by Pizza Hut, and 296,000 tray liners by Subway.

By enlisting these "information multipliers" to creatively promote the U.S. Dietary Guidelines, CNPP has dramatically increased awareness and interest in the guidelines. A 2010 International Food and Information Council (IFIC) study indicated that 82 percent of Americans recognized the Food Pyramid. Of these, 62 percent said that it had positively influenced their eating behavior. Visits to the website MyPyramid.gov increased 44 percent—up to 5.6 million hits a day.

CONCLUSION

What is the solution for the obesity crisis is America? For the past fifteen years people have blamed low-price, easily available food for making Americans fat. Some blame government subsidies to agriculture, supersizing food companies, and even the schools. Others blame the inactivity encouraged by cars, elevators, computers, garage door openers, and PlayStation. If all of these were gone, the environment would clearly be less obesigenic. Would we all revert back to having the sleek, trim figures of people we see in 1950s black-and-white photos? That is less clear.

What is clear is that the stronger the case we make that obesity crisis is the environment's fault, the more we weaken the perceived power of an individual to change it. After all, if the media, government, schools, or food industry is to blame, what can we do?

The solution is not nutrition education, per se, but nutrition empowerment. The nutritional gatekeepers of the family need to realize that they control much more of their family's food decisions than they think. They do it either directly or indirectly. They do it either for the better or for the worse. They do it for the better at home when they replace the cookie jar with a fruit bowl. They do it for the better at restaurants when they model healthy choices by ordering the salad instead of the fries. They do it for the better at school when they give their child a small snack pack of fruit and nuts rather than change for the vending machine.

The U.S. Dietary Guidelines may not be dramatically different than they were twenty years ago. What is different is the way they are being marketed.

REFERENCES

Bouchoux, Ann. 2008. "Promoting Health at the Center for Nutrition Policy and Promotion: An Interview with Brian Wansink, PhD." *Food Insights*, November–December, 1–5.

Bowers, Douglas E. 2000. "Cooking Trends Echo Changing Roles for Women." *Food Review*, 23, 23–29.

Cutler, David M., Edward L. Glaeser, and Jesse M. Shapiro. 2003. "Why Have Americans Become More Obese?" *Journal of Economic Perspectives*, 17, 93–118.

Dietary Guidelines for Americans. 2005. www.health.gov/dietaryguidelines/dga2005/document/pdf/DGA2005.pdf.

French, Simone, Mary Story, and Robert Jeffries. 2005. "Public Health Strategies for Dietary Change: Schools and Workplaces." *Journal of Nutrition*, 135 (4), 910–912.

Mead, Margaret. 1943. "Dietary Patterns and Food Habits." *Journal of the American Dietetic Association*, 19, 1–5.

Polegoto, Rosemary, and Judith L. Zaichlowsky. 1999. "Food Shopping Profiles of Career-Oriented, Income-Oriented, and At-Home Wives." *Journal of Consumer Affairs*, 33 (1), 110–133.

Wansink, Brian. 2003. "Profiling Nutritional Gatekeepers: Three Methods for Differentiating Influential Cooks." *Food Quality and Preference*, 14 (4), 289–297.

———. 2006a. *Mindless Eating: Why We Eat More Than We Think*. New York: Bantam.

———. 2006b. "Nutritional Gatekeepers and the 72% Solution." *Journal of the American Dietetic Association*, 106 (9) (September), 1324–1327.

Wansink, Brian, and Jeffery Sobel 2007. "Mindless Eating: The 200 Daily Food Decisions We Overlook." *Environment & Behavior*, 39, 106–123.

CHAPTER 18

SIMPLIFIED NUTRITION GUIDELINES TO FIGHT OBESITY

JASON RIIS AND REBECCA RATNER

A dizzying array of nutritional information is available to consumers as they make decisions about what foods to consume. Despite the abundant information and perhaps partly because of it, major nutritional problems still exist, the worst of which may be the obesity epidemic. About one-third of Americans are considered obese and a further third are considered overweight (Flegal et al. 2002). Obesity and overweight are associated with considerable morbidity and mortality (Olshansky et al. 2005), and the additional medical costs associated with obesity alone have been estimated at $147 billion per year (Finkelstein et al. 2009).

In this chapter, we describe some of our own research that shows that the nation's main nutrition guideline, the U.S. Department of Agriculture's MyPyramid, could be greatly improved in its ability to influence consumer choice and eventually curb the obesity epidemic. We focus particularly on the benefits that would accrue from drastically simplifying the information presented to consumers. The current guideline is too complex for most consumers to be willing and able to use optimally. Our studies suggest not only that an alternative guideline, the Half Plate, is much easier to remember, but also that consumers find it more motivating. We also offer preliminary evidence that it leads them to make better food choices (in this case, choosing more fruits and vegetables).

We begin the chapter with a brief discussion of some recent work highlighting the virtues of simplicity and the dangers of complexity. We then review research on consumers' use of the nutritional information that appears on product labels, including the impact of nutrition content facts (e.g., fat and calorie content) and product claims (e.g., "low-fat"). The next section describes some recent research on *general food guidelines* (e.g., MyPyramid and various diet plans) and concludes that guidelines can facilitate healthy weight loss and weight maintenance if people actually follow them. Guidelines will greatly differ, however, in consumers' ability and motivation to follow them. The final section presents the major usability and motivational challenges of MyPyramid and our research on the relative advantages of the much simpler Half Plate guideline.

EVIDENCE THAT SIMPLE MAY BE BETTER

In their best-selling book *Made to Stick* (2007), Chip Heath and Dan Heath argue that most "successful" ideas—that is, those that rightly or wrongly become accepted and repeated frequently across cultures—have several features in common. One of these features is simplicity.

Simplicity does not just mean that something can be expressed in a sound bite. Simple ideas are compact, but also they capture the core of what is important. To capture the core, simple ideas must exclude some information. To create a simple idea, one must prioritize, which of course leads to painful decisions about which information to keep and which to leave out. Good simple ideas achieve this prioritization with elegance; they do not simply dumb down more complex ideas. Heath and Heath cite the Golden Rule as an example of a simple idea: "Do unto others as you would have them do unto you." It is compact and yet captures the core idea that many people value and wish their children to value.

Numerous research studies in consumer behavior and psychology indicate that providing people with too much information has serious costs. People get overloaded when they have too much product information; they make more optimal choices when the amount of information provided is appropriately limited (Keller and Staelin 1987). Similar findings emerge when people are given too many options to choose between; having many options to consider can induce choice paralysis (Iyengar and Lepper 2000). Indeed, there are several informational bottlenecks in the human brain that limit people's ability to process information (Marois and Ivanoff 2005).

Although the virtues of simplicity have been documented and may even seem obvious, complexity has a way of taking over in many situations. This is perhaps no more clearly the case than in the domain of consumer electronics. Many consumers find their TV remotes virtually unusable because the two buttons they use most, volume and channel, are surrounded by dozens of other buttons. The phenomenon of "feature creep" emerges whereby new generations of electronic devices gain features, but lose usability. Research suggests that consumers themselves are initially attracted to products that contain an abundance of features, but realize after using the product that too much complexity compromises their experience with the product (Thompson, Hamilton, and Rust 2005). Complexity is often ignored by the engineers who develop electronic products—developers have a much more intimate knowledge of their own products than consumers do, so it can be easy for them to neglect the difficulties that complexity creates for new users, because they themselves do not actually experience these difficulties (Gourville 2006). A similar argument could be made about nutritionists who develop food guidelines and nutrition information. Their richer knowledge of nutrition could lead them to underestimate the difficulty that typical consumers have in processing and remembering nutrition-related information.

In the next section, we consider research that has examined the extent to which consumers do utilize various kinds of nutrition information.

RESEARCH ON PRODUCT LABELS

We will begin this review by considering three kinds of product labels: (1) nutrition content *facts* (such as precise fat and calorie content that must appear on the Nutrition Facts Panel), (2) nutritional *claims* (such as "low-fat"), and (3) third-party nutritional *ratings* (such as the NuVal system that assigns nutritional rating scores to packaged foods).

Studies conducted to test the effects of these types of labels suggest that the provision of nutrition content facts does not strongly influence consumer choice, even when the information is in a relatively simple format. However, simple nutrition claims can be quite powerful, although sometimes with perverse consequences. To our knowledge, there has been no research on nutritional ratings (since they are a relatively new approach), but we will briefly discuss some of the current systems.

Nutrition Content Labels on Products

Since the printing of nutritional content of most packaged foods was mandated in the United States in 1994, there have been several studies of consumer responses to the now prevalent "Nutrition Facts Panel." The panel displays information on nutrients such as calories, total and saturated fats, cholesterol, and sodium in a standardized format. Have the labels helped consumers choose foods that help maintain healthy weight? In fact, there is little evidence that consumers are choosing lower-calorie or lower-fat foods as a result of labeling.

An early study (Moorman 1996) conducted in the periods just before and just after the labels began to appear on packages found that the introduction of labels helped consumers both acquire and comprehend nutritional information. Specifically, consumers surveyed in a supermarket during the post-label period showed more accurate knowledge about the fat content in the foods they purchased than did consumers who were surveyed during the pre-label period.

Other studies have examined whether reading labels translates into improved choice. A correlational study found that people who tended to read nutrition labels were more likely to consume lower-fat foods (Kreuter et al. 1997). This association, however, does not necessarily mean that reading labels is actually the cause of reduced fat consumption. People who tend to read labels may have consumed less fat even if labels were not available. Another study used a large survey panel to investigate such selection effects (Variyam 2008). This study looked at consumption of both packaged foods, which had labels, and restaurant foods, which did not have labels. The results suggested that reading labels did not influence people to consume lower quantities of total dietary fat.

The Nutrition Facts Panel is quite complex, containing more than twenty individual facts for each product. Given that labels do not appear to systematically reduce the fat or calorie content of consumers' grocery choices, some have called for efforts to increase the simplicity and prominence of the labeling. For example, the Nutrition Facts Panel could be changed to make calorie and fat information easier to read (Parker-Pope 2009).

Others have called for labeling to be mandated in restaurant food as well, and several cities and states have taken steps to develop such mandates. New York City was the first jurisdiction to mandate labeling, and since the program began in July 2008, several studies have investigated its impact on consumer choice. The results are not encouraging. For example, one team of researchers collected customers' receipts outside of three fast-food locations in New York City, shortly before and shortly after the labeling mandate went into effect in July 2008 (Downs, Loewenstein, and Wisdom 2009). At two of the three locations, customers did not appear to be making lower-calorie selections after the mandate, but a modest reduction was observed at one restaurant. In another study, researchers collected 1,156 receipts and surveys from adults at fast-food restaurants in low-income neighborhoods in New York City and in a control city (Newark, New Jersey) before and after labeling was introduced in the former (Elbel et al. 2009). Results indicated that labeling did not change mean calories consumed, although the labeling led some consumers to believe that the available calorie information had influenced their food choice.

While studies continue to investigate the effects of these types of labels, it appears that the effects of package and menu labeling are quite modest. Although some consumers attend to the information, it does not appear that most consumers make much use of the information. This may change over time, and further label simplification may help. We believe, however, that the more important opportunities lie in package claims, which go beyond mere labeling to provide consumers with advice about weight-related product virtues, and in guidelines about what constitutes a healthy diet overall.

Nutritional Claims on Products

Front-of-package nutritional claims appear to have a much stronger influence on consumer choice than back-package nutrition content labels (Levy and Fein 1998). This should not be surprising. Shoppers have to make many purchase decisions and they are often rushed. When the part of a product package that they see first (i.e., the front) suggests that the product has desirable properties, many consumers will not scrutinize further.

But what kinds of front-label claims are most effective? Wansink, Sonka, and Hasler (2004) have shown that short product claims are most impactful. Short front-label claims sometimes lead consumers to look more closely at detailed back-label information, giving them a more fact-based impression of the product and a better overall evaluation.

Do such short claims lead to healthier choices? Some simple claims, it seems, actually lead to overeating. Wansink and Chandon (2006) suggest that consumers can place too much weight on claims like "low-fat" and end up eating more calories than they would have if they had been consuming a product that did not have this label. For example, in several studies using packaged snack foods, the researchers gave identical snacks to two groups of consumers. For one group the snack was labeled "low-fat" and for the other it was not labeled this way. The consumers with the low-fat packaging ate an average of fifty-four more calories. The authors attributed this result to the fact that the low-fat label (1) led consumers to believe that the appropriate serving size was larger, and (2) made them feel less guilty about snacking.

Although the labels in this study led to perverse effects, the study does show the potential power of simple front-package labels to influence consumer choice. If the labels had the right simple message, perhaps calorie consumption could be decreased. One type of message that could be included at point-of-purchase involves third-party ratings, as we discuss next.

THIRD-PARTY RATING SYSTEMS ON PRODUCTS

Several large grocery chains have recently implemented major labeling (or rating) systems for store products (through shelf labels) to simplify the decision process for consumers who are searching for healthful products. One of the more prominent such labeling programs, NuVal, was developed by the Yale physician David Katz and has been implemented at some large chains like Meijer. This system considers more than thirty nutritional factors to give all foods a single score between 0 and 100.

Other systems simplify the choice task for consumers by placing special labels on particularly healthy products. For example, the grocery chain Stop & Shop has developed and implemented a system to label foods as "Healthy Ideas" if they meet certain criteria consistent with the U.S. Department of Agriculture (USDA) dietary recommendations. Another simple system, "Smart Choices," used a lower standard of "healthy" and came under considerable criticism. The program was launched in partnership with several of the large food companies, including Kellogg's, Kraft Foods, ConAgra Foods, Unilever, General Mills, PepsiCo, and Tyson Foods. Under the program, these companies could label their products with the Smart Choices logo if they met certain criteria. Some high-calorie foods like heavily sugared cereals can be labeled as Smart Choices, leading Walter Willett, chair of the Department of Nutrition at the Harvard School of Public Health, to describe these as "horrible choices" (Neuman 2009a).

To our knowledge, there is not yet any published research on the relative effectiveness of these different types of third-party labeling (Kennedy 2008). The Food and Drug Administration (FDA) has recently announced its plans to work with industry to develop a consistent approach to front-of-package claims and ratings (Neuman 2009b). We hope that the systems will be evaluated not just on what kinds of foods they recommend, but also on how likely consumers are to actually use them.

RESEARCH ON GENERAL NUTRITIONAL GUIDELINES

Unlike food *labels*, which offer content facts, claims, or ratings for particular products, food *guidelines* give specific recommendations about what kinds of foods, and in what quantities, people ought to eat over the course of a day. We believe that complexity of guidelines is likely to pose an even greater problem for consumers than complexity of product labels. Label information is at least visually available on the product for inspection at the point of purchase, whereas guidelines and recommendations must be actively remembered by the consumer if they are going to be used (Alba, Hutchinson, and Lynch 1991).

We classify nutrition guidelines as being of two main types. The first are public guidelines produced by government agencies (such as the USDA) and by nonprofit organizations (such as the American Heart Association and by Harvard University's School of Public Health). The most prominent of these public guidelines is the USDA's MyPyramid. The second category of nutritional guidelines consists of commercial diet plans such as South Beach, Atkins, and Weight Watchers.

Most research on these guidelines considers the nutritional outcomes that ensue if the guidelines are actually followed. Krebs-Smith and Kris-Etherton (2007) conclude that the major public guidelines are all generally sound with respect to their nutritional advice, but note that their impact will depend largely on how well consumers comply. Similarly, with respect to commercial diet plans, Sacks et al. (2009) have found that, if followed, several popular diets all lead to similar levels of weight loss. Their study of several popular diets (e.g., low-carb, high-protein, low-fat) showed that all such "macronutrient" diets have the same effectiveness— all led to approximately fourteen pounds of weight loss over a six-month period among the overweight and obese participants. Participants in this study received considerable social and educational support, and those who attended more support group sessions lost more weight. These findings highlight the key role of behavioral factors (i.e., compliance with nutrition guidelines) in calorie reduction rather than the macronutrient content of the diets themselves.

In short, these studies suggest that popular diets and guidelines are often nu-tritionally sound. However, the best predictor of whether a guideline will lead to positive nutritional outcomes generally, and weight loss in particular, will be the consumer's ability and inclination to comply with the guideline. In light of this, we will focus in the sections that follow on the nation's foremost dietary guideline, MyPyramid, and suggest that its complexity will limit ease of compliance and therefore limit its impact in battling obesity and overweight.

The USDA MyPyramid

The USDA MyPyramid has a long history. Its most recent precursor, the Food Pyramid, was introduced in 1992 to communicate to the general public the key components of a healthful diet, and a majority of Americans became broadly familiar with it (Britten, Haven, and Davis 2006; Davis, Britten, and Myers 2001). In 2005, the Department of Agriculture introduced MyPyramid as the redesigned, updated national nutrition guideline to replace the one-size-fits-all Food Pyramid. The new MyPyramid guideline is to be obtained by each consumer individually by visiting www.mypyramid.gov. It provides a customized recommended portion size as a function of the consumer's age, gender, and amount of weekly exercise. Each guideline features the same five food groups presented in the original Food Pyramid (grains, vegetables, fruits, milk, and meat/beans), with specific quantities for each (e.g., how many cups of fruits, how many ounces of grains) that the consumer is recommended to consume each day.

Many nutrition scientists have criticized the various iterations of the pyramid, sometimes suggesting that its recommendations are at least partly to blame for the obesity epidemic (Bell, Bell, and Blackburn 2004; Chiuve and Willet 2007). The pyramid guidelines have their defenders too (e.g., Nestle 1998), and Goldberg et al. (2004) have argued that it is not so much the guidelines themselves that are causing obesity, but the fact that Americans are not following them.

Why are Americans not following the guidelines? Part of the reason of course is that people's preferences skew toward less healthy foods so they simply do not want to follow the guidelines. However, people do not like being overweight, and more than half of American adults try to control their weight, spending a total of $50 billion on weight loss products and services each year (Weiss et al. 2006). This suggests that consumer demand for usable guidelines exists.

We argue that the MyPyramid guidelines have many features that make them difficult to use. Consider the information provided in the guideline: A consumer who obtains a customized USDA nutrition profile at www.mypyramid.gov might learn that she should consume five ounces of grains, one and a half cups of fruits, two cups of vegetables, three cups of milk, and five ounces of meats and beans every day. We suggest that there are at least four major factors that will make this guideline very difficult to use:

1. The consumer needs to go online to access the MyPyramid website for her customized recommendation.
2. After she has obtained her guideline, she must remember five different quantities in order to follow the guideline (with both the recommended amounts and units changing between the food groups).
3. She must also know how the foods she eats would be categorized, which for some foods like an apple or a steak is easy, but for other foods like lasagna or cheesecake is difficult.
4. And she must be able to keep track of how much food from each group she is eating over the course of a day.

Crawford (2009) has suggested that the complexity of the guideline is an impediment to its adoption in school settings, but we argue that the cognitive demands of the guideline are nearly prohibitive to all but the most committed adult consumer.

THE PRESENT RESEARCH: SIMPLIFYING THE USDA NUTRITION GUIDELINE

This analysis suggests that a simpler nutrition guideline could have considerable compliance advantages, but to our knowledge, this possibility has never been directly tested. Woolf and Nestle (2008, 263) argue that leading researchers have been making the same basic recommendation for years: "Eat less, move more, eat more fruits, vegetables and whole grains; and avoid junk food." Given such consensus, it seems at least possible that the USDA could offer a much simpler, more basic guideline.

Indeed, such a guideline has been developed. The simple "Half Plate" guideline urges consumers to "Fill half of your plate with fruits and vegetables at every meal." This message, which was developed by Porter Novelli, the same public relations firm that created MyPyramid, captures a key nutritional component of the more complex MyPyramid, which is that roughly half of one's diet should consist of fruits and vegetables. This particular guideline would seem to have considerable weight loss promise as it focuses attention on the two food groups that consumers most neglect (Cerully, Klein, and McCaul 2006). These food groups are low in energy density, and Ello-Martin, Roe, and Rolls (2004) have shown that eating these foods can be a particularly effective route to weight loss.

Given that the Half Plate guideline simplifies the key MyPyramid recommendation about the proportion of one's diet to devote to fruits and vegetables, we sought to compare it in the present research to the MyPyramid guideline on several dimensions of consumer response. In two studies we show that the simpler guideline (1) is much easier to remember, (2) is more motivating, and (3) leads to healthier food choices. It is probably not surprising that the MyPyramid guideline will be harder to remember than the simple Half Plate guideline. But it might be surprising just how much harder it is to remember, and we investigate this in our first study. Our first study also examines whether or not people feel more motivated to follow the Half Plate guideline than the MyPyramid guideline. In Study 2, we examine whether the Half Plate guideline leads to healthier choices. More detail on these and other studies is available in Ratner and Riis (2009).

Study 1: USDA's MyPyramid Versus Half Plate—Memory and Motivation

In this study, participants were randomly assigned to see either the MyPyramid guideline or the Half Plate guideline. Participants in the MyPyramid condition were directed to a screen in which they entered their age, sex, and typical amount of daily exercise—as required on the USDA website—in order to receive their

MyPyramid customized guideline. Participants then saw the same recommended numbers and units for each of five food categories that they would have seen if they had gone to the actual www.mypyramid.gov website (e.g., six ounces of grains, one and a half cups of fruit). Participants in the Half Plate condition read the following nutrition tip: "Fill half of your plate with fruits and vegetables at every meal." Participants were instructed to take as much time as they needed to study the guideline they had seen so that they would be able to describe that guideline to someone else.

Participants next were asked to freely recall the guideline they had just seen. Finally, respondents answered a series of questions about the guideline, including how motivated they were to follow it, how beneficial it was, and how complex it seemed.

Two coders evaluated respondents' open-ended recall of the guideline immediately after exposure to it (98 percent agreement). Discrepancies were resolved by discussion. Only sixteen of the eighty-three respondents (19 percent) in the MyPyramid condition reported their guideline correctly (i.e., correctly recalled quantities and units for all five food categories) immediately after seeing it; twenty-seven respondents (32.5 percent) could recall only one or none of the five numbers in the MyPyramid guideline. In contrast, seventy-one of the eighty-four participants (85 percent) who were shown the Half Plate guideline were able to describe it correctly immediately after seeing it. These large memory differences occurred despite the fact that participants spent on average 30.3 seconds looking at the MyPyramid guideline and only 10.5 seconds looking at the Half Plate guideline $(F(1, 140) = 43.98, p < .0001)$.

Not only was the Half Plate guideline easier to recall, but participants also found it significantly more motivating than the MyPyramid guideline $(Ms = 4.87$ vs. 3.05, $F(1, 155) = 74.14, p < .0001)$, more beneficial $(Ms = 5.42$ vs. 4.90 $F(1, 155) = 5.81$, $p = .017)$, and less complex $(Ms = 1.54$ vs. 2.55, $F(1, 155) = 30.89, p < .0001)$.

From this study, we confirm that the MyPyramid guideline is much harder to remember than a simpler guideline such as Half Plate. We also see that the simpler guideline is preferred by the people who would be using it, which is noteworthy given that they might have found the simplified guideline too "dumbed down" compared to the more complex guideline. To test whether people remember the simpler guideline over a longer time delay and whether the simpler guideline leads people to make healthier food choices, we conducted the next study.

Study 2: USDA's MyPyramid Versus Half Plate—Meal Choice

Participants were randomly assigned to see either the Half Plate or MyPyramid guideline. As in Study 1, those assigned to the MyPyramid guideline entered their age, sex, and typical daily exercise before being presented with their actual MyPyramid personalized recommendation.

Approximately one month later, the participants returned to the lab and were asked to imagine they were at a cafeteria for dinner, on a mundane rather than special occasion, and to "choose six servings" from an eleven-item menu that contained single servings of various items. The menu included five items that were vegetables (e.g., roasted beets, sautéed spinach with garlic, tomato salad with cucumbers) or fruits (fruit salad) and six that were not (e.g., roasted chicken, broiled scallops, chocolate cake). Participants could choose any of the listed items, including as many servings as they wanted of any one item, for a total of six servings.

We were particularly interested in the amount of fruits and vegetables that people would consume following exposure to the two guidelines. We expected the memory and motivational advantages of the Half Plate guideline to lead to greater choice of fruits and vegetables in the Half Plate than MyPyramid condition, and this is indeed what we found. Participants selected more fruits and vegetables if they had been in the Half Plate ($M = 2.59$) than the MyPyramid ($M = 2.29$) condition ($F(1, 285) = 6.57$, $p = .01$). As in Study 1, there were large memory and motivational advantages for Half Plate as well. Approximately one month after exposure to the guideline, 62 percent of those in the Half Plate condition correctly reported that the guideline had recommended a 50 percent allocation to fruits and vegetables. Among those who had been in the MyPyramid condition, only 1 (.7 percent) of the 190 respondents was able to recall all five recommended quantities. As in Study 1, participants in the Half Plate condition felt more motivated than participants in the MyPyramid condition to adhere to the guideline ($Ms = 4.95$ vs. 3.14, $F(1, 376) = 151.08$, $p < .0001$). The Half Plate participants also felt that the guideline would benefit them more than the MyPyramid guideline ($Ms = 5.64$ vs. 4.90, $F(1, 376) = 29.04$, $p < .0001$).

IMPLICATIONS AND RECOMMENDATIONS

Our key recommendation is that the USDA should consider using a very simple guideline as the centerpiece of its consumer efforts. The MyPyramid guideline need not be abandoned, but its detailed recommendations should be deemphasized. We have pointed out several good features of the Half Plate guideline and have shown that thanks to its ease of recall, it does indeed lead consumers to make healthier, fruit-and-vegetable-focused choices and could thus be an effective tool in the fight against obesity and overweight.

The MyPyramid site does provide a lot of useful information and it is encouraging that thousands of people visit the site each day. We doubt, however, that it will be possible to educate enough people sufficiently on the specifics of their personalized guidelines for MyPyramid to play much of a role in reducing obesity. The basic icon is well recognized, even if most people do not make explicit efforts to follow it. But the consumer-facing part of any government effort to reduce obesity should be a simple, straightforward guideline that people can and do make explicit efforts to follow.

A version of Half Plate actually once appeared in the "Tips" section on the

MyPyramid site. We argue that rather than being buried in a column on the website, it could be the centerpiece of the site and indeed of all the government's nutritional communication campaigns.

With respect to product labels, we call for more original research experimenting with different kinds of labels to test the possibility that simple may be better. With respect to Nutrition Fact Panels, there is little evidence to suggest that the introduction of labels in 1994 has had a positive impact on obesity. Increasing the prominence of calorie information on the back of packages would be a possible approach. While early studies of calorie labeling in restaurants have shown little evidence of an effect, the grocery store setting may be more promising as people might make more calorie-sensitive choices when planning meals for the future rather than when choosing for immediate consumption (Trope and Liberman 2003).

In restaurant settings, if calorie labels prove to be insufficient to affect consumer choice, various kinds of calorie "promotions" could be attempted to capture consumer demand for weight loss. Schwartz et al. (2010) have shown that many consumers will, if asked, take smaller meal portions without price discounts in order to control their calorie consumption.

Further, the perverse effects of "low-fat" and "low-calorie" front-package health claims demonstrated by Wansink and Chandon (2006) suggest that explicit calorie labeling could backfire if people feel less guilty about eating foods that have lower calorie totals. But the front-package claims clearly have an impact, and here, too, experimentation may come up with ways to avoid such perverse effects.

As third-party labeling and rating systems become prominent, these will present another opportunity to help consumers make healthier choices. We would like to see research comparing complex versus simple rating systems; we suspect that consumers will respond better to simpler ratings. But the ratings, no matter how simple, need to guide consumers toward healthy choices. The controversy around the Smart Choices program is a reminder that not all simple advice is necessarily good advice. We encourage efforts to develop and evaluate advice that is both good and simple.

We believe that the Half Plate guideline is an example of good and simple advice. This guideline, if promoted, could do a better job than existing, complex guidelines to motivate people to eat more healthful, lower-calorie foods.

REFERENCES

Alba, Joseph W., J. Wesley Hutchinson, and John G. Lynch, Jr. 1991. "Memory and Decision Making." In *Handbook of Consumer Behavior*, ed. T.S. Robertson and H.H. Kassarjian, 1–49. Englewood Cliffs, NJ: Prentice Hall.

Bell, David E., Stacey J. Bell, and George L. Blackburn. 2004. "How Government Shaped the American Diet." Harvard Business School Note 504–064, November 24.

Britten, Patricia, Jackie Haven, and Carole A. Davis. 2006. "Consumer Research for Development of Educational Messages for the MyPyramid Food Guidance System." *Journal of Nutrition Education and Behavior*, 38 (6) (Suppl. S), S108–S123.

Cerully, Jennifer L., William M.P. Klein, and Kevin D. McCaul. 2006. "Lack of Acknowledgement of Fruit and Vegetable Recommendations Among Nonadherent Individuals: Associations with Information Processing and Cancer Cognitions." *Journal of Health Communications*, 11, 103–115.

Chiuve, Stephanie E., and Walter C. Willett. 2007. "The 2005 Food Guide Pyramid: An Opportunity Lost?" *Nature Clinical Practice Cardiovascular Medicine*, 4 (11), 610–620.

Crawford, Patricia. 2009. Presentation to the USDA Dietary Guidelines Advisory Committee Meeting 3. www.cnpp.usda.gov/Publications/DietaryGuidelines/2010/Meeting3/DGACMtg3-Minutes-final.pdf.

Davis, Carole A., Patricia Britten, and Esther F. Myers. 2001. "Past, Present, and Future of the Food Guide Pyramid." *Journal of the American Dietetic Association*, 101 (8), 881–885.

Downs, Julie S., George Loewenstein, and Jessica Wisdom. 2009. "Strategies for Promoting Healthier Food Choices." *American Economic Review*, 99 (2), 159–164.

Elbel, Brian, Rogan T. Kersh, Victoria L. Brescoll, and L. Beth Dixon. 2009. "The Influence of Calorie Labeling on Food Choice: A First Look from Low Income Communities." *Health Affairs*, 28(6): w1110–w21.

Ello-Martin, Julia, Liane S. Roe, and Barbara Rolls. 2004. "A Diet Reduced in Energy Density Results in Greater Weight Loss Than a Diet Reduced in Fat." *Obesity Research*, 12 (Suppl. S), A23–A23.

Finkelstein, Eric A., Justin G. Trogdon, Joel W. Cohen, and William Dietz. 2009. "Annual Medical Spending Attributable to Obesity: Payer- and Service-Specific Estimates." *Health Affairs*, 28, w822–w831.

Flegal, Katherine M., Margaret D. Carroll, Cynthia L. Ogden, and Clifford L. Johnson. 2002. "Prevalence and Trends in Obesity Among US Adults, 1999–2000." *Journal of the American Medical Association*, 288 (14), 1723–1727.

Goldberg, Jeanne P., Marha A. Belury, Peggy Elam, Susan Calvert Finn, Dayle Hayes, Roseann Lyle, Sachiko St. Jeor, Michelle Warren, and Jennifer P. Hellwig. 2004. "The Obesity Crisis: Don't Blame It on the Pyramid." *Journal of the American Dietetic Association*, 104 (7), 1141–1147.

Gourville, John T. 2006. "Eager Sellers and Stony Buyers: Understanding the Psychology of New Product Adoption." *Harvard Business Review*, 84 (6), 98–106.

Heath, Chip, and Dan Heath. 2007. *Made to Stick: Why Some Ideas Survive and Others Die.* New York: Random House.

Iyengar, Sheena S., and Marc Lepper. 2000. "When Choice Is Demotivating: Can One Desire Too Much of a Good Thing?" *Journal of Personality and Social Psychology*, 79, 995–1006.

Keller, Kevin L., and Richard Staelin. 1987. "Effects of Quality and Quantity of Information on Decision Effectiveness." *Journal of Consumer Research*, 14, 200–213.

Kennedy, Eileen. 2008. "Food Rating Systems, Diet Quality, and Health." *Nutrition Reviews*, 66 (1), 21–22.

Krebs-Smith, Susan M., and Penny Kris-Etherton. 2007. "How Does MyPyramid Compare to Other Population-Based Recommendations for Controlling Chronic Disease?" *Journal of the American Dietetic Association*, 107 (5), 830–837.

Kreuter, Matthew W., Laura K. Brennan, Darcell P. Scharff, and Susan N. Lukwago. 1997. "Do Nutrition Label Readers Eat Healthier Diets? Behavioral Correlates of Adults' Use of Food Labels." *American Journal of Preventive Medicine*, 13 (4), 277–283.

Levy, Alan S., and Sara B. Fein. 1998. "Consumers' Ability to Perform Tasks Using Nutrition Labels." *Journal of Nutrition Education*, 30 (4), 210–217.

Lynch, John G., and Thomas K. Srull. 1982. "Memory and Attentional Factors in Consumer Choice: Concepts and Research Methods." *Journal of Consumer Research*, 15, 225–233.

Marois, René, and Jason Ivanoff. 2005. "Capacity Limits of Information Processing in the Brain." *Trends in Cognitive Science*, 9 (6), 296–305.

Moorman, Christine. 1996. "A Quasi Experiment to Assess the Consumer and Informational Determinants of Nutrition Information Processing Activities: The Case of the Nutrition Labeling and Education Act." *Journal of Public Policy and Marketing*, 15, 28–44.

Nestle, Marion. 1998. "In Defense of the USDA Food Guide Pyramid." *Nutrition Today*, 33 (5), 189.

Neuman, William. 2009a. "For Your Health, Froot Loops." *New York Times*, September 5. www.nytimes.com/2009/09/05/business/05smart.html.

———. 2009b. "Food Label Program to Suspend Operations." *New York Times*, October 23. www.nytimes.com/2009/10/24/business/24food.html.

Olshansky, S. Jay, Douglas J. Passaro, Ronald C. Hershow, Jennifer Layden, Bruce A. Carnes, Jacob Brody, Leonard Hayflick, Robert N. Butler, David B. Allison, and David S. Ludwig. 2005. "A Potential Decline in Life Expectancy in the United States in the 21st Century." *New England Journal of Medicine*, 352 (11), 1138–1145.

Parker-Pope, Tara. 2009. "A Makeover for Food Labels." *New York Times*, December 7. http://well.blogs.nytimes.com/2009/12/07/a-makeover-for-food-labels/.

Ratner, Rebecca, and Jason Riis. 2009. "What Good Is a Guideline If People Can't Remember It? An Analysis of the MyPyramid Food Guidance System." In preparation.

Sacks, Frank M., George A. Bray, Vincent J. Carey, Steven R. Smith, Donna H. Ryan, Stephen D. Anton, Katherine McManus, Catherine M. Champagne, Louise M. Bishop, Nancy Laranjo, Meryl S. Leboff, Jennifer C. Rood, Lilian de Jonge, Frank L. Greenway, Catherine M. Loria, Eva Obarzanek, and Donald A. Williamson. 2009. "Comparison of Weight-Loss Diets with Different Compositions of Fat, Protein, and Carbohydrates." *New England Journal of Medicine*, 360 (9), 859–873.

Schwartz, Janet, Jason Riis, Brian Elbel, and Dan Ariely. 2010. "Would You Like to Downsize That Meal? A Nudge Towards Smaller Portions Is More Effective Than Calorie Labeling in Reducing Calorie Consumption in Fast Food Meals." Working paper, Duke University.

Thompson, Debora V., Rebecca W. Hamilton, and Roland T. Rust. 2005. "Feature Fatigue: When Product Capabilities Become Too Much of a Good Thing." *Journal of Marketing Research*, 42, 431–442.

Trope, Yaacov, and Nira Liberman. 2003. "Temporal Construal." *Psychological Review*, 110, 403–421.

Variyam, Jayachandran N. 2008. "Do Nutrition Labels Improve Dietary Outcomes?" *Health Economics*, 17 (6), 695–708.

Wansink, Brian, and Pierre Chandon. 2006. "Can 'Low-Fat' Nutrition Labels Lead to Obesity?" *Journal of Marketing Research*, 43 (4), 605–617.

Wansink, Brian, Stephen T. Sonka, and Claire M. Hasler. 2004. "Front-Label Health Claims: When Less Is More." *Food Policy*, 29 (6), 659–667.

Weiss, Edward C., Deborah A. Galuska, Laura Kettel Khan, and Mary K. Serdula. 2006. "Weight-Control Practices Among U.S. Adults, 2001–2002." *American Journal of Preventive Medicine*, 31 (1), 18–24.

Woolf, Steven H., and Marion Nestle. 2008. "Do Dietary Guidelines Explain the Obesity Epidemic?" *American Journal of Preventive Medicine*, 34 (3), 263–265.

CHAPTER 19

SHRINKING LIBERTY TO COMBAT EXPANDING WAISTLINES

PETER A. UBEL

As has been widely reported, people in most developed countries are getting increasingly fat (Thoms 2007; Tuckman 2003; Wang and Beydoun 2007). Obesity is spreading like an epidemic (Christakis and Fowler 2007). While the consequences of this epidemic are not completely known, some problems are already evident. Obesity leads to many serious health problems, including heart disease, sleep apnea, degenerative arthritis, and diabetes. Those people who have diabetes from obesity must worry about suffering from its complications, which include blindness, kidney failure, and stroke (U.S. Department of Health and Human Services 2001). Obesity also carries adverse social and economic consequences. Obese people earn less money than nonobese people and are less happy (Cawley 2004; Oswald and Powdthavee 2007; Zagorsky 2004). Finally, obesity is harmful to people who are not obese. Think of how much people suffer when their loved ones die prematurely because of obesity.

Given the increasing prevalence of obesity and the negative consequences of obesity, we need to ask ourselves what, if anything, governments should do to combat obesity. The goal of this chapter is to view the tension between libertarianism and paternalism through the lens of the obesity epidemic.

HARMING OTHERS THROUGH OBESITY

In considering what, if anything, society should do to combat obesity, we should consider who, if anyone, is being harmed by the epidemic. The best way to start is to examine whether obesity creates what economists call externalities—harms to third parties. When a factory dumps toxic waste into a river, this waste is an externality—it harms people downstream. Because free markets do not do a good job of preventing externalities from happening, even most libertarians agree that some kind of government intervention should be considered to contain or compensate the harms of externalities.

If obesity creates externalities, then a strong case can be made for combating obesity with public money and government power. For example, efforts to combat tobacco use have been strengthened, morally and politically, by evidence of the harms created by exposure to secondary smoke. Similarly, the regulation of alcohol is more defensible because of the harms of drunk driving.

What evidence is there that obesity creates externalities? For starters, some economists have argued that obesity creates financial burdens for nonobese people (Finkelstein, Ruhm, and Kosa 2005). For example, in the United States, health insurance companies do not typically charge more money to obese people. Since obese people are sicker than nonobese people and incur more health-care expenses, nonobese people essentially subsidize the health-care costs of obese people (Bhattacharya and Sood 2004). This externality is also relevant in countries with nationalized health insurance, where the greater health expenses of obese people are borne by the general public.

Obesity also creates externalities whenever life insurance companies fail to charge higher premiums to obese people. If life insurance premiums do not adequately account for the reduced life expectancy of obese people, then nonobese people will be forced to subsidize the life insurance costs of their obese peers.

Despite the insurance costs associated with obesity, it is not yet clear whether obesity, in total, creates financial burdens for nonobese people. For instance, by dying at younger ages, obese people draw less upon their old-age pensions. In addition, by dying young, they save money on health care in later years (Van Baal et al. 2008).

What about nonfinancial externalities? When an obese person gets sick or dies at a young age, friends and relatives suffer emotionally, and this suffering could be viewed as an externality. In addition, recent evidence suggests that obesity is socially contagious (Christakis and Fowler 2007). This contagion could be viewed as another externality—by gaining weight, an obese person has increased the likelihood that a close friend will also become obese. Obesity, according to this view, harms nonobese people by causing them to become obese.

Taken together, the case for regulating obesity—based on the externalities it creates—is weak. Obesity does not appear to be a tremendous financial burden to nonobese people. And if we believe the limited evidence that obesity is socially contagious, we cannot call that an externality unless we can convince ourselves that obesity harms those people who are obese.

To judge whether the government should intervene, in any manner, to combat the obesity epidemic, we need to explore whether obesity is harmful to those who become obese or simply, as some prominent libertarians argue, a harmless consequence of people's rational choices.

RATIONAL OBESITY

On the surface, obesity appears to be an obvious harm. Obesity causes people to experience pain, disability, and premature mortality. The existence of these harms, however, does not prove that obesity, on balance, harms obese people. We know, for instance, that snowboarding can lead to serious injury and even death, but it is still possible (even likely) that the benefits of snowboarding outweigh these harms. Indeed, some experts contend that obesity is largely a rational choice and therefore in people's best interests (Philipson and Posner 2003). If people enjoy Doritos and graham crackers, perhaps the benefits of such consumption (the pleasure of tasting these foods) outweigh the health effects of these foods. Indeed, among those experts who believe that consumers are largely rational most of the time, the choice to spend money on Coca Cola rather than orange juice merely reflects the behavior of people who are maximizing their best interests, in alignment with their individual preferences.

Writing in a Department of Agriculture publication called *Amber Waves*, a group of market enthusiasts opined that the expanding girth of the American populace "may be a rational response to changing technology and prices" (Kuchler et al. 2005). They point out that many people work in sedentary jobs, and therefore the only way for them to stay thin is to exercise (which many people do not enjoy) or to eat less (which is also unpleasant). They contend that people have decided that—with pills to lower their cholesterol and balloons to open their clogged arteries—obesity is not so much a health problem as it is a lifestyle choice, and an obese life, full of delicious foods and reclining chairs, is simply better than the alternative.

The more convinced we are that obesity is the result of rational choices—of people's freedom to pursue their individual versions of the good life—the less inclined we should be to call upon the government to combat obesity.

However, I am not convinced that people are as rational as some libertarians have claimed. As I explain below, I think obesity results in large part from unconscious decisions and from limited will power, meaning that most people with obesity have not maximized their happiness by becoming obese.

"DECIDING" TO BE OBESE

At the most basic level, obesity results from consuming more calories than one burns. Thus, theoretically people can control their body weight by adjusting how much they eat and exercise. With the cause of obesity so obvious (taking in too many calories) and the cure so apparent (eat less and exercise more), it is not surprising that rational choice theorists have called the word overweight a "misnomer" (Philipson and Posner 2003).

I do not consider obesity to be either rational or a choice. To begin with, the number of calories that people consume in a given day is a result of many unconscious factors. For example, one group of researchers convinced workers at a day-care center to vary the number of children that they placed around the snack table each day. The researchers observed the children and discovered that, as the number of children around the table increased, so too did their snack consumption (Lumeng and Hillman 2007). Studies of adults reveal the same finding (Clendenen, Herman, and Polivy 1994). When in large groups, people not only eat faster, but remain at the dinner table longer, too. As a result, the number of calories people consume at any given meal is not determined solely by their appetite or their caloric needs, but also influenced, unconsciously, by the social context of the meal.

The amount of food people eat is also influenced by a host of other unconscious forces. If people happen to select large dinner plates from the shelves rather than medium-sized plates, they will eat more food (Wansink 2006), because people tend to empty their plates of whatever food is placed upon them. Bigger plates lead to bigger meals.

Even the flavor of food can be influenced by unconscious forces. This finding was demonstrated by a group of marketing researchers who invited people into their research offices, purportedly to test the flavor of several crackers. The researchers portrayed one brand of crackers as having eleven grams of good fat and two grams of bad fat. They described the other brand as having two grams of good fat and eleven of bad. No matter which cracker they labeled as being high in good fat (and they varied which cracker was "healthy"), people described that healthy cracker as being less tasty (Raghunathan, Naylor, and Hoyer 2006).

A large portion of the calories people eat is not a result of rational deliberation. But that does not mean that people have no ability to control their intake. Many people are quite disciplined about their eating. If they gain weight, they will cut out desserts or eat smaller portion sizes for a while. Does that mean that those people who persist in being obese have chosen to remain obese? Or are they simply too weak to control their appetites?

SELF-CONTROL AND DISCOUNTING OF THE FUTURE

Some people are far more future-oriented than others. When deciding between a small short-term gain and a larger long-term one, they will wait for the long-term benefits. Given a choice between $10,000 today versus $15,000 in a year, these people will wait one year. Other people, by contrast, will opt for near-term gains. They will take the $10,000 right now.

Economists have a way of characterizing why some people would choose the early $10,000 and some would wait one year to receive $15,000. They contend that these people have different underlying preferences for immediate versus delayed consumption—they have different *discount rates*—the person willing to wait longer has a lower discount rate (Vuchinich and Simpson 1998).

Rationally speaking, then, obese people may simply have higher discount rates than nonobese people. They shrug off the risk of early mortality in favor of the more immediate joys of fatty food. Indeed, this view is supported by the fact that people with low incomes are typically more obese than those with higher incomes (Schoenborn 2002). People with low incomes, according to this logic, have less reason to care about their future than people with higher incomes.

In strict neoclassical economics, there is no such thing as an irrational discount rate. In holding this open-minded view, in fact, economists hark back to the philosopher David Hume, who famously wrote: "'Tis not contrary to reason to prefer the destruction of the whole world to the scratching of my finger" (1739). Less eloquent shades of this view can be seen in Becker, Grossman, and Murphy's theory of rational addiction; they write: "This paper relies on a weak concept of rationality that does not rule out strong discounts of future events" (1991).

The problem with this kind of discount rate agnosticism, however, is that it ignores the role that self-control problems play in people's near- versus long-term behaviors. Imagine you are choosing between receiving $100 in one year or $110 in one year and one day. If you are like most people, you will choose the larger sum of money, figuring that a 10 percent increase is a nice reward for waiting just one day. Now consider a different choice, between receiving $100 today and $110 tomorrow. In this situation, the majority of people choose the *smaller* sum of money (Laibson 1997). Most people are willing to wait one day in the distant future to make $10, but they are not willing to do that today. They have a high discount rate in the short run and a low one in the long run. Which of these discount rates reflects their true preferences? Can we even talk about rational discount rates when people are so inconsistent?

Indeed, these inconsistencies raise what I call, to paraphrase Matthew Rabin and Ted O'Donoghue, "the March 1st problem" (O'Donoghue and Rabin 2007). If you ask me on January 1 what I hope to do on March 1, I will tell you that I hope to exercise, eat well, be patient with my kids, be efficient at work, and watch no more than thirty minutes of TV. If you ask me the same question on January 2, or February 3, or February 15, I will give you the same answer. I have strong feelings about how I want to behave on March 1, and those feelings exist every day of the year—until March 1 arrives, when I blow off exercise, stuff down a triple-cheeseburger, snap at my kids, surf the web at work instead of rewriting this article, and zone out in front of an NBA match-up between two teams I do not even care about. By March 2, I not only regret what I did on March 1, but I plan tomorrow and the next day and indeed next year on March 1 to behave better.

Which self deserves priority? The one that reigns one day a year, on March 1, or the one that states its preferences the other 364 days?

INTERNALITIES

Social psychology research has demonstrated that people have limited ability to control their impulses. When people are tired or unhappy or hungry, their self-control declines. For instance, researchers have given people brief tasks that require them to exert will power—such as writing down any thought that comes to mind but doing their best, during this writing time, not to think about white bears. Then the researchers give these same people another task—such as asking them to solve an unsolvable puzzle. People who have spent energy trying not to think about white bears give up faster at their next task, compared to people who performed the writing task without having to shut white bears out of their minds (Baumeister et al. 1998).

According to the rational choice view, poor people have high obesity rates because they have less to live for and therefore have chosen to pursue near-term over long-term gains. Research on will power suggests a more plausible alternative: poor people face more daily stress than other people, and this stress depletes their available reserves of will power.

Drawing upon the long history of work in externalities, behavioral economists have begun referring to self-control problems as "internalities" (Herrnstein et al. 1993). If your short-term self decides to gorge on a pint of ice cream, then it is harming your long-term self. The short-term self gets all the benefits—the pleasures of a full belly and a tasty dessert, while the long-term self bears all the harmful consequences—the clogged arteries and the worn-out joints.

In situations involving externalities, most people think that government regulation or intrusion is justified. The government can tax companies for polluting, to give them an incentive to reduce pollution. Or they can regulate the quantity of particles they can emit from any given chimney. For the same reason that the government can intrude to reduce the harms brought upon people by externalities, many of us who work in behavioral economics believe the government should act to reduce the harms brought upon people by internalities.

THE CONDITIONS FOR GOVERNMENT INVOLVEMENT

When should the government get involved in people's daily lives? One reason would be if there are important externalities involved, harms that befall the general public because of something that given individuals are doing. Arguably, a second reason government should get involved is to fight internalities. People do not always make the rational decisions they would strive to make. And they do not control many of the impulses they would like to control. This creates harm to their own selves, internalities, that the government may have a legitimate role in fighting.

I have briefly argued that obesity creates internalities. As a result, we should consider the pros and cons of the government intervening to combat obesity. In doing this, we need to ask a question—can government improve this situation? It is important to explore what the government's options are when combating obesity, and weigh the likely costs and benefits of these various alternatives, before deciding if any of these alternatives are justified.

At the paternalistic extreme, governments could decide to use the full powers of their coercion to enforce appropriate body weight among their citizens. The government could combat the obesity epidemic by jailing people once they became overweight, by denying them retirement or health benefits, or by taking away their right to vote. Such policies, of course, would be a ludicrous way to combat obesity. We all recognize that obesity is not the kind of problem that warrants the activation of a police state.

Closer to the libertarian extreme, governments could decide to eliminate any activities they currently engage in that distort food markets and thereby contribute to the obesity epidemic. For example, the U.S. government offers farm subsidies to corn growers, thereby reducing the price of high-fructose corn syrup, the main sweetener in products like cereal and soda pop. I think that such subsidies should be phased out, at a rate that does not create sudden crises in farming communities. I see no moral justification for these subsidies and in fact think that they cause real moral harms. I recognize that farmers and their communities will ultimately suffer from the loss of these subsidies, just as any group suffers when it loses government support. I also recognize the difficulty of overcoming powerful lobbying interests, including the powerful influence that Iowa primary voters have over American presidential politics. Nevertheless, I hope that these subsidies can be reduced, because public support for these subsidies is waning.

But eliminating these subsidies alone will not do much to reduce obesity. Millions of years of evolutionary programming stand in the way of such easy progress.

EVOLUTION AND DIETING

Only 5 percent of people who try to lose weight manage to do so in a sustained manner (Kolata 2007). This extremely low success rate is not merely the fault of calorie imbalance, laziness, or weak wills. Instead, it is a result of mixing dieting with evolution. To understand how evolution has conspired against diet success, consider our time as hunters and gatherers, living out on the tundra under constant threat of starvation (Polivy and Herman 2006). In times of plenty, our ancestors would gorge themselves on their kill, storing the meat in their fat cells rather than letting it rot on the bone. In between successful hunts, however, it was important to stave off starvation. Consequently, evolution favored those individuals who could conserve energy and thereby hold on to the calories they had already consumed. Dieters will recognize the unfortunate result of these evolutionary pressures. When they diet, they do not seem to lose as much weight as they are supposed to.

Consider what dieters have been told by their doctors, or what they have heard on television, about the tiny changes that influence how much people weigh. Weight gain, they have been told, can result from a handful of extra crackers a day, those fifty extra calories adding up over the years to thousands of calories. If this is true, they are told, then the flip side should hold: if they simply cut out a few crackers a day, they will lose weight.

In response to such exhortations, people eliminate crackers from their diet, but nothing happens. They cut out snacks, but lose nary a pound. They drop one of their three daily meals, and they *still* do not lose weight. The poor dieters do not know what to think. The calorie in/calorie out theory does not seem to fit their experience.

Dieters have every right to bemoan their caloric struggles, because evolutionary pressures have made human beings into prolific hoarders of calories. When we diet, our bodies respond as they did back on the tundra when our seasonal food supplies dwindled. They go into starvation mode. To cope with this seeming starvation, our evolutionary programming kicks in to slow down our metabolism. We might drop our calorie intake by 10 percent and still not lose any weight, because our metabolism has dropped by the same amount.

To lose substantial weight, then, requires an even bigger drop in consumption. That will take enormous willpower, however, because our evolutionary programming—which, remember, thinks we are starving—has also tweaked our brain chemistry to fixate our attention on finding food. This programming was quite helpful in our tundra days, of course. But it backfires in a world where food is easy to come by. As a result of this programming, dieters obsess about food. They even experience a shift in their dietary preferences. A sugary meal that before their diet would have struck them as cloying will now taste great.

When evolving on the tundra, no survival advantages accrued to people who were good at losing weight. Humans did not evolve to be successful dieters. On the contrary, as evolutionary psychologists Polivy, Herman et al. put it, "Dieting is precisely the sort of threat that we have evolved to combat" (1993).

BACK TO POLICY OPTIONS

It is important to keep these evolutionary forces in mind when we consider the costs and benefits of policy alternatives. Consider, for example, some less coercive (but nevertheless paternalistic) options that governments could pursue to combat obesity. Governments could combat obesity by creating financial incentives to influence behavior. The government could offer tax rebates to people with healthy body weights, much the way health insurers offer rebates to people who do not smoke. It could subsidize healthy foods, or tax unhealthy ones, in order to encourage people to eat more wisely. Or it could subsidize the cost of fitness centers, and of transportation to and from such centers, for low-income people whose neighborhoods are not suitable for outdoor exercise.

Financial incentives like these, when not too extreme, are a soft form of paternalism (Ubel 2009). They influence people's behavior without restricting their options. (Of course, when people are poor or when the financial penalty is steep, such incentives can be quite coercive.) Financial incentives also take account of people's rational and irrational natures. If people were completely rational, they would not need to be dissuaded from fatty food (or cigarettes) through taxes. And if they were completely irrational, such financial incentives would not have any effect on their behavior!

Another approach strikes me as reasonable: to use government resources to make fruits and vegetables more affordable for people in low-income neighborhoods. For example, the New York City government announced in 2007 that it was hoping to pass "green cart legislation" to increase the number of food carts offering fresh fruits and vegetables to residents of low-income neighborhoods ("Mayor Bloomberg"

2007). Most New Yorkers did not perceive this policy as an example of unacceptable government coercion. I, nevertheless, would like to see good evidence that such a program actually benefits people before making it a permanent part of the budget. Given what I have written above about the challenge of fighting obesity, I am skeptical that the mere presence of affordable apples will reduce people's inclination to grab a box of Chicken McNuggets.

A third and even less coercive approach would influence obesity rates through information: the government would regulate industries so that consumers received consistent and explicit information about the products they buy. This informational approach often puts libertarians in an awkward position. They are opposed to government bureaucracy and thus instinctively oppose any regulations that would require the makers of consumer goods to give information to consumers. They would argue that governments should not intrude by forcing McDonald's to display the number of calories in a Big Mac or requiring manufacturers to tell consumers how many grams of trans fat there are in a frozen dinner. Such regulations restrict market liberty and create expenses for food manufacturers. Libertarians find this coercive and objectionable.

On the other hand, libertarian philosophy is based in large part on the moral value of letting people make informed choices about their lives. And how can people make such choices if companies are not willing to provide information about their products? Indeed, one could argue that Food and Drug Administration food label regulations in the United States have made the food market more like a true free market by arming consumers with information that they can use to make purchasing choices.

Along these lines, New York City has implemented a new policy requiring chain restaurants to prominently display caloric information on their menus and menu boards ("Board of Health" 2007). This regulation, opposed strongly by chain restaurants when first proposed, aims to help consumers decide how much food they really want to consume.

I expect that many people are comfortable using the power of regulation to give consumers helpful information. I am skeptical, however, that such information will have a substantial impact on people's decisions. Dry, numeric information about calorie counts simply cannot compete with glossy pictures of juicy burgers.

That suggests a fourth approach that policy-makers could take—leading consumers to make better choices not through incentives or coercion, but through emotional or even unconscious psychological forces (Thaler and Sunstein 2008). Such an approach would go beyond tedious statistical displays of data about carbohydrates and fat calories to labeling food with evocative images that create aversions to food that are not healthy. Think how effective the skull-and-crossbones label has been in keeping people from ingesting poisonous materials. The word "poison," in large font, would never have had as much impact as that picture. If we want to discourage Burger King customers from ordering Whoppers and encourage them to eat the healthier items on the menu, we need to appeal not only to their intellect, but also to their emotions.

The government can play the role of persuader rather than rely only on coercion. In doing so, it should take advantage of what behavioral scientists have learned about human nature. We know that a dry appeal to the rational risks of smoking did not stop most adolescents from lighting up. Far more effective was the Truth Campaign, an uninformative ad campaign that played off teenagers' emotions by appealing to their suspicion that adults at tobacco companies are trying to manipulate them. If experts are convinced about what is in people's best interest, they should find persuasive ways to convince people to behave accordingly.

HELPING THE NEXT GENERATION

Given my nihilism about the government's ability to help obese people lose weight, I believe the most promising options will focus on reducing the chance that nonobese people will become obese. Our goal as a society should be to create environments in which people do not get obese in the first place (Hayne, Moran, and Ford 2004). We should work to create neighborhoods and park systems that make it easy for people to get outside and walk or play. We should encourage employers to create opportunities for employees to exercise during working hours. And we should exert most of our efforts toward children—to find ways to prevent the next generation from supersizing itself.

In targeting our efforts at children, we need to assess whether changes in school lunch programs and gym classes help kids develop healthier habits. No simple jiggering of the school lunch menu will take care of childhood obesity. We should pour funding into research on how to use the schools to develop healthy habits among children and their parents. And if we find successful ways to do so, we should set up strong incentives for local school programs to implement these techniques.

CONCLUSION

In touching upon the topic of obesity, I have tried to lay out some fundamental issues that help societies deliberate about how to set the proper balance between liberty and well-being. Obesity threatens the well-being of society. Obesity results from many forces, including not only people's deliberate decisions about how much to eat and exercise, but also many unconscious forces that influence these same habits, as well as limitations of self-control that hinder people's abilities to pursue their own best interests.

Given the harms of obesity, societies ought to explore a range of policies that offers a chance of reducing the toll obesity takes on their citizens.

REFERENCES

Baumeister, Roy F., Ellen Bratslavsky, Mark Muraven, and Dianne M. Tice. 1998. "Ego Depletion: Is the Active Self a Limited Resource?" *Journal of Personality and Social Psychology*, 74 (5), 1252–1265.

Becker, Gary S., Michael Grossman, and Kevin M. Murphy. 1991. "Rational Addiction and the Effect of Price on Consumption." *American Economic Review*, 81 (2), 237–241.

Bhattacharya, Jay, and Neeraj Sood. 2004. "Health Insurance, Obesity, and Its Economic Costs." *The Economics of Obesity: A Report on the Workshop Held at USDA's Economic Research Service*. Washington, DC: Economic Research Service, USDA.

"Board of Health Votes to Invite Public Comment on New Calorie Listing Proposal for Chain Restaurants." 2007. Press Release, New York City Department of Health and Mental Hygiene, www.nyc.gov/html/doh/html/pr2007/pr089-07.shtml.

Cawley, John. 2004. "The Impact of Obesity on Wages." *Journal of Human Resources*, 39 (2), 451–474.

Christakis, Nicholas A., and James H. Fowler. 2007. "The Spread of Obesity in a Large Social Network Over 32 Years." *New England Journal of Medicine*, 357 (4), 370–379.

Clendenen, Vanessa I., C. Peter Herman, and Janet Polivy. 1994. "Social Facilitation of Eating Among Friends and Strangers." *Appetite*, 23, 1–13.

Finkelstein, Eric, Christopher J. Ruhm, and Katherine M. Kosa. 2005. "Economic Causes and Consequences of Obesity." *Annual Review of Public Health*, 26, 238–257.

Hayne, Cheryl, Patricia A. Moran, and Mary M. Ford. 2004. "Regulating Environments to Reduce Obesity." *Journal of Public Health Policy*, 25 (3–4), 391–407.

Herrnstein, Richard J., George F. Lowenstein, Drazen Prelec, and William Vaughan Jr. 1993. "Utility Maximization and Melioration: Internalities in Individual Choice." *Journal of Behavioral Decision Making*, 6, 149–185.

Hume, David. 1739. *A Treatise of Human Nature*. London: Penguin.

Kolata, Gina. 2007. *Rethinking Thin: The New Science of Weight Loss—And the Myths and Realities of Dieting*. New York: Farrar, Straus & Giroux.

Kuchler, Fred, Elise Golan, Jayachandran N. Variyam, and Stephen R. Curtchfield. 2005. "Obesity Policy and the Law of Unintended Consequences." *Amber Waves*, June.

Laibson, David. 1997. "Golden Eggs and Hyperbolic Discounting." *Quarterly Journal of Economics*, 62, 443–477.

Lumeng, Julie C., and Katherine H. Hillman. 2007. "Eating In Larger Group Increases Food Consumption." *Archives of Disease in Childhood*, 92(5), 384–387.

"Mayor Bloomberg and Speaker Quinn Announce Green Cart Legislation to Improve Access to Fresh Fruits and Vegetables in Neighborhoods With Greatest Need." 2007. News from the Blue Room, www.nyc.gov/portal/site/nycgov/menuitem.c0935b9a57b-b4ef3daf2f1c701c789a0/index.jsp?pageID=mayor_press_release&catID=1194&doc_name=http%3A%2F%2Fwww.nyc.gov%2Fhtml%2Fom%2Fhtml%2F2007b%2Fpr467-07.html&cc=unused1978&rc=1194&ndi=1.

O'Donoghue, Ted, and Matthew Rabin. 2007. "Incentives and Self-Control." In *Advances in Economics and Econometrics: Theory and Applications*, ed. Richard Blundell, Whitney Newey, and Torsten Persson, 215–245. Cambridge, UK: Cambridge University Press.

Oswald, Andrew, and Nattavudh Powdthavee. 2007. "Obesity, Unhappiness, and the Challenge of Affluence: Theory and Evidence." Bonn, Germany: Institute for the Study of Labor.

Philipson, Thomas J., and Richard A. Posner. 2003. "The Long-Run Growth in Obesity as a Function of Technological Change." *Perspectives in Biology & Medicine*, 46 (3), S87–S107.

Polivy, Janet, and C. Peter Herman. 2006. "An Evolutionary Perspective on Dieting." *Appetite*, 47 (1), 30–35.

Raghunathan, Rajagopal, Rebecca W. Naylor, and Wayne D. Hoyer. 2006. "The Unhealthy = Tasty Intuition and Its Effects on Taste Inferences, Enjoyment, and Choice of Food Products." *Journal of Marketing*, 70 (4), 170–184.

Schoenborn, Charlotte A. 2002. "Body Weight Status of Adults: United States, 1997–98." *Advance Data*, 330, 1–15.

Thaler, Richard R., and Cass R. Sunstein. 2008. *Nudge: Improving Decisions About Health, Wealth and Happiness*. New Haven, CT: Yale University Press.

Thoms, Jessica. 2007. "Global Obesity: A BIG Disease Is Growing." *Faces*, 23 (7), 22–25.

Tuckman, Jo. 2003. "U.S. Lifestyles Blamed for Obesity Epidemic Sweeping Mexico: Latin American Countries Succumb to Fast Food and Sedentary Behaviour." *Guardian*, August 11. www.guardian.co.uk/world/2003/aug/11/foodanddrink.mexico.

Ubel, Peter. 2009. *Free Market Madness: Why Human Nature Is at Odds with Economics—and Why It Matters*. Boston: Harvard Business Press.

U.S. Department of Health and Human Services. 2001. "The Surgeon General's Call to Action to Prevent and Decrease Overweight and Obesity." U.S. Department of Health and Human Services, Public Health Service, Office of the Surgeon General. Rockville, MD.

van Baal, Pieter H.M., Johan J. Polder, G. Ardine de Wit, Rudolf T. Hoogenveen, Talitha L. Feenstra, Hendriek C. Boshuizen, Peter M. Engelfriet, and Werner B.F. Brouwer. 2008. "Lifetime Medical Costs of Obesity: Prevention No Cure for Increasing Health Expenditure." *Public Library of Science*, 5 (2), e29.

Vuchinich, Rudy E., and Cathy A. Simpson. 1998. "Hyperbolic Temporal Discounting in Social Drinkers and Problem Drinkers." *Experimental and Clinical Psychopharmacology*, 6, 292–305.

Wang, Youfa, and May A. Beydoun. 2007. "The Obesity Epidemic in the United States—Gender, Age, Socioeconomic, Racial/Ethnic, and Geographic Characteristics: A Systematic Review and Meta-Regression Analysis." *Epidemiologic Reviews*, 29, 6–28.

Wansink, Brian. 2006. *Mindless Eating: Why We Eat More Than We Think*. New York: Bantam.

Zagorsky, Jay L. 2004. "Is Obesity as Dangerous to Your Wealth as to Your Health?" *Research on Aging*, 26 (1), 130–152.

CONTROLLING OBESITY: LESSONS LEARNED FROM TOBACCO CONTROL AND TOBACCO MARKETING RESEARCH

BARBARA LOKEN, K. VISWANATH, AND
MELANIE A. WAKEFIELD

During the past twenty-five years, the proportion of overweight and obese adults and children worldwide has increased at an alarming rate, leading to calls for renewed research and funding to address and reduce this trend. In the United States, according to the Centers for Disease Control and Prevention in 2008 (CDC 2008), thirty-two states had obesity prevalence rates greater than 25 percent and only one state (Colorado) had an obesity prevalence of less than 20 percent. In fact, in the United States, the magnitude of the obesity threat to public health has led to calls for a national comprehensive prevention program similar to the strategies used in tobacco control (Emery et al. 2007). Recently, the National Cancer Institute (NCI 2008) published a monograph titled *The Role of the Media in Promoting and Reducing Tobacco Use*, which synthesized the scientific literature on media communications in tobacco promotion and tobacco control, bridging disciplines of marketing, psychology, communications, statistics, epidemiology, and public health. The monograph is comprehensive in scope and represents the work of numerous scientific editors, authors, and external peer reviewers. Given the long history of research and evaluation of tobacco control campaigns and the successes in reducing tobacco use in many countries, key lessons and conclusions from this distillation of research on tobacco control can be useful for researchers and policy-makers in other areas of public health, such as obesity.

In this chapter, we derive a few of these lessons from conclusions of the NCI monograph on tobacco. These lessons are particular to media communications, but extend beyond the impact of persuasive communications experiments, addressed in other chapters of this volume. The media communications addressed in the NCI monograph include forces both promoting tobacco use (e.g., marketing by the tobacco industry) and reducing tobacco use (e.g., media use in public health campaigns), as well as the role of news and entertainment media, public relations efforts, and tobacco industry media efforts to influence tobacco control media and ballot initiatives.

The prevention of tobacco use and the prevention of obesity have many common elements. One common denominator is the clear effect on health behaviors and increased risk of numerous life-threatening diseases from both cigarette smoking and behaviors associated with obesity. Also common to both tobacco control and obesity control policy is the importance of reducing risks to children and youth (Bauman 2004; Economes et al. 2007; NCI 2008). The need to curb tobacco use and obesity during the developmental years is critical to long-range success in curbing smoking and obesity and highlights the importance of role models and development of normative behaviors and expectations in promoting healthy rather than unhealthy behaviors. Prevention of cigarette smoking and prevention of obesity are also similar in the dominance of many of the relevant industries and in the prevalence of marketing dollars devoted to competitor behaviors. Many of the tobacco and food industries have sizable budgets that dwarf the budgets of public health media campaigns (French, Story, and Jeffrey 2001; NCI 2008). Another common element for both tobacco control and obesity control is the importance of long-range campaigns across entire populations as well as specialty programs for key segments of high-risk populations.

Five lessons learned from the NCI monograph will be discussed in this chapter: (1) understanding the effectiveness of mass media campaigns and the role of multicomponent community campaigns, (2) understanding the relative exposure of health-related versus non–health-related marketing messages, (3) understanding the effectiveness of message content and message type, (4) determining the role of news and entertainment media, and (5) evaluating partnerships with industry and understanding corporate social responsibility initiatives.

EFFECTIVENESS OF MASS MEDIA CAMPAIGNS

Mass Media Campaigns Can Be Effective

The NCI monograph (NCI 2008, Chapter 12) reviewed findings from both field experiments (twenty-five studies for youth smoking, thirty-nine studies for adult smoking) and population studies of state and national tobacco control mass media campaigns (fifty-two cross-sectional and five longitudinal studies) in which media were a major component, to determine their overall effectiveness. These studies were conducted by numerous investigators in many countries (e.g., Biglan et al. 2000; Farrelly et al. 2005; Flay et al. 1995; Flynn et al. 1997; Hafstad et al. 1997; Meshack et al. 2004; Perry et al. 1992; Slater et al. 2006; Vartiainen et al. 1998). The most frequently used medium for conveying antismoking messages was television, but radio, print, and billboards were also frequently used. Further, media were often combined with other components such as school and community programs. As described in the NCI monograph, overall, studies of campaign effectiveness show evidence for changes in youth smoking attitudes, reductions in smoking uptake, and progress in adult cessation.

So the good news is that public health campaigns can work, as observed by others across several public health domains (Hornik 2002). While there is considerable variability in the success of past physical activity (e.g., Cavill and Bauman 2004) and nutrition (Matson-Koffman et al. 2005) campaigns, both the research on tobacco control and the successes of recent obesity campaigns, such as the CDC's VERB campaign (Berkowitz et al. 2008; Huhman et al. 2007) are encouraging and highlight some of the essential components that are needed for a successful campaign.

Mass Media Work Best When Combined With Other Community Components

Reviews of literature on tobacco control campaigns (NCI 2008, Chapters 11 and 12) suggest that comprehensive programs, in which a variety of community-wide programs are engaged, often yield more success than media-alone campaigns. For example, the controlled field experiments for youth and adults indicated that media programs were generally effective and that they tended to be most effective in the context of more comprehensive campaigns that also included other components. Some of these field experiments showed a dose-response relationship between an increased number of program components and smoking reduction. A comprehensive campaign, analogous to integrative marketing communications approaches but more extensive in outreach, is more likely to provide consistent messages and sufficient exposure in multiple contexts within the community (e.g., leisure, workplace, and/ or school) in multiple forms, and sufficient exposure across time may be needed in order to produce sizable and significant population effects. While evaluations of nutrition and physical activity campaigns that include mass media alone are scarce, the evidence currently available seems to suggest, similar to evidence from tobacco control campaigns, that a multicomponent approach may work best (Cavill and Bauman 2004; Kahn et al. 2002). The VERB campaign uses commercial marketing techniques and a sizable advertising budget to achieve its objectives of increasing physical activities in children ages nine to thirteen, combining this extensive media reach with community-level programs (Huhman et al. 2007). A second-year campaign evaluation of VERB revealed sizable exposure rates, significant population levels of physical activity (among youth), and evidence for a dose-response relationship between campaign exposure and behavioral change (i.e., greater amounts of exposure were associated with greater amounts of behavioral change).

The importance of multicomponent programs is also evidenced by the success in both nutrition and physical activity research of environmental "prompts" at the point of purchase or point of choice. Literature reviews of signs labeling healthy choices in supermarkets, restaurants, and vending machines, and signs in shopping malls urging people to use the stairs instead of the elevators, show these prompts to be generally effective in promoting behavioral change, at least in the short term (French, Story, and Jeffery 2001; Marcus et al. 2006; Matson-Koffman et al. 2005). Research also indicates that nutrition campaigns are more effective when environmental changes facilitate nutritious food choices (e.g., by making fruits and vegetables readily available; Matson-Koffman et al. 2005; Pomerleau et al. 2005; Snyder 2007). Research is unclear about whether campaigns are more effective when combining both nutrition and physical activity (versus only nutrition or only physical activity). However, it seems reasonable to suggest that whatever the key message of an obesity campaign, it will be more successful to the extent that community-wide efforts to change normative behaviors are expended and environmental supports, such as access to green space and presence of sidewalks, are in place.

UNDERSTANDING THE RELATIVE EXPOSURE OF HEALTH-RELATED AND NON–HEALTH-RELATED MARKETING MESSAGES

In addition to giving health messages greater exposure through sizable media budgets and comprehensive media campaigns, attention must be given to competitor messages and promotional expenditures of competitive industries (in which unhealthy messages are promoted).

Tobacco Marketing Expenditures Are a Competitive Force for Tobacco Control Campaigns

As reported in the NCI monograph (2008), the tobacco industry's advertising and promotional efforts, regarded as highly effective by the advertising industry, have represented a major hurdle for tobacco control efforts. *Advertising Age* rated the Marlboro Man as the top advertising icon of the twentieth century, and Marlboro was ranked as the third-best advertising campaign of the century (Volkswagen and Coca-Cola were first and second). Campaigns for four other cigarette brands were on the top 100 list of *Advertising Age* campaigns. In 2006, *Business Week* rated Marlboro as the twelfth most valued global brand, with a brand equity value of $21.4 billion. Based on marketing expenditure data, the NCI monograph concluded that cigarettes are one of the most heavily marketed products in the United States. Most of the promotional budgets (about 75 percent) are allocated to price discounts, about $10 billion in 2005. Since the 1998 master settlement agreement, marketing at the point of purchase has increased in importance; tobacco has a strong presence in convenience stores, where 60 percent of all cigarettes in the United States are sold.

Obesity-Promoting Marketing Expenditures Are a Competitive Force for Obesity Control Campaigns

What does this mean for the study of obesity? First, it means determining which industries are contributing to unhealthy food choices and sedentary behaviors, the amount of marketing expenditures devoted to messages promoting determinants of obesity (e.g., consumption of unhealthy foods) and, in some cases, whether companies are willing or interested in making needed investments to promote healthier alternatives (e.g., increased nutrition in food brands). For obesity, an additional consideration studied by researchers is the extent to which children and adolescents are exposed to advertising for unhealthy foods and the role these ads play in food choices. Recent research that examined 170 top-rated television shows for nine months during 2003–2004 found that food advertising made up over one-quarter of TV ads viewed by adolescents (Powell, Szczypka, and Chaloupka 2007), most commonly fast food, sweets, and beverage products, and that most food products advertised were high in fat, sugar, or sodium. Research in 2008 found that sugared cereals were heavily promoted to children (Harris et al. 2009). Establishing whether and/or to what extent exposure to advertisements for unhealthy foods impacts consumption of unhealthy food is important for children and adults, across multiple contexts. Online food marketing to children and adolescents is also a growing concern (Moore and Rideout 2007). While some companies are stepping up efforts toward self-regulation of junk food marketing, more research is needed to determine whether these efforts are successful or not in changing the types of food products promoted to youth.

Environmental Barriers to Curbing Obesity

Finally, a key issue in obesity policy is the need to remove environmental barriers to healthy eating and physical activity. Policy-makers and researchers (e.g., French, Story, and Jeffery 2001) have called for a reduction in the marketing of unhealthy food products in schools and workplaces (e.g., vending machines), an increase in availability of healthy food choices (e.g., fruits and vegetables, whole grains), and an increase in availability of physical activity (e.g., more walking paths).

DEVELOPING EFFECTIVE MESSAGE CONTENT AND MESSAGE TYPE

Tobacco Control and Emotionally Arousing Ads

Research in media communications places an emphasis on message content and message type, including the types of messages that are most effective in changing both behavior and proximal measures such as recall, belief and attitude change, and intention to change. Tobacco-control advertisements have varied considerably from one campaign to the next with respect to message content and message type, so it is difficult to assess across studies the extent to which each of these types of ads is successful. One of the few consistent findings, however, is that ads that elicited strong emotions performed better than ads that did not elicit strong emotions (e.g., Biener, Gilpin, and Albers 2004; Biener, McCallum-Keeler, and Nyman 2000; Farrelly et al. 2002; Pechmann and Reibling 2006; Wakefield et al. 2005). Persuasion and information-processing research finds that ads that evoke high arousal yield greater attention to the ad, and affective responses are important in understanding precursors to behavior change. In a review of tobacco control messages (NCI 2008), negative emotional arousal was more likely than either neutral or humor responses to affect indicators of message processing (such as recall of the advertisement, thinking more about it, discussing it). In fact, in the context of tobacco control advertising, the emotions triggered by the ads were more important than demographic factors such as race, ethnicity, nationality, and age group. Common themes of effective tobacco control advertisements depicted harms resulting from smoking or secondhand smoke in an authentic manner and/or depicted tobacco industry awareness of the dangers of smoking.

Obesity Control and Emotionally Arousing Ads

In the context of obesity research, we would expect that strong emotional responses to ads might also be more likely to engage audiences, although whether the arousal of positive or negative affect is more effective for nutrition and physical activity messages at a population level is important to assess. In addition, determining whether other types of messages, message framing, and message positioning effectively engender these responses across different target segments (Keller and Lehmann 2008) is an issue that needs addressing at the population level.

NEWS AND ENTERTAINMENT MEDIA

News Media Influence Health Behaviors

In the area of tobacco control and public health in general, the news media have often been used to frame messages about health or other tobacco-related issues (NCI 2008, Chapter 9). As a result, news coverage has served as a potential source of influence on both tobacco policy and individual smoking behavior (e.g., Asbridge 2004; Cummings, Sciandra, and Markello 1987; Laugesen and Meads 1991; Niederdeppe et al. 2007; Pierce and Gilpin 2001; Smith et al. 2008). For example, following news coverage of the 1964 U.S. surgeon general's report on smoking and health, research suggests an increase in smoke-free policies (Warner 1977). People are primed or more sensitive to other messages in their environments after hearing television news stories on health issues. Coverage of obesity issues in the news media may be, in some cases, even more important than paid advertising and promotion. It can set in motion changes at the community, state, and national levels, and news is known to set the agenda for public discourse.

Entertainment Media Influence Health Behaviors

Entertainment media, such as movies and television, provide powerful modeling that may be linked to either healthy or unhealthy behavior. In the tobacco area, entertainment media, particularly movies, have been instrumental in promoting pro-smoking messages to youth (e.g., Dalton et al. 2003; Dixon 2003; Dixon et al. 2001; Pechmann and Shih 1999; Sargent et al. 2005). As of the mid-2000s, tobacco depictions occurred in about 75 percent or more of box office hits, and exposure to them has been causally linked to increased smoking initiation among youth (NCI 2008, Chapter 10). In the case of obesity, reducing the number of depictions of role models consuming unhealthy foods in TV, movies, and video games is, of course, important, especially for children and adolescents. Further, increases in exposure to healthy (relative to unhealthy) foods may help to normalize healthy food choices among children (Dixon et al. 2007). Researchers have also examined whether reductions in the number of hours of screen time (television viewing and computer use) are linked to reductions in sedentary behavior; the evidence is mixed (Robinson 1999). All these efforts are important in understanding the role of entertainment media, role model product endorsement, and product placement as contributing sources of exposure to obesity-relevant behaviors.

DIFFERENT GOALS FOR PUBLIC-HEALTH-SPONSORED CAMPAIGNS AND COMMERCIAL CAMPAIGNS

Corporate Social Responsibility Initiatives

For companies in today's marketplace, engaging in social cause efforts, such as public health campaigns and partnerships with nonprofit industries, is considered important to the overall functioning of a company's brands and perhaps even a necessity (Bhattacharya and Sen 2004). This trend has benefited both companies and causes and is likely to continue in the years to come. Nevertheless, it is important to remember that the goals of a corporate social responsibility (CSR) initiative are not necessarily identical or even hospitable to the goals of a public health campaign. One of the important considerations in evaluating commercially driven obesity campaigns and developing partnerships with commercially driven companies in promoting anti-obesity campaigns is whether the primary goals of the campaign represent health behavioral outcomes. The primary goals of corporate image campaigns and corporate sponsorship initiatives are generally to define and improve a corporate reputation, attract a target segment of consumers, and strengthen a corporate image (Bloom et al. 2006; Gurhan-Canli and Fries 2010). Since these goals are not related to health promotion or obesity prevention, consumer skepticism and suspicion about company motives can ensue (Gurhan-Canli and Fries 2010). Research yields mixed findings about the conditions under which corporate image campaigns heighten or reduce consumer skepticism about company motives (NCI 2008, Chapter 6).

Tobacco Companies' Responses to Consumer Skepticism

The public's high level of industry distrust appears to be a contributing factor in the tobacco industry's development of corporate image campaigns with messages focusing on charitable causes and prevention of youth smoking. Skepticism by consumers was justified in that at times corporate spending on charitable campaigns vastly exceeded the amount actually given to the charities (NCI 2008, Chapter 6). Further, tobacco industry documents indicated that despite the companies' insistence on the sincerity of their efforts to prevent youth smoking, assessments of youth smoking intentions and behavior were not measured by the companies (Wakefield, McLeod, and Perry 2006). Instead, survey measures focused on consumers' perceptions of the company (such as whether the public's perceptions of the company as dishonest and culpable for adolescent smoking were reduced). Indeed, the public perceived the company as less dishonest, less culpable, more socially responsible, and more favorable as a function of exposure to the antismoking campaign. Independent studies conducted outside the industry evaluated the effectiveness of the antismoking campaigns of the tobacco industry on youth smoking intentions and behavior, and found them largely ineffective (e.g., NCI 2008; Wakefield et al. 2006). In fact, intentions to smoke in the next five years among eighth graders increased as a result of exposure to the tobacco industry's youth-directed campaign, and likelihood of smoking in the past month among tenth and twelfth graders increased with exposure to the parent-directed campaign.

Obesity Promotion and Industry Responses

The industries backing tobacco use and nutrition or physical activity are different in many respects. The number of industries producing tobacco is comparatively small, and the number of tobacco products is narrow, relative to the food, exercise, and weight loss industries. The food industry includes not only food manufacturers, but also restaurants, vendors, and grocers, adding to the diversity of marketing of foods and beverages that contribute to the obesity epidemic. In addition, tobacco industries do not have a healthy alternative to tobacco products other than ceasing to produce them, whereas many food industries have alternatives. Positive examples abound of food industry changes that have positively influenced consumers' health choices, such as General Mills's directive to change all its cereals to whole grain and the milk industry's efforts to promote substitution of high-fat with low-fat milk. So fundamental to partnerships with industry is determining the extent to which the goals of the company are congruent or incongruent with the goals to promote the healthy behavior. When the goals of the company and the social cause are incongruent, or the goals of the company are chiefly for image-enhancement, barriers to health behavior change may exist. Partnerships with the Fruit and Vegetable Growers Association may yield less conflict of interest than partnerships that encourage 100-calorie, after-school snacks or quick weight loss products. With regard to building an evidence base of findings on obesity, it might also be important to evaluate the effects of industry-related efforts separately from public-health-related efforts.

CONCLUSION

A database of evaluations of nutrition and physical activity campaigns and environmental supports is increasing (for reviews see Bauman et al. 2006; Kahn et al. 2002; Matson-Koffman et al. 2005; Pomerleau et al. 2005). In the case of tobacco marketing, the cumulative evidence from multiple types of studies, investigators from different disciplines, and data from many countries leads to the conclusion of a causal link between tobacco advertising and promotion and increased use of tobacco; and the total weight of evidence from cross-sectional, longitudinal, and experimental studies leads to concluding a causal link between exposure to depictions of tobacco use in movies and the initiation of smoking among youth (NCI 2008). These links are important in influencing policy decisions such as tobacco tax increases and stricter enforcement of youth access to tobacco products.

The public health behaviors associated with obesity are complex (Norman et al. 2007; Snyder 2007). While cigarette consumption has multiple determinants, and multiple strategies exist for promoting smoking cessation, obesity is best viewed as an outcome of several behaviors, including making healthy eating choices and engaging in regular physical activity, in addition to the possible role of genetics. The particular food choices that prevent obesity and the levels of physical activity needed to prevent obesity vary, depending on the particular market segment. For example, children have different nutritional needs than adults, and older adults have different physical capabilities and nutritional requirements than younger adults (Marcus et al. 2006). In addition to these complexities, public health guidelines on ideal levels of physical activity or the most acceptable amounts of nutritional intake (e.g., number of fruits and vegetables, number of servings of fiber and grains) continue to evolve over time as more studies linking food choices and activity to obesity are obtained (Marcus et al. 2006).

Addressing these complexities is furthered by research with strong research designs, both in field experiments and population-level studies, that contribute to an evidence base on the many steps required to curb the obesity trend. At a basic level, field studies in obesity prevention have been evaluating several of these steps, such as determining the role of overexposure to unhealthy food messages and unhealthy foods (Emery et al. 2007; French, Story, and Jeffery 2001; Powell, Szczypka, and Chaloupka 2007), exploring message content and message type (Berkowitz et al. 2008), determining the impact of availability of healthy foods on food choice (Pomerleau et al. 2005; Snyder 2007), increasing understanding of the role of sedentary behavior and how to increase activity (Berkowitz et al. 2008; Economes et al. 2007; Huhman et al. 2007; Kahn et al. 2002), determining the impact of environmental supports on physical activity (Matson-Koffman et al. 2005), and determining the effectiveness of Internet-based interventions on diet and physical activity (Norman et al. 2007; Winett et al. 2005). More research is needed at a *population* level to determine the degree of media exposure required to produce significant change, the most effective mix of persuasive communications and community-level components, the most appropriate methods for reducing availability of unhealthy options, and the degree of environmental supports needed to produce change. Analysis of the competitive information environment and assessing appropriate controls and covariates for obesity campaign evaluations are also important (Emery et al. 2007; Snyder 2007). An obesity prevention evidence base can also be used to further the understanding of the density of advertising of obesity-promoting versus obesity-reducing products and services and finding high-risk populations (Marcus et al. 2006; Tirodkar and Jain 2003). Research is needed to understand the links between obesity-related messages in news and entertainment media and public response. Finally, given the importance of the obesity trend worldwide, international dissemination of effective prevention strategies and targeting of high-risk populations is needed (Bauman et al. 2006).

REFERENCES

Asbridge, Mark. 2004. "Public Place Restrictions on Smoking in Canada: Assessing the Role of the State, Media, Science, and Public Health Advocacy." *Social Science and Medicine*, 58 (1), 13–24.

Bauman, Adrian. 2004. "Commentary on the VERB Campaign: Perspectives on Social Marketing to Encourage Physical Activity Among Youth." *Preventing Chronic Disease*, 1 (3), 1–3.

Bauman, Adrian E., David E. Nelson, Michael P. Pratt, Victor Matsudo, and Stephanie Schoeppe. 2006. "Dissemination of Physical Activity Evidence, Programs, Policies, and Surveillance in the International Public Health Arena." *American Journal of Preventive Medicine*, 31 (4S), S57–S65.

Berkowitz, Judy M., Marian Huhman, Carrie D. Heitzler, Lance D. Potter, Mary Jo Nolin, and Stephen W. Banspach. 2008. "Overview of Formative, Process, and Outcome Evaluation Methods Used in the VERB Campaign." *American Journal of Preventive Medicine*, 34 (6S), S222–S229.

Bhattacharya, C.B., and Senkar Sen. 2004. "Doing Better at Doing Good: When, Why, and How Consumers Respond to Corporate Social Initiatives." *California Management Review*, 47 (1), 9–24.

Biener, Lois, Ming Ji, Elizabeth A. Gilpin, and Alison B. Albers. 2004. "The Impact of Emotional Tone, Message, and Broadcast Parameters in Youth Anti-Smoking Advertisements." *Journal of Health Communication*, 9 (3), 259–274.

Biener, Lois, Garth McCallum-Keeler, and Amy L. Nyman. 2000. "Adults' Response to Massachusetts Anti-Tobacco Television Advertisements: Impact of Viewer and Advertisement Characteristics." *Tobacco Control*, 9 (4), 401–407.

Biglan, Anthony, Dennis V. Ary, Keith Smolkowski, Terry Duncan, and Carol Black. 2000. "A Randomized Controlled Trial of a Community Intervention to Prevent Adolescent Tobacco Use." *Tobacco Control*, 9 (1), 24–32.

Bloom, Paul N., Steve Hoeffler, Kevin L. Keller, and Carlos E. Basurto Meza. 2006. "How Social-Cause Marketing Affects Consumer Perceptions." *Sloan Management Review*, 47 (2), 49–55.

Cavill, Nick, and Adrian Bauman. 2004. "Changing the Way People Think About Health-Enhancing Physical Activity: Do Mass Media Campaigns Have a Role?" *Journal of Sports Science*, 22, 771–790.

Centers for Disease Control and Prevention. 2008. "U.S. Obesity Trends: Trends by State, 1985–2008." www.cdc.gov/obesity/data/trends.html.

Cummings, K. Michael, Russell Sciandra, and Samuel Markello. 1987. "Impact of a News-paper Mediated Quit Smoking Program." *American Journal of Public Health*, 77 (11), 1452–1453.

Dalton, Madeline A., James D. Sargent, Michael L. Beach, Linda Titus-Ernstoff, Jennifer J. Gison, M. Bridget Ahrens, Jennifer J. Tickle, and Todd F. Heatherton. 2003. "Effect of Viewing Smoking in Movies on Adolescent Smoking Initiation: A Cohort Study." *Lancet*, 362 (9380), 281–285.

Dixon, Helen G. 2003. "Portrayal of Tobacco Use in Popular Films: An Investigation of Audience Impact." PhD diss., University of Melbourne.

Dixon, Helen G., David J. Hill, Ron Borland, and Susan J. Paxton. 2001. "Public Reaction to the Portrayal of the Tobacco Industry in the Film *The Insider*." *Tobacco Control*, 10 (3), 285–291.

Dixon, Helen G., Maree L. Scully, Melanie A. Wakefield, Victoria M. White, and David A. Crawford. 2007. "The Effects of Television Advertising for Junk Food Versus Nutritious Food on Children's Food Attitudes and Preferences." *Social Science and Medicine*, 65 (7), 1311–1323.

Economes, Christina D., Raymond R. Hyatt, Jeanne P. Goldberg, Aviva Must, Elena N. Naumov, Jessica J. Collins, and Miriam E. Nelson. 2007. "A Community Intervention Reduces BMI Z-Score in Children: Shape Up Somerville First Year Results." *Obesity*, 15 (5), 1324–1336.

Emery, Sherry L., Glen Szczypka, Lisa M. Powell, and Frank J. Chaloupka. 2007. "Public Health Obesity-Related TV Advertising." *American Journal of Preventive Medicine*, 33 (4S), S257–S263.

Farrelly, Mathew C., Kevin C. Davis, M. Lyndon Haviland, Peter Messeri, and Cheryl G. Healton. 2005. "Evidence of a Dose-Response Relationship Between 'Truth' Antismoking and Youth Smoking Prevalence." *American Journal of Public Health*, 95 (3), 425–431.

Farrelly, Mathew C., Cheryl G. Healton, Kevin C. Davis, Peter Messeri, James C. Hersey, and M. Lyndon Haviland. 2002. "Getting to the Truth: Evaluating National Tobacco Countermarketing Campaigns." *American Journal of Public Health*, 92 (6), 901–907.

Flay, Brian R., Todd Q. Miller, Donald Hedeker, Ohid Siddiqui, Cynthia F. Britton, Bonnie R. Brannon, C. Anderson Johnson, William B. Hansen, Steve Sussman, and Clyne Dent. 1995. "The Television, School, and Family Smoking Prevention and Cessation Project: 8. Student Outcomes and Mediating Variables." *Preventive Medicine*, 24 (1), 29–40.

Flynn, Brian S., John K. Worden, Roger H. Secker-Walker, Phyllis L. Pirie, Gary J. Badger, and Joseph H. Carpenter. 1997. "Long-Term Responses of Higher and Lower Risk Youths to Smoking Prevention Interventions." *Preventive Medicine*, 26 (3), 289–294.

French, Simone A., Mary Story, and Robert W. Jeffery. 2001. "Environmental Influences on Eating and Physical Activity." *Annual Review of Public Health*, 22, 309–335.

Gurhan-Canli, Zeynep, and Anne Fries. 2010. "Branding and Corporate Social Responsibility." In *Brands and Brand Management: Contemporary Research Perspectives*, ed. Barbara Loken, Rohini Ahluwalia, and Michael J. Houston, 91–110. New York: Psychology Press.

Hafstad, A., L.E. Aaro, A. Engeland, A. Andersen, F. Langmark, and B. Stray-Pedersen. 1997. "Provocative Appeals in Anti-Smoking Mass Media Campaigns Targeting Adolescents: The Accumulated Effect of Multiple Exposures." *Health Education Research*, 12 (2), 227–236.

Harris, Jennifer L., Marlene B. Schwartz, Kelly D. Brownell, Vishnudas Sarda, Megan E. Weinberg, Sarah Speers, Jackie Thompson, Amy Ustjanauskas, Andrew Cheyne, Eliana Bukofzer, Lori Dorfman, and Hannah Byrnes-Enoch. 2009. "Cereal FACTS: Evaluating the Nutrition Quality and Marketing of Children's Cereals." Rudd Center for Food Policy and Obesity, Yale University, October.

Hornik, Robert, ed. 2002. *Public Health Communication: Evidence for Behavior Change*. New York: Lawrence Erlbaum.

Huhman, Marian E., Lance D. Potter, Jennifer C. Duke, David R. Judkins, Carrie D. Heitzler, and Faye L. Wong. 2007. "Evaluation of a National Physical Activity Intervention for Children." *American Journal of Preventive Medicine*, 32 (1), 38–43.

Kahn, Emily B., Leigh T. Ramsey, Ross C. Brownson, Gregory W. Heath, Elizabeth H. Howze, Kenneth E. Powell, Elaine J. Stone, Mummy W. Rajab, and Phaedra Corso. 2002. "The Effectiveness of Interventions to Increase Physical Activity." *American Journal of Preventive Medicine*, 22 (4S), 73–107.

Keller, Punam A., and Donald R. Lehmann. 2008. "Designing Effective Health Communications: A Meta-Analysis." *Journal of Public Policy and Marketing*, 27 (2), 117–130.

Laugesen, Murray, and Chris Meads. 1991. "Advertising, Price, Income, and Publicity Effects on Weekly Cigarette Sales in New Zealand Supermarkets." *British Journal of Addiction*, 86 (1), 83–89.

Marcus, Bess H., David M. Williams, Patricia M. Dubbert, James F. Sallis, Abby C. King, Antronette K. Yancey, Barry A. Franklin, David Buchner, Stephen R. Daniels, and Randal P. Claytor. 2006. "Physical Activity Intervention Studies: What We Know and What We Need to Know." *Circulation*, 114, 2739–2752.

Matson-Koffman, Dyann M., J. Nell Brownstein, Jennifer A. Neiner, and Mary L. Greaney. 2005. "A Site-Specific Literature Review of Policy and Environmental Interventions That Promote Physical Activity and Nutrition for Cardiovascular Health: What Works?" *American Journal of Health Promotion*, 19 (3), 167–193.

Meshack, A.F., S. Hu, U.E. Pallonen, A.L. McAlister, N. Gottlieb, and P. Huang. 2004. "Texas Tobacco Prevention Pilot Initiative: Processes and Effects." *Health Education Research*, 19 (6), 657–668.

Moore, Elizabeth S., and Victoria J. Rideout. 2007. "The Online Marketing of Food to Children; Is It All Just Fun and Games?" *Journal of Public Policy and Marketing*, 26 (2), 202–220.

National Cancer Institute (NCI). 2008. *The Role of the Media in Promoting and Reducing Tobacco Use: Tobacco Control Monograph No. 19*, ed. Ronald M. Davis, Elizabeth A. Gilpin, Barbara Loken, K. Viswanath, and Melanie A. Wakefield. Bethesda, MD: U.S. Department of Health and Human Services, National Cancer Institute. NIH Pub. No. 07–6242. www.cancercontrol.cancer.gov/tcrb/monographs/19/index.html.

Niederdeppe, Jeff, Mathew C. Farrelly, Kristin Y. Thomas, Dana Wenter, and David Weitzenkamp. 2007. "Newspaper Coverage as Indirect Effects of a Health Communication Intervention: The Florida Tobacco Control Program and Youth Smoking." *Communication Research*, 34 (4), 382–405.

Norman, Gregory J., Marion F. Zabinski, Marc A. Adams, Dori E. Rosenberg, Amy L. Yaroch, and Audie A. Atienza. 2007. "A Review of eHealth Interventions for Physical Activity and Dietary Behavior Change." *American Journal of Preventive Medicine*, 33 (4), 336–345.

Pechmann, Cornelia, and Ellen T. Reibling. 2006. "Antismoking Advertisements for Youths: An Independent Evaluation of Health, Counter-Industry, and Industry Approaches." *American Journal of Public Health*, 96 (5), 906–913.

Pechmann, Cornelia, and Chuan-Fong Shih. 1999. "Smoking Scenes in Movies and Anti-Smoking Advertisements Before Movies: Effects on Youth." *Journal of Marketing*, 63 (3), 1–13.

Perry, Cheryl L., Steven H. Kelder, David M. Murray, and Knut I. Klepp. 1992. "Community-Wide Smoking Prevention: Long-Term Outcomes of the Minnesota Heart Health Program and the Class of 1989 Study." *American Journal of Public Health*, 82 (9), 1210–1216.

Pierce, John P., and Elizabeth A. Gilpin. 2001. "News Media Coverage of Smoking and Health Is Associated with Changes in Population Rates of Smoking Cessation but Not Initiation." *Tobacco Control*, 10 (2), 145–153.

Pomerleau, Joceline, Karen Lock, Cecile Knai, and Martin McKee. 2005. "Interventions Designed to Increase Adult Fruit and Vegetable Intake Can Be Effective: A Systematic Review of the Literature." *Journal of Nutrition*, 135, 2486–2495.

Powell, Lisa M., Glen Szczypka, and Frank J. Chaloupka. 2007. "Adolescent Exposure to Food Advertising on Television." *American Journal of Preventive Medicine*, 33 (4 Suppl.), S251–S256.

Robinson, Thomas N. 1999. "Reducing Children's Television Viewing to Prevent Obesity: A Randomized Control Trial." *Journal of the American Medical Association*, 282, 1561–1567.

Sargent, James D., Micheal L. Beach, Anna M. Adachi-Mejia, Jennifer J. Gibson, Linda T. Titus-Ernstoff, Charles P. Carusi, Susan D. Swain, Todd F. Heatherton, and Madeline A. Dalton. 2005. "Exposure to Movie Smoking: Its Relation to Smoking Initiation Among U.S. Adolescents." *Pediatrics*, 116 (5), 1183–1191.

Slater, Michael D., Kathleen J. Kelly, Ruth W. Edwards, Pamela J. Thurman, Barbara A. Plested, Thomas J. Keefe, Frank R. Lawrence, and Kimberly L. Henry. 2006. "Combining In-School and Community-Based Media Efforts Reducing Marijuana and Alcohol Uptake Among Younger Adolescents." *Health Education Research*, 21 (1), 157–167.

Smith, Katherine C., Melanie A. Wakefield, Yvonne M. Terry-McElrath, Frank J. Chaloupka, Brian Flay, Lloyd Johnston, Ann Saba, and Catherine Siebel. 2008. "Relationship Between Newspaper Coverage of Tobacco Issues and Perceived Smoking Harm and Smoking Behavior Among American Teens." *Tobacco Control*, 17 (1), 17–24.

Snyder, Leslie B. 2007. "Health Communication Campaigns and Their Impact on Behavior." *Journal of Nutrition Education and Behavior*, 39(2S) (March–April), S32–S40.

Tirodkar, Manasi, and Anjali Jain. 2003. "Food Messages on African American Television Shows." *American Journal of Public Health*, 93 (3), 439–442.

Vartiainen, Erkki, Meri Paavola, Alfred McAlister, and Pekka Puska. 1998. "15-Year Follow-Up of Smoking Prevention Effects in the North Karelia Youth Project." *American Journal of Public Health*, 88 (1), 81–85.

Wakefield, Melanie, George I. Balch, Erin Ruel, Yvonne Terry-McElrath, Glen Szczypka, Brian Flay, Sherry Emery, and Katherine Clegg-Smith. 2005. "Youth Responses to Anti-Smoking Advertisements from Tobacco Control Agencies, Tobacco Companies, and Pharmaceutical Companies." *Journal of Applied Social Psychology*, 35 (9), 1894–1910.

Wakefield, Melanie, Kim McLeod, and Cheryl L. Perry. 2006. "'Stay Away From Them until You're Old Enough to Make a Decision': Tobacco Company Testimony About Youth Smoking Initiation." *Tobacco Control*, 15 (Suppl. IV), iv44–iv53.

Wakefield, Melanie, Yvonne Terry-McElrath, Sherry Emery, Henry Saffer, Frank J. Chaloupka, Glen Szczypka, Brian Flay, Patrick M. O'Malley, and Lloyd D. Johnston. 2006. "Effect of Televised, Tobacco Company-Funded Smoking Prevention Advertising on Youth Smoking-Related Beliefs, Intentions, and Behavior." *American Journal of Public Health*, 96 (12), 2154–2160.

Warner, Kenneth E. 1977. "The Effects of the Anti-Smoking Campaign on Cigarette Consumption." *American Journal of Public Health*, 67 (7), 645–650.

Winett, Richard A., Deborah F. Tate, Eileen S. Anderson, Janet R. Wojcik, and Sheila G. Winett. 2005. "Long-Term Weight Gain Prevention: A Theoretically Based Internet Approach." *Preventive Medicine*, 41, 629–641.

ABOUT THE EDITORS AND CONTRIBUTORS

EDITORS

Rajeev Batra is Sebastian S. Kresge Professor of Marketing and Co-Director of the Yaffe Center for Persuasive Communication at the Stephen M. Ross School of Business, University of Michigan. His research interests include the strategy and tactics of building brands; global branding and advertising; marketing issues in emerging markets; emotional advertising; consumers' attitude structure toward brands and brand personality; repetition effects; and advertising budgeting.

Punam Anand Keller is Charles Henry Jones Third Century Professor of Management at the Tuck School of Business, Dartmouth College. Her current research focus is designing and implementing communication programs. Her research is supported by the National Cancer Institute, the Center for Disease Control, and the National Endowment for Financial Education. She served as president of the Association for Consumer Research in 2008–2009.

Victor J. Strecher is Professor of Health Behavior and Health Education and Director of Cancer Prevention and Control in the University of Michigan's Comprehensive Cancer Center. Dr. Strecher also founded the University of Michigan's Center for Health Communications Research (CHCR): a multidisciplinary team of behavioral scientists, physicians, computer engineers, instructional designers, graphic artists, and students from a wide variety of disciplines.

CONTRIBUTORS

Imène Becheur is Assistant Professor and Researcher at the Wesford School of Business in Grenoble, France.

Jonah Berger is Assistant Professor of Marketing at the Wharton School at the University of Pennsylvania.

Pierre Chandon is Professor of Marketing at INSEAD, France.

Alexander Chernev is Associate Professor of Marketing, Kellogg School of Management, Northwestern University.

Darren W. Dahl is Fred H. Siller Professor in Applied Marketing Research, Sauder School of Business, University of British Columbia.

Gavan J. Fitzsimons is F.M. Kirby Research Fellow and Professor of Marketing and Psychology at Fuqua School of Business, Duke University.

Kelly Geyskens is Assistant Professor of Marketing in the Department of Marketing at Maastricht University, The Netherlands.

Jakob D. Jensen is Assistant Professor in the Department of Communication at Purdue University.

Seung-A Annie Jin is Assistant Professor in the Department of Communication, Boston College.

Brian Keefe is a master's student in the Department of Communication at George Mason University.

Myoung Kim is a doctoral student in the Department of Consumer Science, School of Human Ecology, at the University of Wisconsin–Madison.

Gary L. Kreps is University Distinguished Professor and Chair of the Department of Communication at George Mason University, where he holds the Eileen and Steve Mandell Endowed Chair in Health Communication and directs the Center for Health and Risk Communication.

Christian Ledford is a PhD student in the Department of Communication at George Mason University, where she is preparing her dissertation on persuasion in the physician-patient relationship.

Donald R. Lehmann is George E. Warren Professor of Business and the Chair of the Marketing Division at Columbia Business School, Columbia University.

Barbara Loken is Professor in the Department of Marketing at the Carlson School of Management, University of Minnesota.

Brent McFerran is Assistant Professor of Marketing, Stephen M. Ross School of Business, University of Michigan.

Colleen McHorney (PhD) is Senior Director at Merck U.S., Outcomes Research, where she leads all of Merck's adherence scientific work.

Andrea C. Morales is Associate Professor of Marketing at W.P. Carey School of Business, Arizona State University.

Anirban Mukhopadhyay is Associate Professor of Marketing at Hong Kong University of Science and Technology, Clear Water Bay, Kowloon, Hong Kong.

Daniel J. O'Keefe is the Owen L. Coon Professor in the Department of Communication Studies at Northwestern University.

Lindsay P. Rand is a graduate of Stanford University with a degree in psychology.

Rebecca Ratner is Associate Professor of Marketing at the Robert H. Smith School of Business at the University of Maryland.

Jason Riis is Assistant Professor of Business Administration in the marketing unit at Harvard Business School.

Michael L. Rothschild is Emeritus Professor at the Wisconsin School of Business, University of Wisconsin–Madison.

John J. Sailors is Assistant Professor of Marketing at the University of St. Thomas.

Norbert Schwarz is the Charles Horton Cooley Collegiate Professor of Psychology; Research Professor at the Institute for Social Research; Research Professor in the Program in Survey Methodology; and Professor of Marketing, Ross School of Business—all at the University of Michigan.

Ian Skurnik is Associate Professor in Business Administration at the Darden School of Business, University of Virginia

Jeff Stone is Associate Professor of Social Psychology in the Psychology Department at the University of Arizona.

Peter A. Ubel (MD) is the John O. Blackburn Professor of Business Administration and Public Policy at Duke University.

Pierre Valette-Florence is Professor of Marketing and Quantitative Methods at IAE de Grenoble Domaine Universitaire in France.

Melinda M. Villagran is Associate Professor, Director of Military Programs in Strategic Communication, and a Research Fellow at the Center for Health and Risk Communication at George Mason University in Fairfax, Virginia. She is also a Research Associate at the Center for Infrastructure Protection at George Mason University School of Law.

K. Viswanath is Associate Professor in the Department of Society, Human Development, and Health at the Harvard School of Public Health.

Melanie A. Wakefield is Director and NHMRC Principal Research Fellow at the Centre for Behavioural Research in Cancer, Cancer Control Research Institute, Australia.

Brian Wansink is John S. Dyson Professor of Marketing and of Nutritional Science at Cornell University, where he directs the Cornell Food and Brand Lab. From 2007 to 2009 he was the executive director of the U.S. Department of Agriculture's Center for Nutrition Policy and Promotion, the federal agency in charge of developing the 2010 U.S. Dietary Guidelines and promoting the Food Guide Pyramid (MyPyramid.gov).

Melinda Weathers is a doctoral student in the Department of Communication at George Mason University.

Nancy Wong is Associate Professor in the Department of Consumer Science, School of Human Ecology, at the University of Wisconsin–Madison.

Carolyn Yoon is Associate Professor of Marketing at the Stephen M. Ross School of Business at the University of Michigan.

Xiaoquan Zhao is Assistant Professor in the Department of Communication at George Mason University.

NAME INDEX

SUBJECT INDEX

T - #0459 - 101024 - C0 - 229/152/23 - PB - 9780765627186 - Gloss Lamination